100 Pearls in Clinical Diagnostic Radiology

100 Pearls in Clinical Diagnostic Radiology

Harold D. Rosenbaum, M.D.

Professor and Chairman
Department of Diagnostic Radiology
University of Kentucky Medical Center
Lexington, Kentucky

University Park Press • Baltimore

University Park Press
International Publishers in Medicine and Human Services
300 North Charles Street
Baltimore, Maryland 21201

Sponsoring editor: Larry W. Carter
Production editor: Michael Treadway
Cover and text design by: Caliber Design Planning, Inc.

Typeset by: Waldman Graphics, Inc.
Manufactured in the United States of America by: Halliday Lithograph

Library of Congress Cataloging in Publication Data

Rosenbaum, Harold D.
100 pearls in clinical diagnostic radiology.

1. Diagnosis, Radioscopic—Case studies. I. Title.
II. Title: One hundred pearls in clinical diagnostic radiology. [DNLM: 1. Radiography—Case studies. WN 240 R813z]
RC78.R685 1984 616.07'572 84-3503
ISBN 0-8391-1979-8

Contents

Preface

An analytical approach to the radiologic manifestations of health and disease has much merit, especially if one is to understand the pathologic mechanisms that generate x-ray findings. Nevertheless, many conditions lead to radiologic changes that are so characteristic they can be diagnosed immediately and with confidence solely from their x-ray manifestations. No need exists for piecemeal analytical dissection. Other pathologic conditions cause sufficiently typical radiologic changes as to leave little room for diagnostic doubt if appropriate clinical findings also exist. These appearances, often called "pearls" by both learners and teachers of diagnostic radiology, are truly "Aunt Minnies" and can become as familiar to the experienced radiologist as one's spouse, children, or intimate friends. They are the stuff of this book.

This volume contains 100 radiologic pearls. These cases have been selected with no purpose other than to represent examples of the varied disease processes encountered in the practice of radiology. The 100 presentations have been selected from more than 500 cases that have been prepared at the University of Kentucky Medical Center. This material is used in the instruction of diagnostic radiology residents and medical students. Students and staff members of other departments of the Medical Center also spend considerable time viewing these pearls, which are displayed, five at a time, on a row of twenty viewboxes in the Department of Diagnostic Radiology.

A brief history is presented with each case. The clinical data are restricted, in general, to that needed for a confident diagnosis. Additional radiographs may be included to amplify or to confirm the diagnosis. Although angiographic, radioisotopic, computed tomographic, ultrasonographic, or even magnetic resonance images may be shown or mentioned, the primary purpose of this book is to illustrate diagnostic plain film findings. Each presentation concludes with no more than four pertinent references and sources for further reading.

I must acknowledge my indebtedness to many individuals. Prominent among this group are the residents and faculty members of the Department of Diagnostic Radiology at the University of Kentucky Medical Center. Many others have been indispensable. These include Mr. Del Henderson, our Department Administrator, who assisted in many ways both large and small. Essential and professionally skilled help was obtained from Mr. Jerry Fischer, Photographer in the Department of Diagnostic Radiology, and from Mrs. Frances Woods, who provided incomparable secretarial excellence. I also cannot forget representatives of University Park Press, particularly Mr. Larry Carter, Ms. Berta Steiner, and Mr. Michael Treadway.

100 Pearls in Clinical Diagnostic Radiology

Case 1

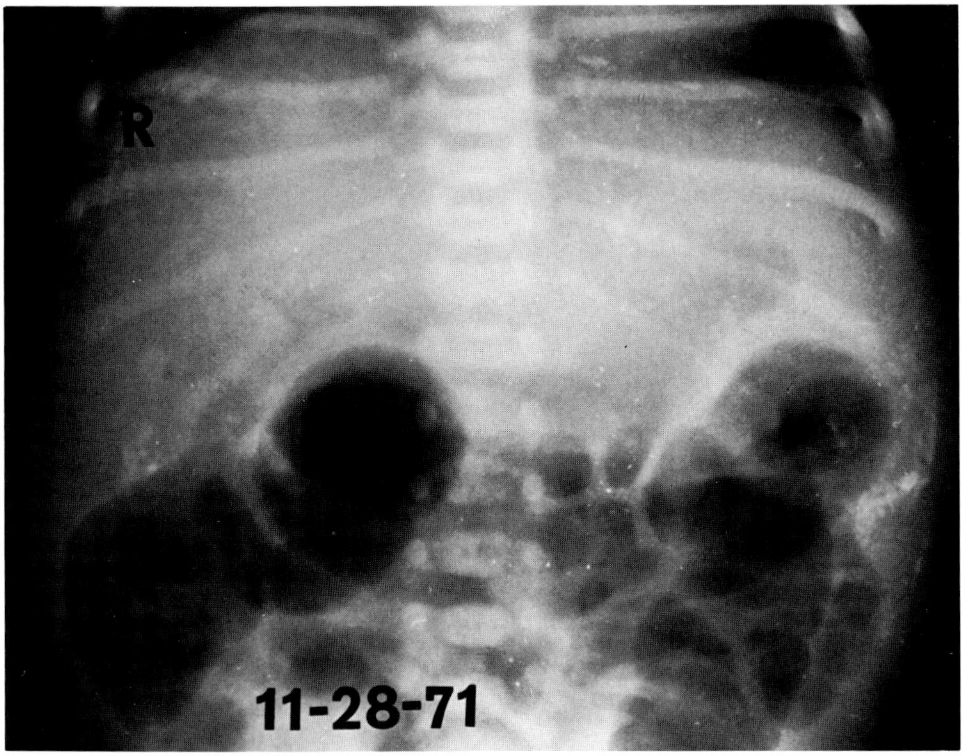

A

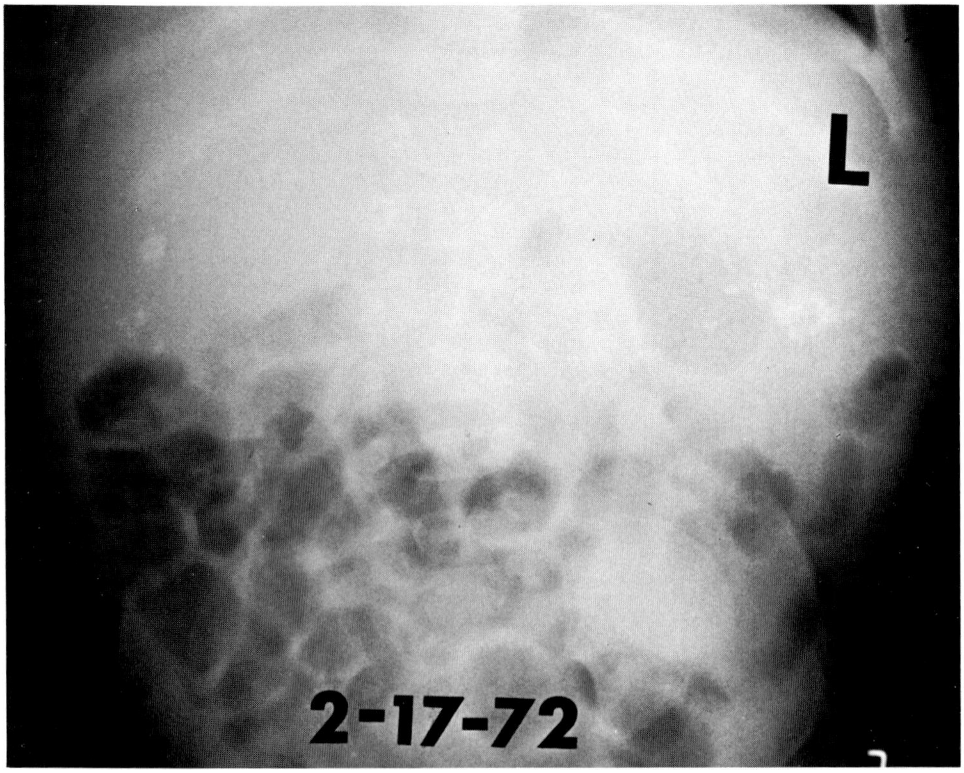

B

Meconium Peritonitis

Clinical Information

This 1-day-old infant was admitted to the hospital because of vomiting and a distended abdomen. A perforation of the transverse colon was repaired at surgery. There was gross contamination of his peritoneal cavity with meconium. The patient progressed satisfactorily after surgery, although he had bilateral clubbed feet and hip dislocations. The mother's pregnancy had been complicated by polyhydramnios.

Roentgen Findings

A flat film of the abdomen on admission (A) shows rather striking intestinal distention. In addition, there are abundant flecks and plaques of calcification scattered throughout the abdominal cavity. They are located on the peritoneal surfaces and are particularly abundant overlying the liver in the upper abdomen. A follow-up film (B) shows no intestinal distention. Some of the calcifications have disappeared but some remain. No evidence of growth arrest lines is seen on either film.

Comments

Calcification on the peritoneal surfaces in the newborn is diagnostic of meconium peritonitis. This condition is often seen in association with bowel rupture, as was true in this case, but it may be encountered in an otherwise normal newborn. It is presumed that the calcification results from contamination of the peritoneal cavity with meconium, which is irritating. This leads to an inflammatory reaction, which heals with the deposition of calcium. The calcium can appear rather rapidly, probably within 1–2 weeks. It may disappear as quickly, particularly if the calcification is not abundant, although in many patients a much longer period, even up to 1 or more years, passes before no x-ray evidence of the calcium can be seen. Calcification has been seen in the scrotum (1), since the processus vaginalis is open at this age. The meconium can lead to very large, walled-off, noncommunicating pseudocysts in the peritoneal cavity (3).

The cause of the intestinal perforation may not be evident. Perhaps a fetal vascular accident or volvulus is involved. It is difficult to explain how the gut reconstitutes its continuity when no other abnormalities are demonstrable at birth. It is said that 15% of patients with cystic fibrosis have meconium peritonitis, although this figure is probably too high. It is more likely that about 15% of patients with meconium peritonitis have cystic fibrosis. These patients often show growth arrest lines (4). The insult of bowel rupture during pregnancy is alleged to account for these lines. Other types of intestinal obstruction in the newborn are not generally associated with this finding, although growth arrest lines have been seen in infants with erythroblastosis fetalis or congenital syphilis.

The calcification that develops in meconium peritonitis is dystrophic in nature. Its appearance on an x-ray examination is unmistakable (2). The flecks of calcification vary in quantity but are always located on the serosal surfaces of the abdominal cavity. It is important not to misinterpret intraluminal calcified meconium, which occasionally is seen, for peritoneal calcification.

Source Materials

1. Berdon WE, Baker DH, Becker J, DeSanctis P. Scrotal masses in healed meconium peritonitis. N Engl J Med 277:585, 1967.
2. Finkel LI, Slovis TL. Meconium peritonitis, intraperitoneal calcifications and cystic fibrosis. Pediatr Radiol 12:92, 1982.
3. Fujioka M, Bowen A'D. Cystic meconium peritonitis. Radiology 140:380, 1981.
4. Wolfson JJ, Irgell RR. Anticipated meconium peritonitis from metaphyseal bands. Radiology 92:1055, 1969.

Case 2

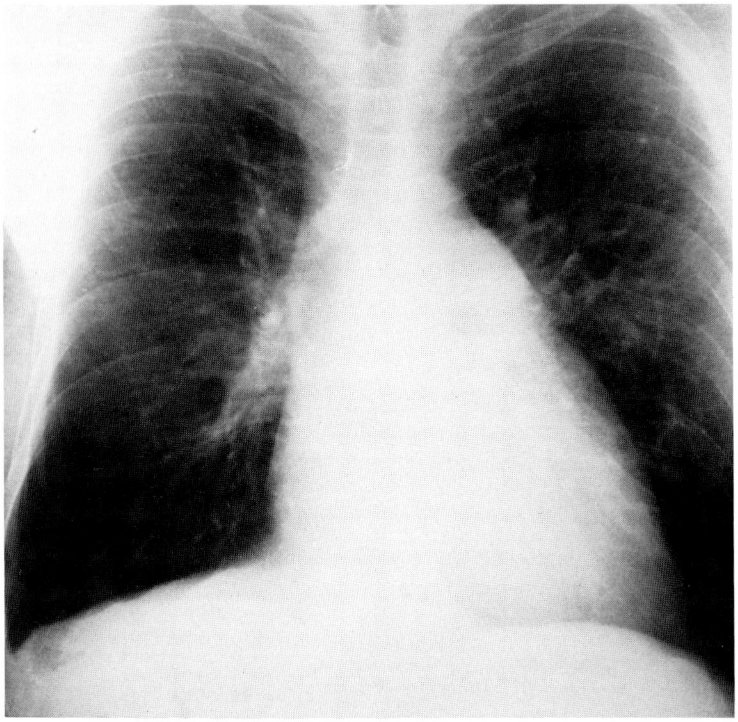

A

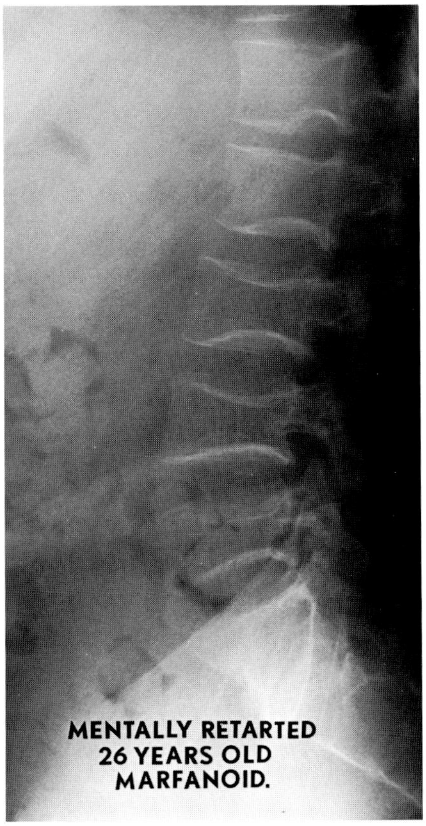

B

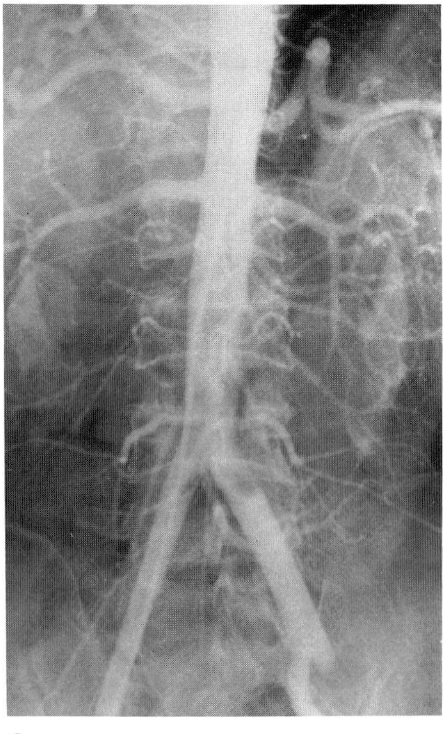

C

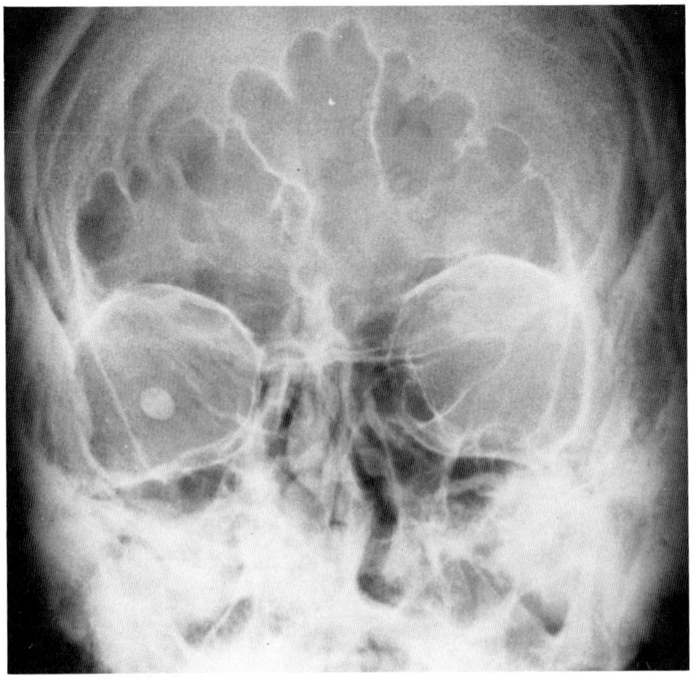

D (another patient)

Homocystinuria

Clinical Information

This 26-year-old white, mentally retarded male with laboratory evidence of homocystinuria suffered a stroke at 10 months of age. There was a history of repeated pulmonary infarcts. Shortly before admission he developed a cold left leg. A large thrombus was surgically removed from his left iliac arteries with return of good circulation to this extremity. Two years later he suffered another pulmonary infarction, developed cor pulmonale, and died. Two brothers were similarly affected.

Roentgen Findings

A posteroanterior film of the chest (A) exposed 2 years before death shows prominence of the pulmonary arteries and an enlarged heart, with a configuration consistent with right ventricular enlargement. The lateral lumbar spine film (B) reveals rather marked osteoporosis with biconcave deformities of the vertebral bodies. An aortogram (C) shows thrombi in the distal aorta and iliac arteries with total occlusion of the left external iliac.

Comments

Homocystinuria was first described in 1962. It is an uncommon autosomal recessive trait characterized by a deficiency of cystathionine synthetase, which is required to convert homocystine and serine into cystathionine (1). This leads to excessive levels of homocystine and methionine in the urine and the blood. Excess quantities of these amino acids are thought to produce the manifestations of this disease. They apparently interfere with the formation of normal collagen. These amino acids have been shown to produce toxic effects on the blood vessels of animals.

There is a less common pyridoxine-sensitive form of homocystinuria that is responsive to a soybean-based dietary regime. Fifty percent of patients show some improvement, which may become evident radiologically. Individuals who are pyridoxine-resistant, as was this patient, do not respond to such treatment but may respond to betaine (4).

Patients with homocystinuria are usually (85%) mentally retarded and have repeated arterial and venous thromboemboli. The vascular complications of homocystinuria are particularly treacherous and are said to have been caused by so small an insult as venipuncture. Patients with homocystinuria also exhibit rather striking osteoporosis (3). These three features—mental retardation, thrombi, and osteoporosis—help distinguish this disease from Marfan's syndrome, although there are other differences. Both conditions lead to an asthenic habitus and ectopic lens. The lens tends to dislocate downward in homocystinuria but upward in Marfan's syndrome. Film D shows calcification of a subluxed lens in another patient with homocystinuria. Patients with Marfan's syndrome have increased joint mobility, whereas the opposite is the case in homocystinuria, which leads to a reduced range of joint motion. Laboratory studies reveal abnormalities with homocystinuria that are absent in Marfan's syndrome. Patients with either condition may have arachnodactyly. Homocystinurics do not exhibit aortic dissection. Newborns with homocystinuria have shown bone changes in the wrist similar to those that may occur with phenylketonuria, although infants born of mothers with homocystinuria are less likely to be abnormal than are infants born of mothers with phenylketonuria (2).

Source Materials

1. Brill PW, Mitty HA, Gaull GE. Homocystinuria due to cystathionine synthase deficiency: Clinical-roentgenologic correlations. AJR 121:45, 1974.
2. Kurczynski TW, Muir WA, Feisher LD, et al. Maternal homocystinuria: Studies of an untreated mother and fetus. Arch Dis Child 55:721, 1980.
3. Thomas PS, Carson NAJ. Homocystinuria—The evolution of skeletal changes in relation to treatment. Ann Radiol 21:95, 1978.
4. Wilcken DEL, Wilcken B, Dudman NPB, Tyrrell PA. Homocystinuria—The effects of betaine in the treatment of patients not responsive to pyridoxine. N Engl J Med 309:448, 1983.

Case 3

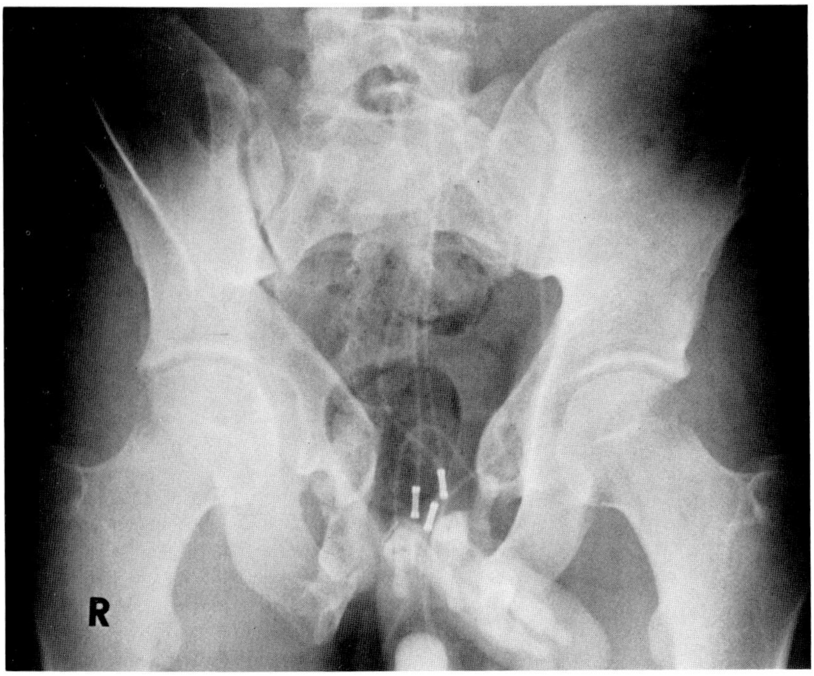

A

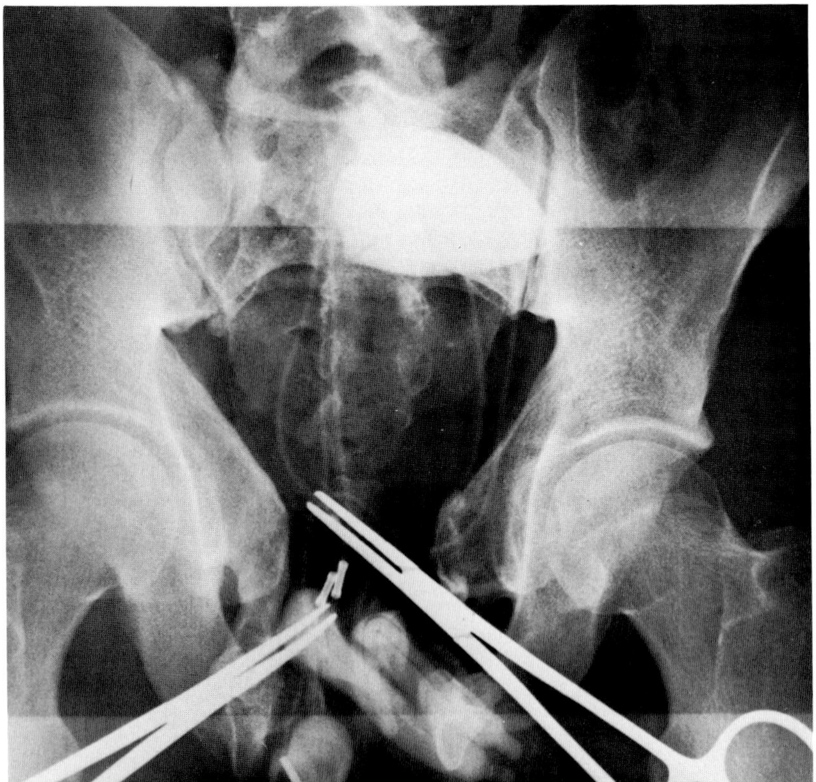

B

Inflatable Penile Implant with Leak

Clinical Information

This 25-year-old male had been impotent since a severe pelvic injury was sustained during the Vietnam War. An inflatable penile implant was inserted, which, after some complications were corrected, was effective.

Roentgen Findings

The pubic bones are separated as a result of the war injury (A). Portions of an inflatable penile implant are evident, but no radiopaque fluid is present in the reservoir. This indicates a leak, which was repaired. An intraoperative film after the repair with the penis semierect is shown in B.

Comments

Good results are obtained with an inflatable penile implant in about 90% of impotent male patients (1, 2). The advantages of an inflatable implant over rigid or flexible implants utilized in the past are a normal-appearing penis in the nonerect stage, a more nearly normal erection, and greater satisfaction of the patient's sexual partner. This device is somewhat difficult to implant and is liable to mechanical failure. There are four parts to the inflatable implant. A reservoir, which contains absorbable radiopaque fluid, is inserted within the prevesical space immediately behind the rectus muscle. The reservoir is connected by a single tube to an inflate-deflate pump, which is inserted in the scrotum. The reservoir also connects through tubing with two soft silicone cylinders, one in each of the two corpora cavernosa. The patient obtains an erection at will by pumping fluid from the reservoir into the silicone cylinders. He has similar control over termination of the erection.

Many conditions can lead to an inability to achieve an erection. Bilateral renal transplants, trauma, and certain medications can cause impotence. Perhaps the most common cause is psychogenic. Patients with psychogenic impotence can be distinguished because they continue to exhibit normal nocturnal penile tumescence. Neurogenic impotence can be identified with a sacral latency test, which reveals loss of integrity of the sacral neural pathways. About 25% of all patients with impotence have vascular insufficiency, which can be demonstrated by selective internal iliac arteriography. Atherosclerotic disease is the most common offender. Some patients show a vascular steal from the internal pudendal to the profunda femoralis arteries. Erection is achieved in this situation, but it is immediately lost with commencement of sexual thrusting. Angioplasty or endarterectomy might be employed in these patients, but no controlled series is as yet available (4). A Doppler probe has been used to record blood pressure in the major artery to the penis. Blood flow to the penis has also been studied with isotopes. About 50% of patients who desire penile implants have diabetes, which may cause either vasculogenic or neurogenic impotence.

Radiologic studies can diagnose many complications of an inflatable implant although wound infection, which occurs in 3–4% of these patients, is not demonstrable on an x-ray examination (3, 4). A single film in an oblique projection with the device inflated is usually adequate, although anteroposterior films in both inflated and deflated states may be needed. Radiology can show malposition of the pump or reservoir, fluid leaks, kinking of the tubing, buckling of a cylinder, or ballooning of a section of one of the cylinders. A portion of the proximal part of one or both cylinders may fold upon itself.

Source Materials

1. Beaser RS, Van der Hoek C, Jacobson AM, et al. Experience with penile prostheses in the treatment of impotence in diabetic men. JAMA 248:943, 1982.
2. Kessler R. Surgical experience with the inflatable penile prosthesis. J Urol 124:611, 1980.
3. Kossoff J, Krane RJ, Naimark A. Inflatable penile implant for impotence: Radiologic evaluation. AJR 136:1109, 1981.
4. Miller K, Kaplan L, Weitzman AF, et al. The radiology of male impotence. RadioGraphics 2:131, 1982.

Case 4

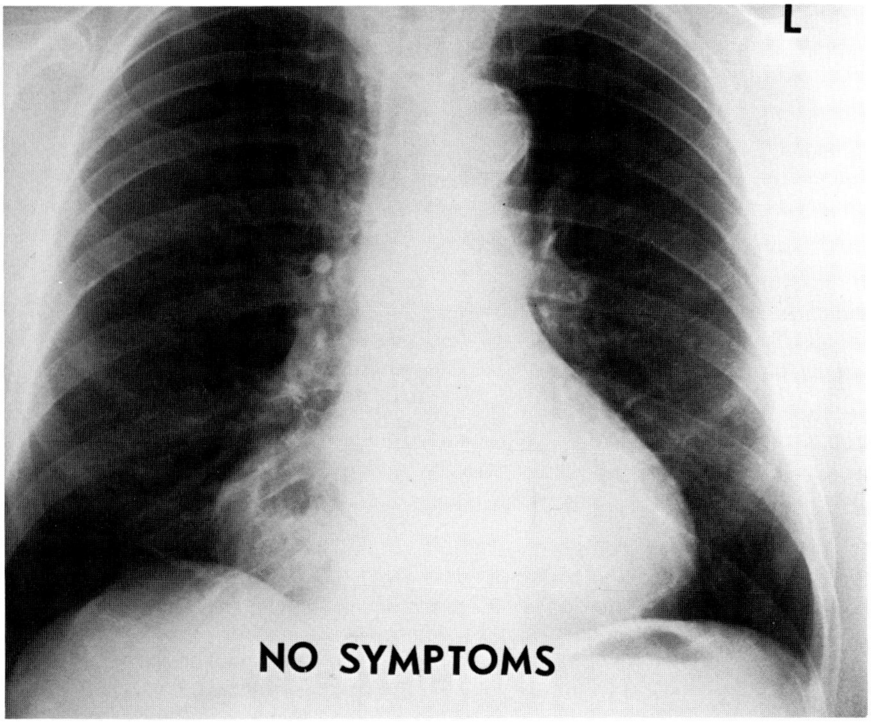

A

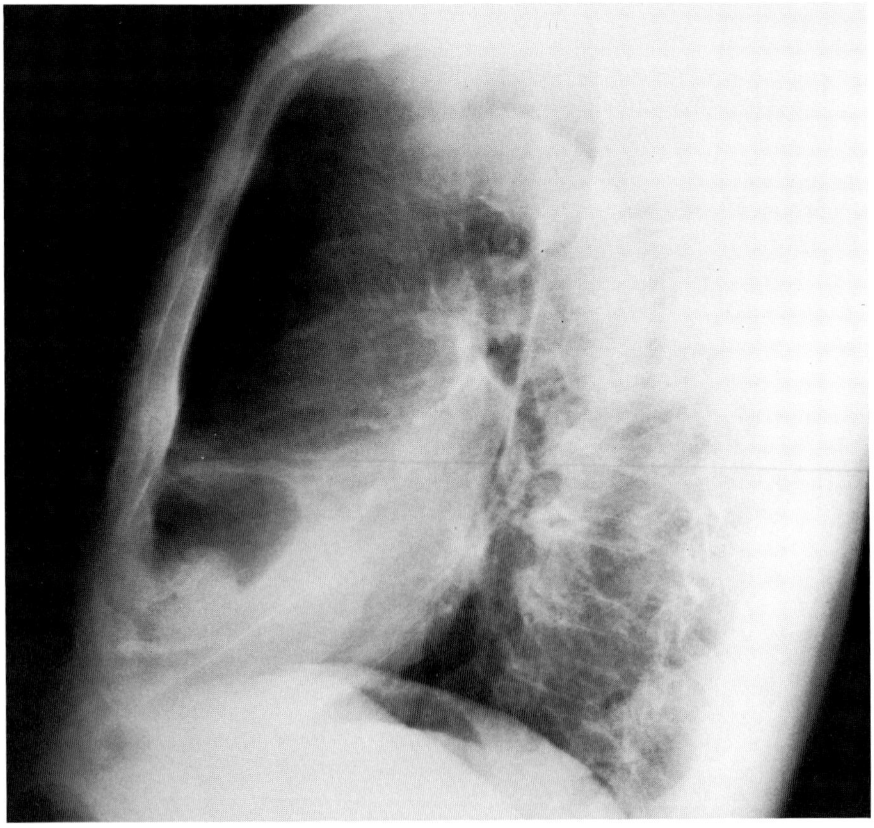

B

Morgagni Hernia

Clinical Information

This 50-year-old man had no symptoms. The chest films were obtained during a general physical evaluation. No treatment was recommended for the Morgagni hernia.

Roentgen Findings

Posteroanterior (A) and lateral (B) films of the chest show a rounded soft tissue density in the right cardiophrenic angle just behind the right side of the sternum. The density contains gas, which appears to be within a loop of bowel. The lateral film reveals a rounded density within the gas, which probably represents fecal material. No other abnormalities are seen.

Comments

The foramina of Morgagni are two small triangular areas, one on each side of the midline immediately behind the sternum. These potential openings are sites of muscular weakness situated between diaphragmatic muscle fibers that originate from the xiphisternum medially and others that arise laterally from the seventh ribs. They are normally filled with no tissue other than fat and are covered with a layer of pleura above and a layer of peritoneum below. Peritoneal contents can herniate upward into the thoracic cavity through these foramina, particularly when the openings are larger than usual. Such hernias have been called Morgagni hernias, Larrey's hernias, retrosternal hernias, or simply anterior diaphragmatic hernias. A soft tissue density located just above the diaphragm in the right retrosternal area that contains gas suggesting a loop of bowel is diagnostic of a Morgagni hernia, particularly when fecal material appears to be present. These hernias are much less frequent than hernias through a posterolateral defect (Bochdalek) in the diaphragm. Morgagni hernias are nearly always on the right side because the left side is protected by the heart and pericardium. The hernial contents are usually omentum or large intestine. Occasionally other abdominal organs are present. Morgagni hernias are usually first discovered in adults around the age of 50, although they have been seen in children (2). Bochdalek hernias are much more commonly encountered in newborns and infants.

No sex predominance has been seen with Morgagni hernias. No cause for the herniation, other than the size of the defect, has been discovered. Morgagni hernias are usually asymptomatic, although these patients occasionally complain of retrosternal pain or dyspepsia. Strangulation or intestinal obstruction is rare. In their absence no treatment is indicated. Either complication obviously requires surgical intervention. An abdominal approach is usually employed.

The only significant differential diagnostic possibilities from a radiologic viewpoint are a pericardial cyst or a fat pad. The presence of gas within the lesion rules out these two considerations. Enlarged nodes of Hodgkin's disease are occasionally present in this location. It is possible to diagnose a Morgagni hernia with a barium enema even in the absence of gas within the hernia, as occurs when it is filled with omentum. The barium enema will show the midtransverse colon to peak upwardly toward the defect due to traction from the herniated omentum. The distal stomach and duodenum may also be displaced upwardly. The "sign of the cane" has been described (1) in Morgagni hernias. This sign depends upon the fact that these hernias carry peritoneum upward as they pass into the thoracic cavity. The lateral chest film may show the properitoneal fat line to be continuous from the anterior abdominal wall and to surmount the hernia, which leads to an appearance that suggests a candy cane.

Source Materials

1. Lanuza A. The sign of the cane: A new radiologic sign for the diagnosis of small Morgagni hernias. Radiology 101:293, 1971.
2. Merten DF, Bowie JD, Kirks DR, Grossman H. Anteromedial diaphragmatic defects in infancy: Current approaches to diagnostic imaging. Radiology 142:361, 1982.
3. Paris F, Tarazona V, Casillas M, et al. Hernia of Morgagni. Thorax 28:631, 1973.
4. Patton I, Harris WC. Herniation through the foramen of Morgagni. Br J Radiol 34:368, 1961.

Case 5

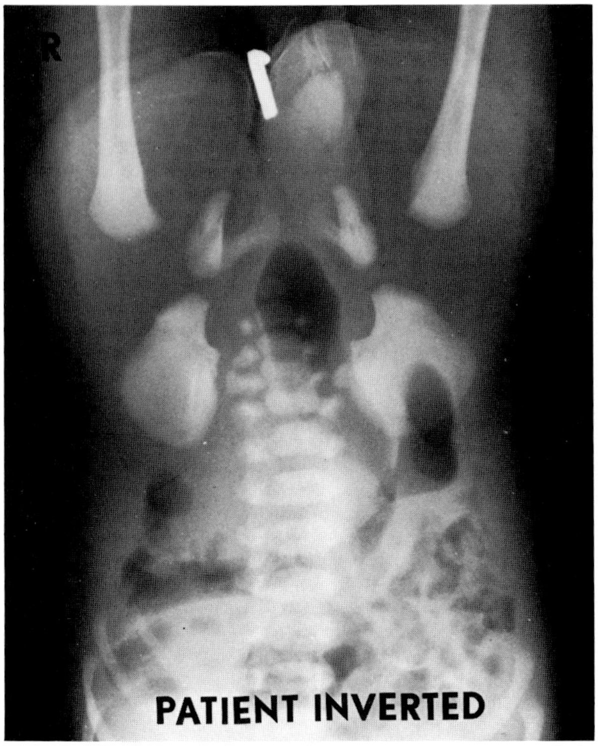

A

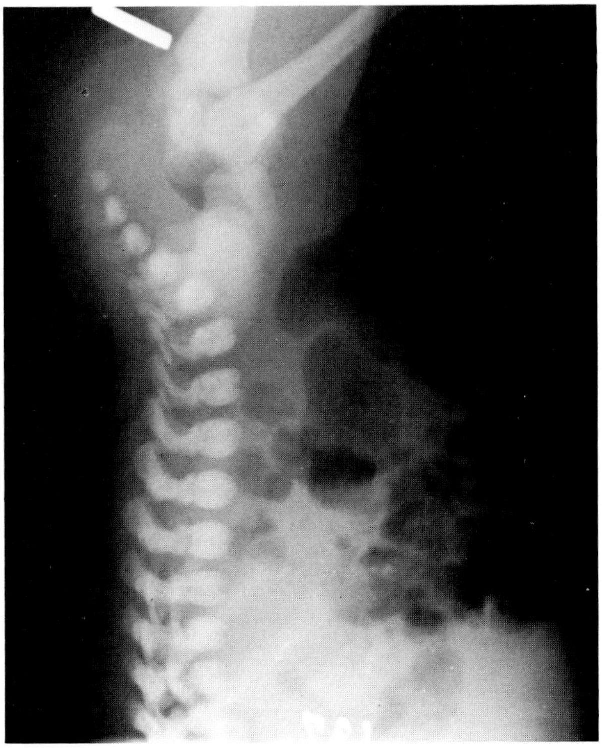

B

Imperforate Anus

Clinical Information

This 1-month-old white male was referred for evaluation of an imperforate anus and a perineal fistula. He did well after surgical intervention.

Roentgen Findings

Inverted anteroposterior (A) and lateral (B) films of the abdomen with a marker over the anal dimple show more than 2.5 cm separation between the end of the column of gas in the colon and the marker. This incorrectly suggests a high imperforate anus. No sacral anomalies are evident.

Comments

Imperforate anus is a general term for various anomalies at the distal end of the gastrointestinal tract. There frequently are other anomalies, particularly involving the genitourinary tract and the spine. Fistulization is usually present from the distal end of the colon to the perineum or lower genitourinary tract. An imperforate anus occurs about once in every 5000 births. There is significant separation between the end of the gut and the perineum in so-called high defects. In these patients there is failure of descent of the hindgut through the levator ani sling, which is hypoplastic or absent. A high arrest is virtually always associated with a rectovaginal or high rectourethral fistula. These patients often have fecal incontinence after definitive surgical repair following a required initial colostomy. In so-called low arrest the colon has passed through the levator ani sling, which is well developed and functional. There almost always is an associated low rectovaginal, low rectourethral, or perineal fistula. Low lesions are handled by immediate repair, generally with good results.

It is possible to diagnose a high from a low arrest from physical examination (3). Low arrest shows an anal dimple, perineal fistula, corrugated perineum, or perineal pearls in both males and females. Separate urethral and vaginal openings with a hymen in a female also indicate a low lesion. A high lesion is indicated by only a cloaca or no hymen in the female and a smooth perineum in both sexes. There is a very high association of other anomalies with an imperforate anus. Most investigators have reported that high lesions in both sexes and low lesions in males are commonly associated with spinal and genitourinary anomalies (1). These reports indicate females with a low lesion do not have an increased incidence of such anomalies. At least one study reported females with a low lesion to have about as many of these anomalies as males (4). The frequent association of imperforate anus with other anomalies has led to various acronyms, the most common of which is VATER (*V*ertebral, *A*nal, *T*racheo-*E*sophageal, and *R*adial and/or *R*enal) syndrome.

Inverted radiographs with a marker over the anal dimple can be misleading. It was said that separation of more than 1.5 cm indicates a high lesion. Errors occur, as in this case, because air may not have reached the distal end of the gastrointestinal tract; there may be additional anomalies; straining of the infant can change the location of the termination of the air; there may be impaction of meconium at the distal end of the intestinal tract or distal rectal spasm; a line drawn from the pubis to the coccyx may or may not represent the true position of the levator ani sling; and, lastly, compression by the levator ani muscle can give a false impression of a long, narrow fistulous tract. It has been suggested by some that a transperineal percutaneous injection of a water-soluble contrast agent may provide valuable information. Others disagree. Sonography can be helpful (2). Air within the male bladder or the female vagina is evidence of an internal fistula with a high lesion. An intravenous pyelogram will show urinary tract and spinal anomalies.

Source Materials

1. Berdon WE, Baker DH, Santulli TV, Amoury R. The radiologic evaluation of imperforate anus. An approach correlated with current surgical concepts. Radiology 90:466, 1968.
2. Oppenheimer DA, Carroll BA, Schochat SJ. Sonography of imperforate anus. Radiology 148:127, 1983.
3. Seibert JJ, Golladay ES. Pictorial essay. Clinical evaluation of imperforate anus: Clue to type of anal-rectal anomaly. AJR 133:289, 1979.
4. Thompson W, Grossman H. The association of spinal and genitourinary abnormalities with low anorectal anomalies (imperforate anus) in female infants. Radiology 113:693, 1974.

Case 6

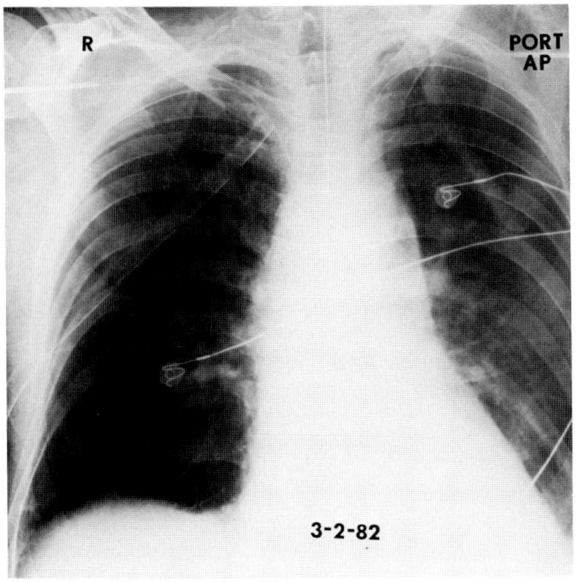

A

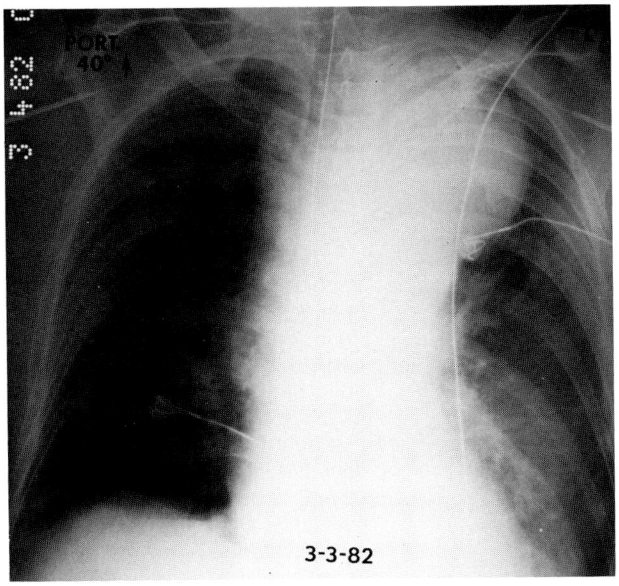

B

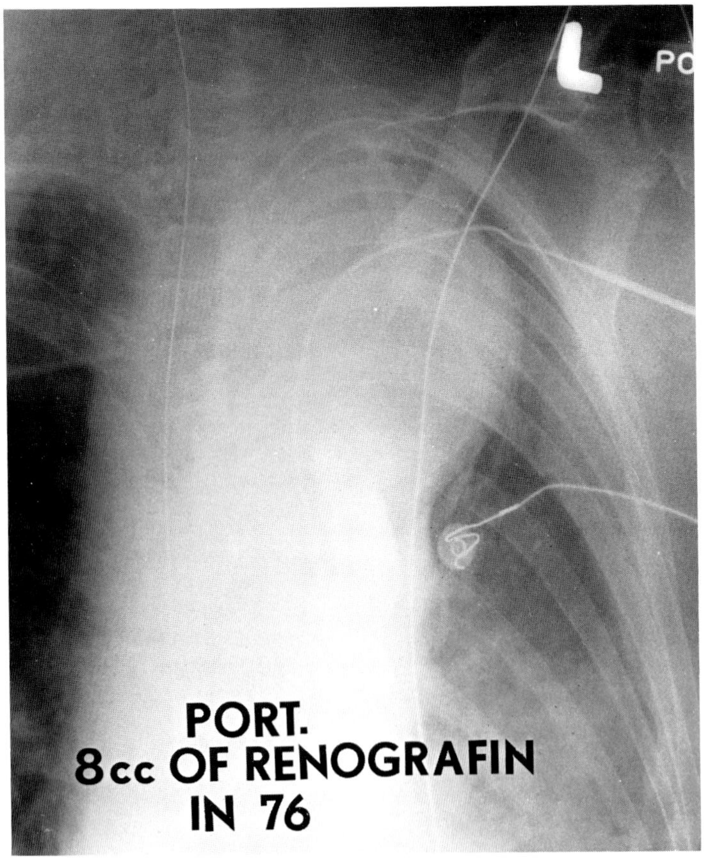

C

Central Venous Catheter Complication

Clinical Information

This 54-year-old male was being treated for complications following perforation of a duodenal ulcer. Bilateral central venous catheters were introduced. Transbronchial aspiration on 3-3-82 revealed a sterile hematoma. The left-sided catheter was withdrawn. The hematoma resolved.

Roentgen Findings

Film A shows a normally placed right central venous catheter with its tip in the superior vena cava. The left-sided catheter terminates in an aberrant location. Its tip is superimposed upon the aortic knob. Film B shows a large left-sided mediastinal density. Injection of contrast agent through the left-sided catheter (C) reveals its extravascular location.

Comments

Central venous catheterization was introduced and became very popular during the third quarter of the 20th century. It has proved to be particularly valuable for pressure monitoring, hyperalimentation, and the introduction of fluids and blood. The two most popular routes are through a subclavicular subclavian or an internal jugular venipuncture. The complication rate of the latter is about 1%, and that of the former approximately 6%, although a subclavian puncture has been used more frequently.

The most frequent complication associated with a central venous catheter is pneumothorax (3, 4). It accounts for almost a third of all such problems. The pneumothorax is usually unilateral, although it can be bilateral or even under tension. Pneumothorax results from laceration of the parietal pleura. There may be an associated pneumomediastinum. About 30% of the complications of these procedures are due to malposition of the central venous catheter (2). The aberrant location often indicates perforation. Structures in the involved region may be affected. About 20% of these complications follow puncture of the subclavian artery, which can lead to an extrapleural hematoma. Aortic dissections have also occurred. Perforation of a vein may occur in long-standing catheterization with erosion of the catheter tip through the vessel wall, although it also can be seen immediately after the catheter is introduced. The tip of the catheter may be in the mediastinum or the pleural space. Hydrothorax or hydromediastinum from infusion of parenteral fluids can occur. Hemothorax or a sizeable hemomediastinum due to bleeding is less common (1). Chylothorax has been reported. Termination of the catheter in the jugular vein with retrograde infusion of a toxic substance can lead to adverse results.

Most of the complications that attend insertion of a central venous catheter can be prevented by determining that the catheter tip is properly positioned in the distal superior vena cava. Respiratory-related pressure fluctuations recorded through the central venous catheter can be helpful, although false positive readings occur in about 25% of these patients. Consequently, there is some risk when only these fluctuations are used for monitoring. A chest film to show the catheter in a proper position without evident abnormality is the most satisfactory method of monitoring. Complications that may be detected can at times be lethal.

Source Materials

1. Arbitman M, Kart BH. Hydromediastinum after aberrant central venous catheter placement. Crit Care Med 7:27, 1979.
2. Dunbar RD, Mitchell R, Lavine M. Aberrant locations of central venous catheters. Lancet 1:711, 1981.
3. Feliciano DV, Mattox KL, Graham JM, et al. Major complications of percutaneous subclavian vein catheters. Am J Surg 138:869, 1979.
4. Mitchell SE, Clark RA. Complications of central venous catheterization. AJR 133:467, 1979.

Case 7

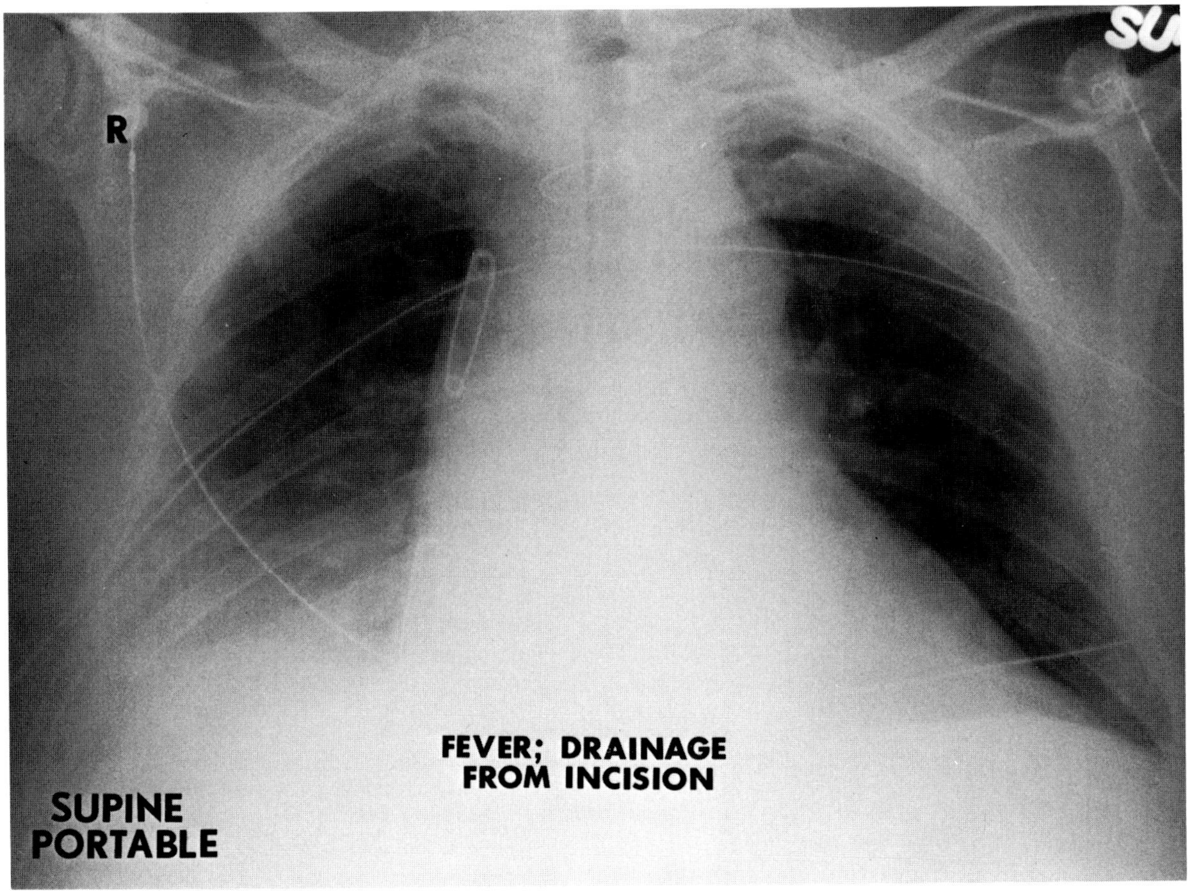

Dehiscence of Median Sternotomy

Clinical Information

This 68-year-old white male had an aortic valve prosthesis inserted at the same operation during which an aneurysm of the ascending aorta was resected. He developed atelectasis, which required reintubation and mechanical ventilatory assistance. A serosanguinous drainage was noted at the sternotomy incision 8 days postoperatively. At the same time the chest film showed a midsternal radiolucent stripe. The sternum was rewired, but the patient died 3 days later from arrhythmias and septic shock.

Roentgen Findings

A supine portable film is underexposed. The prosthetic aortic valve is not visible. Wire sutures in the sternum are faintly seen. They are unchanged in orientation from that noted on previous films. A narrow vertical midline radiolucent stripe is visible from the top of the manubrium down to at least the middle of the sternum.

Comments

Complications of a median sternotomy (3) include brachial plexus injury, fractures of first and sometimes second ribs, infection, and dehiscence. Dehiscence occurs in 2–5% of these patients. It is a serious complication. Factors that predispose toward dehiscence are hemorrhage, external cardiac massage, assisted respiration, poor surgical technique, an off-center cut in the sternum, inadequate fixation, excessive use of electrocautery or bone wax, reopening the wound to control hemorrhage, and infection. Almost every factor, except advanced age, that gives the patient a poor outlook is associated with an increased incidence of dehiscence. This helps account for the high mortality of about 50% that is associated with this complication. Careful supervision is all that is indicated when only a narrow radiolucent stripe is seen by x-ray. If the median sternotomy wound is more widely separated, appropriate therapy involves antibiotics and reopening the wound with debridement. The sternum is closed after reoperation with a reinforcing pattern that is more sturdy than simple interrupted wire sutures.

Dehiscence must be recognized promptly. Radiologic evidence of median sternotomy dehiscence may be seen before clinical signs are noted (1, 4). Sternal dehiscence in most cases is not due to wire breakage. Rather, the wires pull through the sternum. This may lead to a change in their shape or orientation. They often rotate. A thin vertical lucent cleft or stripe at the site of the incision is very common. This may be very narrow and can exist without subsequent major dehiscence. A vertical stripe is seen with increased frequency when only one manubrial suture is used. Disagreement exists as to how frequently a vertical stripe is followed by a major dehiscence. At any rate, the appearance of such a radiologic finding is significant and warrants close monitoring of the patient.

Source Materials

1. Berkow AE, Demos TC. The midsternal stripe and its relationship to postoperative sternal dehiscence. Radiology 121:525, 1976.
2. Carter AR, Sostman HD, Curtis AM, Swett HA. Thoracic alterations after cardiac surgery. AJR 140:475, 1983.
3. Goodman LR, Kay HR, Teplick KD, Mundth ED. Complications of median sternotomy: Computed tomographic evaluation. AJR 141:225, 1983.
4. Ziter FMH Jr. Major thoracic dehiscence. Radiographic considerations. Radiology 122:587, 1977.

Case 8

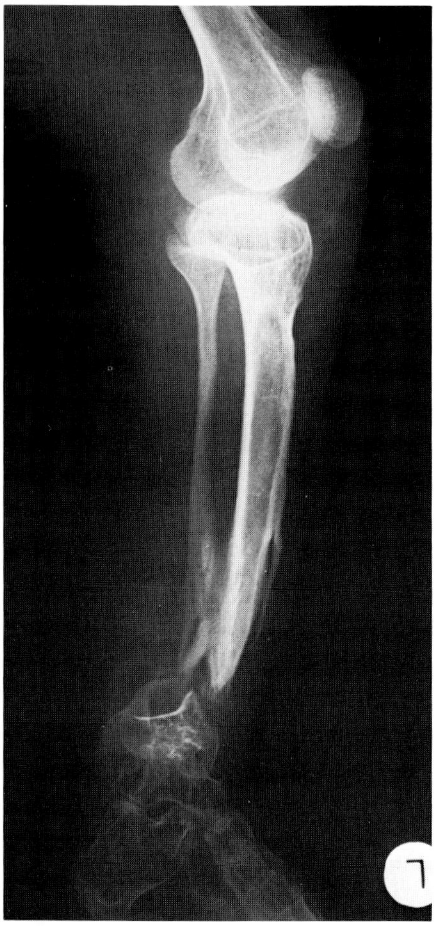

A

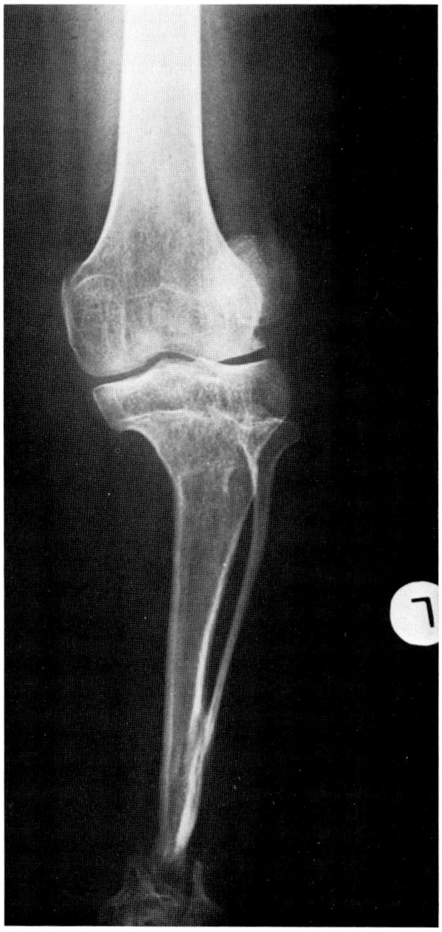

B

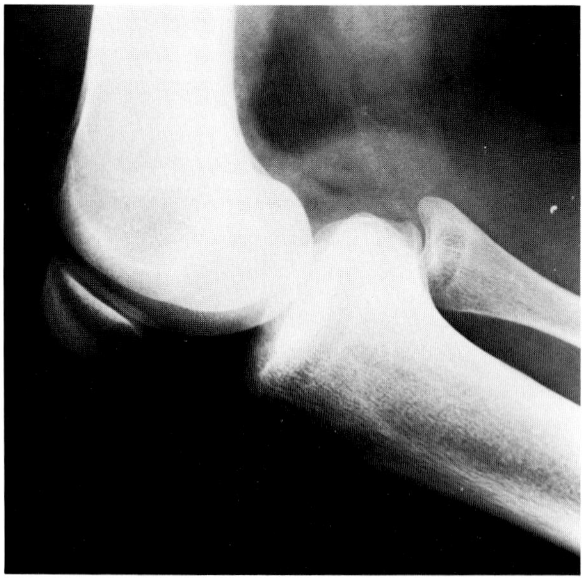

C

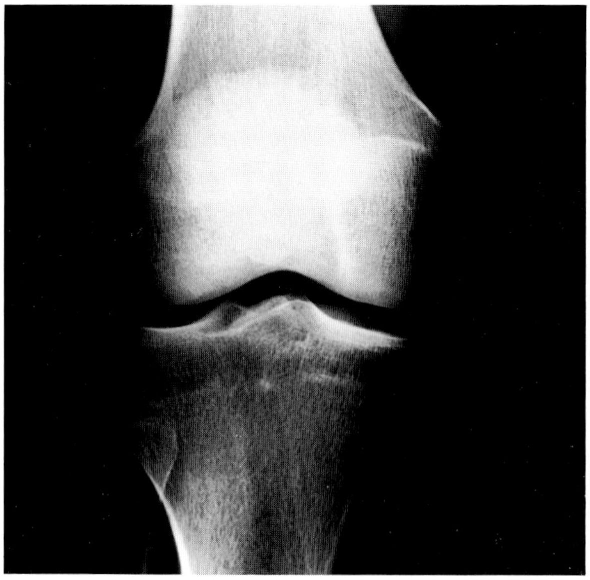

D

Congenital Pseudarthrosis of the Leg

Clinical Information

This 20-year-old white female student, admitted for a dislocated left patella, was known to have congenital pseudarthrosis of the left tibia and fibula. She had undergone five unsuccessful bone grafts. The subluxed patella was reduced. She could walk with a supportive brace, although the left lower extremity was 6 inches shorter than the right.

Roentgen Findings

The left patella is subluxed laterally (A, B). There is anterior bowing of the left leg with osteoporosis of both bones, which taper ("pencil pointing") on both sides of a false joint in the distal third of the leg. Deformities on both sides of the pseudarthrosis have resulted from the previous operations. The left leg is shortened, and the bones of the left leg are smaller than those on the right (C, D). The bones of the left hind foot are considerably deformed (A).

Comments

Bony pseudarthrosis may be apparent at birth, particularly if the tibia is affected (2, 3). In other instances, pseudarthrosis may not become evident for a few months or years after birth. The history will distinguish such pseudarthroses from the nonunion that can follow severe fractures. Also, post-traumatic pseudarthrosis does not exhibit the degree of bony tapering seen with congenital pseudarthrosis. About half of the patients with congenital pseudarthrosis have neurofibromatosis. A portion of the remainder suffer from fibrous dysplasia. There are a fair number of patients in whom neither fibrous dysplasia nor neurofibromatosis is evident. It is possible that these cases represent a forme fruste of neurofibromatosis. None of the patients with pseudarthrosis show distinctive histologic findings in the affected bones. All demonstrate a total lack of callus formation and tapered bone ends at the site of the false joint (1). Such pseudarthroses most often involve the bones of the leg, particularly of the tibia, but other bones, such as those in the upper extremities, have been affected. The ribs also have been involved. It is likely that reported cases of congenital pseudarthrosis of the clavicle represent a different entity (4).

There have been many theories proffered to explain the etiology of this condition. These include intrauterine trauma, mechanical compression of the fetal extremity, defective nutrient arteries, and endocrine disturbances. In actual fact no good evidence exists to support any of these theories. Treatment is unsatisfactory. Many of these patients undergo repeated unsuccessful bone grafts. Fewer than half ever show satisfactory healing. The prognosis is worse if the pseudarthrosis is congenital rather than first appearing in childhood. Onset of the pseudarthrosis before 2 years of age has a less hopeful outlook than a later onset. There is some evidence to indicate results are likely to be better if the bone graft is stabilized with internal fixation.

Congenital pseudarthrosis is characterized by deossification, bony tapering, and bowing in addition to the false joint. In patients who experience a juvenile onset of this condition, the actual pseudarthrosis is often preceded by anterior bowing. Anterolateral bowing of the tibia is much more ominous than posteromedial bowing. The medullary canal slowly becomes narrowed and cystic areas form within the bone. The latter phenomenon often betokens impending fracture and subsequent nonunion.

Source Materials

1. Andersen KS. Radiological classification of congenital pseudarthrosis of the tibia. Acta Orthop Scand 44:719, 1973
2. Brown GA, Osebold WR, Ponseti IV. Congenital pseudarthrosis of long bones. A clinical, radiographic, histologic, and ultrastructural study. Clin Orthop 128:228, 1977.
3. Campanacci M, Nicoll EA, Pagella P. Differential diagnosis of congenital pseudarthrosis of the tibia. Int Orthop 4:283, 1981.
4. Manashil G, Laufer S. Congenital pseudarthrosis of the clavicle: Report of three cases. AJR 132:678, 1979.

Case 9

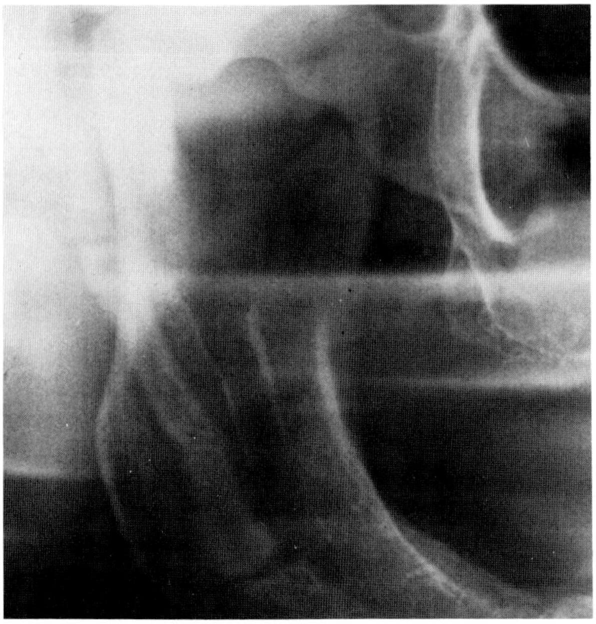

A

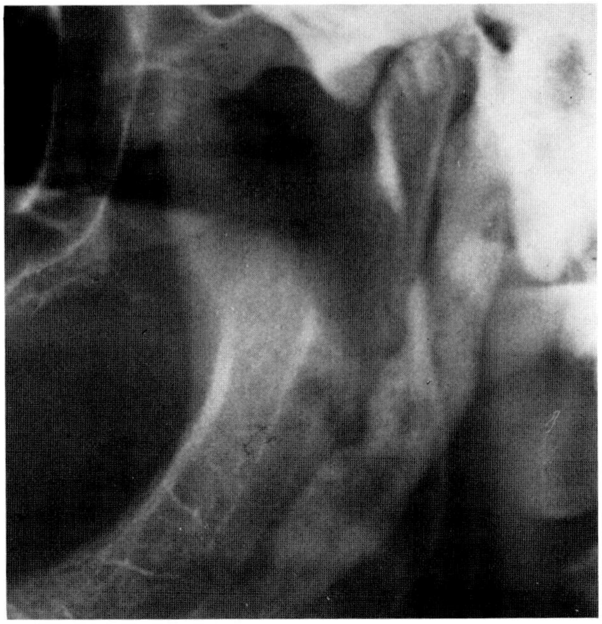

B

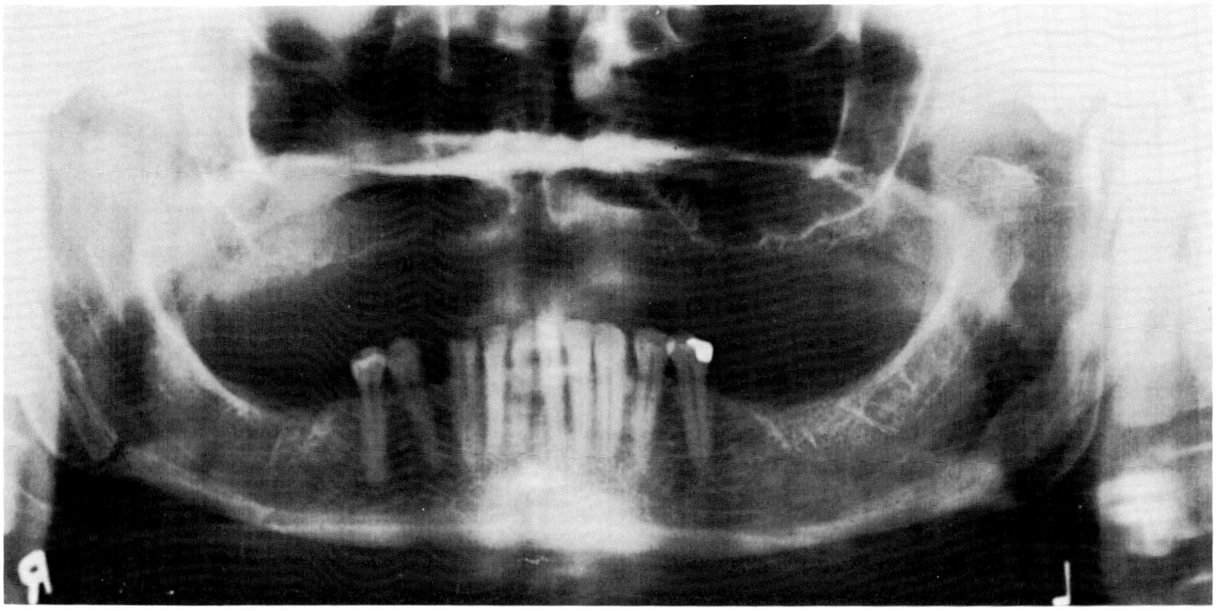

C

Eagle Syndrome

Clinical Information

This 43-year-old man had complained of neck pain since a tonsillectomy 15 years previously. The pain was worse on the left side and was exaggerated by turning his head toward the left. Surgical removal of elongated styloid processes and ossified stylohyoid ligaments, first on the left and subsequently on the right, resulted in complete relief of his distress.

Roentgen Findings

Panoramic views (A–C) of the mandible and surrounding areas show many missing teeth. Both styloid processes are elongated and fused to long, ossified stylohyoid ligaments. The entire stylohyoid apparatus on the left is markedly thickened, and the right shows multiple articulations.

Comments

Films of the neck or mandible often reveal an elongated styloid process attached to an elongated, calcified stylohyoid ligament on one or both sides. The observation is especially frequent when panoramic views are available. This radiologic finding is often present without related symptoms. Indeed, many believe it is without clinical significance. Nevertheless, there are two groups of patients in whom this radiologic appearance is associated with symptoms, which can be relieved by surgical removal of the elongated stylohyoid apparatus. The most distressing symptom in one group is nagging pharyngeal pain that radiates toward the ear. A feeling of a foreign body in the area is often noted. These patients may also have dysphagia. All individuals with these symptoms have had a previous tonsillectomy with the formation of abundant scar tissue, which can be palpated in the tonsillar fossa. Such palpation reproduces the patient's symptoms.

The second group of patients suffer from carotidynia, which is manifested by pain in the distribution of the carotid artery. It is believed that symptoms in these patients result from compression of the external carotid artery by a stiff, elongated, and possibly deviated stylohyoid chain. Complaints of this type increase in frequency with the patient's age. Almost all symptomatic individuals are beyond 30 years of age. Perhaps muscular or ligamentous inelasticity and increasing stiffening of portions of the apparatus cause the complaints.

The stylohyoid apparatus on each side includes the lesser cornua of the hyoid bone, its related stylohyoid ligament, and the styloid process itself. This combination of structures arises from four distinct embryologic segments of the second branchial arch. The stylohyoid ligament often becomes calcified, and articulations may develop between it and other portions of the stylohyoid chain. A few muscles and ligaments attach to the stylohyoid apparatus, which lies behind the pharyngeal wall near the palatine fossa. It is situated between the external carotid artery laterally and the internal carotid artery medially. The jugular vein runs along its medial aspect, as do the hypoglossal, facial, and glossopharyngeal nerves.

As indicated above, there is controversy concerning the clinical significance of the rather frequent x-ray finding of an enlarged, elongated, calcified stylohyoid apparatus. This x-ray appearance obviously has no significance in the absence of symptoms. There are other causes for pain in this area, such as trauma, infection, or malignancy. It has been said that 50% of patients with symptoms due to these causes also have an elongated stylohyoid apparatus. Despite these contentions, it is difficult to deny the significance of an elongated, calcified stylohyoid chain when typical symptoms that can be reproduced by pressure palpation are relieved by its surgical removal.

Source Materials

1. Eagle WW. Elongated styloid processes. Report of two cases. Arch Otolaryngol 25:584, 1937.
2. Gossman JR Jr, Tarsitano JJ. The styloid-stylohyoid syndrome. J Oral Surg 35:555, 1977.
3. Lorman JG, Biggs JR. The Eagle syndrome. Am J Roentgenol 140:881, 1983.
4. Stafne EC, Hollinshead WH. Roentgenographic observations on the stylohyoid chain. Oral Surg 15:1195, 1962.

Case 10

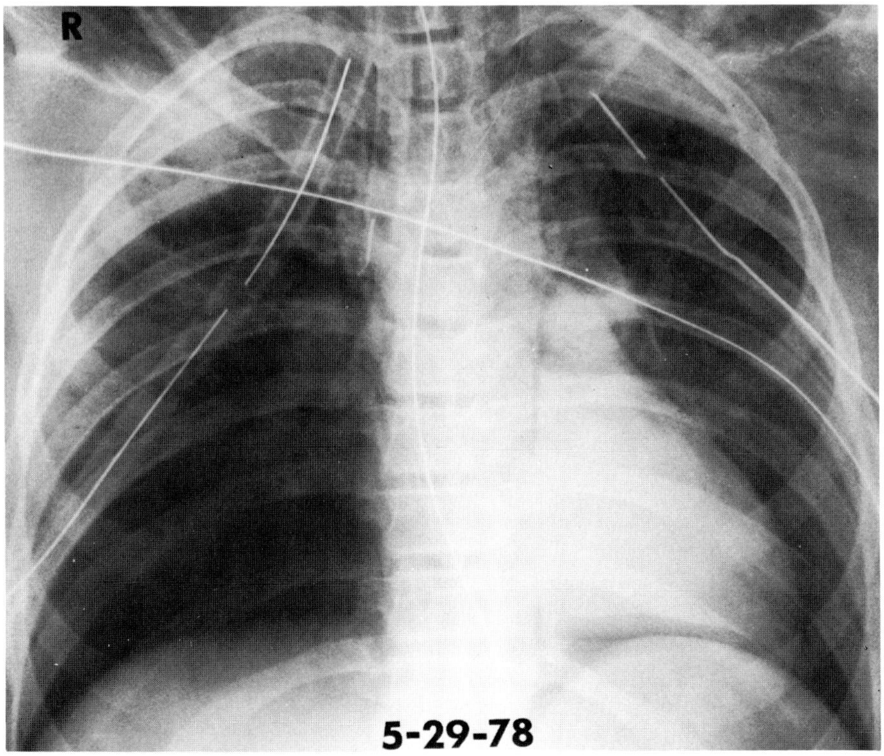

A

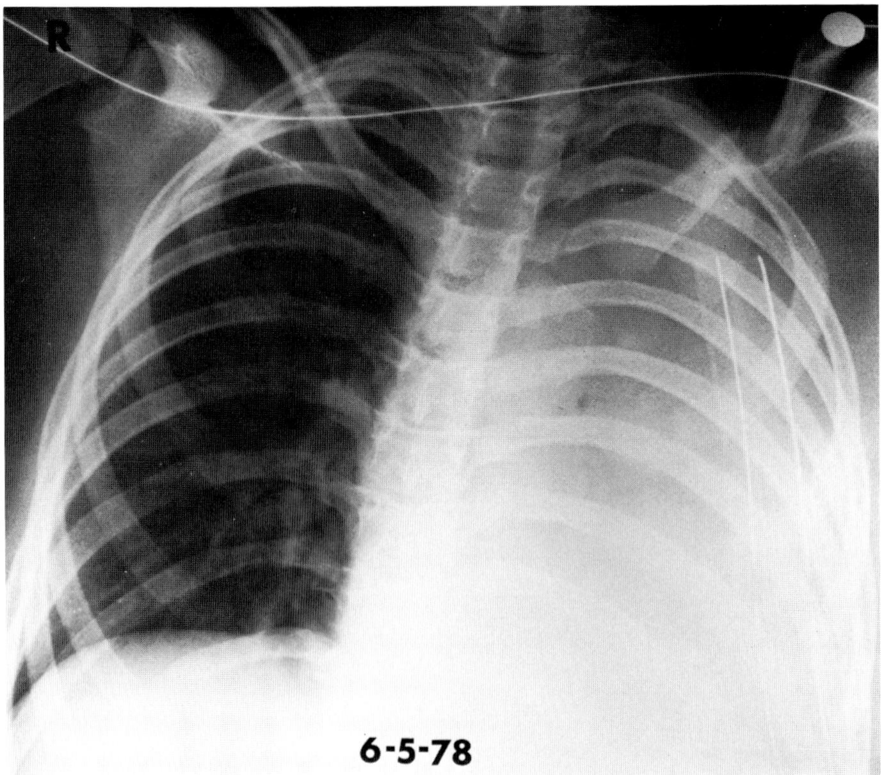

B

Ruptured Bronchus

Clinical Information

This 23-year-old male was involved in an automobile accident on 5-29-78. Bronchoscopy 6 days later revealed laceration of the left mainstem bronchus, which was repaired with a return of normal radiologic findings in the left lung.

Roentgen Findings

A supine chest film (A) obtained shortly after the accident shows bilateral chest tubes and a nasogastric tube in place, subcutaneous emphysema, pneumomediastinum, left basilar pneumothorax, fractures of the left first rib and left clavicle, bilateral pulmonary contusions, and partial left lower lobe collapse. A radiograph exposed six days later (B) reveals that the right-sided abnormalities, pneumothorax, pneumomediastinum, and subcutaneous emphysema have disappeared. The right-sided chest tube has been removed and a second tube added on the left. Nevertheless, the mediastinum has shifted toward that side, and the left hemithorax is now almost completely radiopaque, indicative of left lung collapse. This progression of x-ray changes is consistent with rupture of the left mainstem bronchus.

Comments

Bronchial rupture is most often due to a motor vehicle accident with deceleration. The rupture can be caused by direct compression of the bronchus between the sternum and the vertebral column; by forced expiration against a closed glottis, which increases intrabronchial pressure; or by a shearing force created by sudden deceleration of the lung, which pulls against a fixed trachea. This injury nearly always occurs within an inch of the carina. The distal trachea is involved in about 20% of the cases. The right mainstem bronchus is injured slightly more frequently than the left. Bilateral injury or rupture beyond the mainstem bronchi is rare. A bronchus can be completely transected, or there may only be a break in a portion of the bronchial wall.

Hemoptysis and dyspnea are common symptoms, although complaints due to other multiple injuries often predominate. Indeed, bronchial rupture may cause no symptoms initially. This injury is associated with a mortality of about 30%, although perhaps half of these deaths can be attributed to other trauma. Delay in diagnosis seriously worsens the prognosis. Only 30% are diagnosed correctly within the first 24 hours. The diagnosis is delayed for a month in an equal number. Bronchial rupture is frequently missed entirely until autopsy. The only reasonable treatment is surgical repair, even if the diagnosis is much delayed. Untreated patients that survive may develop bronchial stenosis and subsequent pulmonary collapse.

The diagnosis of bronchial rupture can be strongly suggested from x-ray findings and the patient's clinical course, although bronchoscopy is required for confirmation. Massive pneumothorax is common (3, 4). It tends to be progressive and usually fails to respond to tube thoracostomy. X-ray findings can be minimal or absent. Bronchography is probably contraindicated immediately after the accident, since it may further compromise respiration. The upper ribs are fractured in approximately 90% of these patients. This is indicative of the severity of the injury. Massive atelectasis as well as mediastinal and cervical emphysema are common. A linear air collection may parallel the damaged bronchus. The development of persistent massive atelectasis in spite of adequate chest tube drainage, as demonstrated by this patient, suggests the diagnosis. Complete transection of a bronchus can lead to the "fallen lung" sign, which is pathognomonic (2). The portion of the lung served by the transected bronchus loses its anchoring support and, in the presence of the pneumothorax, falls away from the hilum.

Source Materials

1. Harvey-Smith W, Bush W, Northrop C. Traumatic bronchial rupture. AJR 134:1189, 1980.
2. Kumpe DA, Oh KS, Wyman SM. A characteristic pulmonary finding in unilateral complete bronchial transection. AJR 110:704, 1970.
3. Wiot JF. Tracheobronchial trauma. Semin Roentgenol 18:15, 1983.
4. Woodring JH, Fried AM, Hatfield DR, et al. Fractures of first and second ribs: Predictive value for arterial and bronchial injury. AJR 138:211, 1982.

Case 11

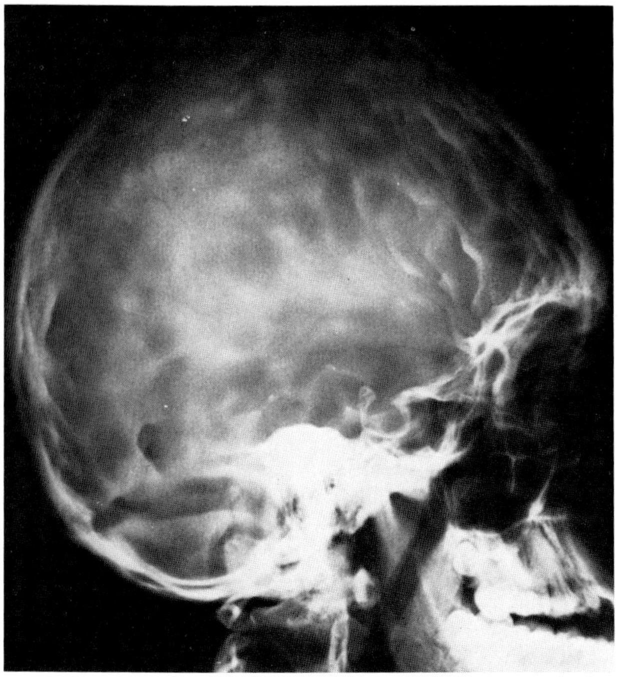

A

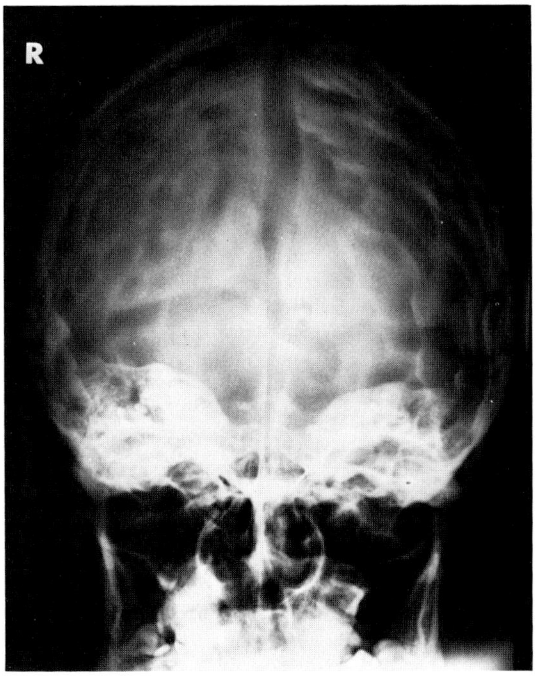

B

Crouzon's Syndrome (Craniofacial Dysostosis)

Clinical Information

This 20-year-old white female was admitted to the hospital with a primary complaint of persistent headaches. She had an odd-shaped head, a protuberant mandible, hypertelorism, prominent eyes, and divergent strabismus. Several family members were similarly affected.

Roentgen Findings

The cranial vault is shortened anteroposteriorly and lengthened superoinferiorly (A, B). There are exaggerated digital impressions visible on the inner table of the skull. The grooves that accommodate the sagittal and lateral venous sinuses are very prominent. These findings are indicative of premature closure of all the cranial sutures. The midface is small and somewhat depressed and the orbits are shallow. Protuberance of the mandible has resulted from the relatively small size of the maxillae. These findings in concert with the clinical appearance are indicative of Crouzon's syndrome, which is also called craniofacial dysostosis (more correctly dysplasia) or dysmorphism.

Comments

X-ray findings of craniosynostosis and midface hypoplasia with an appropriate facial appearance and a family history indicative of dominant inheritance are diagnostic of Crouzon's syndrome (1). This condition becomes evident very early in life, usually within the first 3 years. All of the cranial sutures need not be closed, although such is frequently the case. The premature synostosis usually involves sutures at the base of the skull as well as those in the cranial vault. The deformity that results depends upon which sutures are affected. The pathogenesis of premature craniosynostosis is not known, although there is evidence that the dura is an important determinant (4). Optic nerve atrophy, which may lead to blindness and possibly mental retardation, can be occasioned by the increased intracranial pressure secondary to the premature craniosynostosis. Vision is affected in 80% of adult patients with Crouzon's syndrome.

Hypoplasia of the maxillary and zygomatic bones causes the characteristic shallow orbits, frequent proptosis, prognathism, and "parrot beak" profile. Hypertelorism is usually present. Other associated anomalies, including choanal atresia and ear anomalies, are common. Linear craniectomies along or parallel to the closed sutures are indicated to prevent damage to the cranial nerves (3). This surgery should be performed as soon as possible because the brain grows very rapidly during the first year of life. Severe exophthalmos may be ameliorated by orbital decompression. Subsequent surgical therapy directed toward the facial bones is largely cosmetic.

Characteristic x-ray findings of Crouzon's syndrome include mandibular prognathism, midface hypoplasia, a flattened nasal arch, protuberant eyes, hypertelorism, and evidence of craniosynostosis. The orbits frequently are shallow. They may be oval and slant upward and outward due to bilateral coronal suture synostosis. The paranasal sinuses, as in this case, are usually small and underdeveloped. Bone scanning may be helpful in identifying sutures that are prematurely fused or are fusing (2). No significant differential diagnostic possibilities exist in the presence of consistent physical, radiologic, and familial evidence. Apert's syndrome can be identified by the presence of syndactylism. Differentiating clinical findings exist in several other syndromes that feature craniosynostosis as a portion of their presentation.

Source Materials

1. Cohen MM Jr. Genetic perspectives in craniosynostosis and syndromes with craniosynostosis. J Neurosurg 47:886, 1977.
2. Gates GF, Dore EK. Detection of craniosynostosis by bone scanning. Radiology 115:665, 1975.
3. Hoffman HJ, Hendrick EB. Early neurosurgical repair in craniofacial dysmorphism. J Neurosurg 51:796, 1979.
4. Smith DW, Töndury G. Origin of the calvaria and its sutures. Am J Dis Child 132:662, 1978.

Case 12

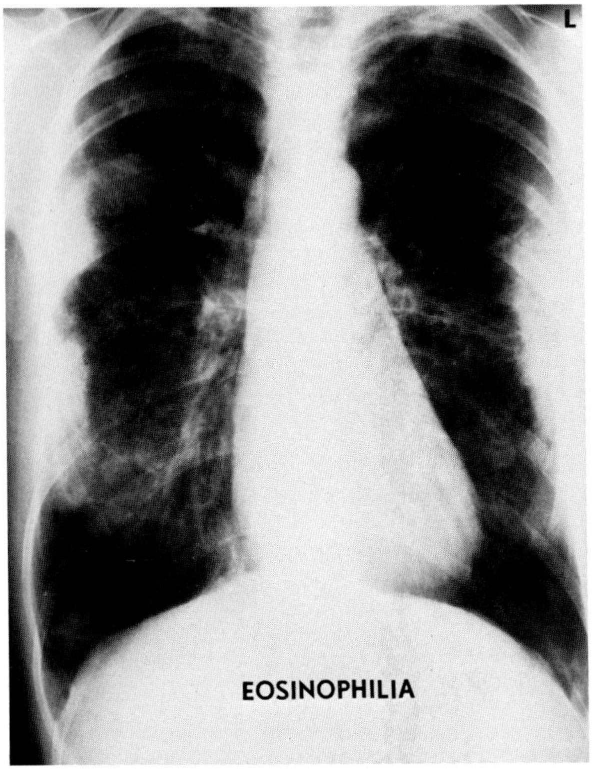

A

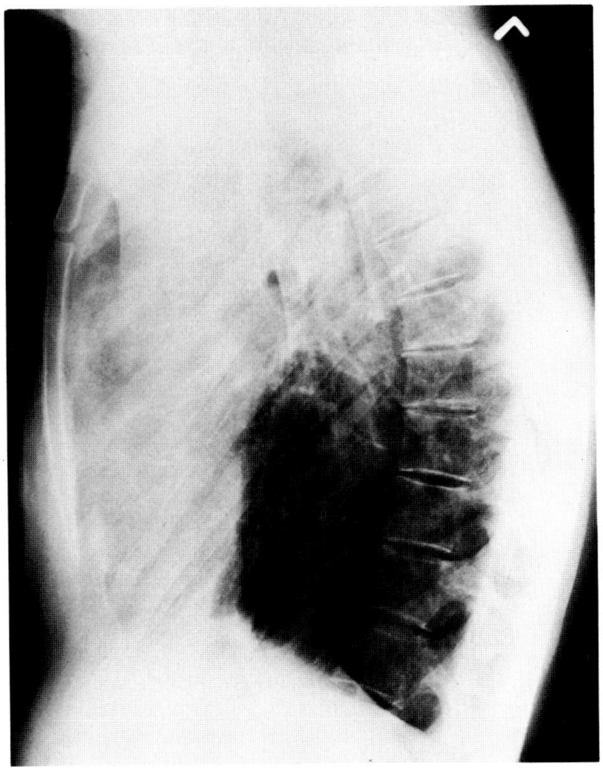

B

Chronic Eosinophilic Pneumonia

Clinical Information

This 41-year-old white female had a history of asthma. She was admitted to the hospital with symptoms of fever, cough, chest pain, and peripheral eosinophilia. A lung biopsy confirmed the radiologic diagnosis of chronic eosinophilic pneumonia. Her pulmonary infiltrates responded promptly and satisfactorily to steroid therapy.

Roentgen Findings

Posteroanterior (A) and lateral (B) films of the chest show multiple soft, fluffy pulmonary infiltrates in the periphery of the lung fields. The peripheral location is particularly evident in the axillary portions of the lungs. Both nipple shadows are well seen. No pleural effusion is evident.

Comments

Several conditions can lead to pulmonary parenchymal disease associated with blood eosinophilia (2). These include simple pulmonary eosinophilia (Loeffler's syndrome), which is characterized by mild symptoms and migratory pulmonary infiltrates; tropical eosinophilia due to microfilaria; pulmonary eosinophilia with asthma, which usually is a manifestation of one type of aspergillosis; and vascular conditions such as polyarteritis nodosa and Wegener's granulomatosis, as well as chronic eosinophilic pneumonia.

Chronic eosinophilic pneumonia can result from specific etiologies such as certain parasites, bacteria, drugs, or antigens, although no specific cause is evident in a considerable proportion of these patients. One-third of affected individuals have asthma. About two-thirds will have a typical x-ray appearance, which is characterized by fluffy infiltrates located in the peripheral portions of the lungs. These have been described as the photographic negative of the appearance seen with classical pulmonary edema (4). Approximately 70% of patients with chronic eosinophilic pneumonia have peripheral blood eosinophilia. The usual symptoms include a high fever, night sweats, chest pain, and shortness of breath. Extensive weight loss is common. Sinusitis is relatively frequent. The pulmonary infiltrates and the symptoms characteristically respond extremely favorably to steroid therapy, although chronic eosinophilic pneumonia can be progressive and lead to pulmonary insufficiency, which may be fatal. Response to steroid therapy may begin within an hour of its institution. The promptness of this response is almost diagnostic. Steroids are much more rapidly effective in this disease than with pulmonary infiltrates caused by other etiologies. The densities occasionally return when steroid treatment is withdrawn. In such instances the recurrent infiltrates often reappear in the same location and present the same appearance as originally. Pulmonary function tests in patients with progressive disease typically show restrictive changes. Lung biopsies reveal an eosinophilic exudate in both the interstitial and the alveolar tissues.

Typical x-ray findings with blood eosinophilia justify a confident diagnosis. Biopsy is not needed in such circumstances. Pleural effusion is uncommon. The infiltrates have sometimes been described as presenting a "ground glass" appearance. They usually lie against the pleurae, do not have a segmental or lobar distribution, and are most commonly seen in the apical and axillary portions of the lungs. The infiltrates can, when located in the lung bases, mimic a loculated effusion. About 10% of these patients exhibit characteristic radiologic densities in the absence of blood eosinophilia and still prove on biopsy to have chronic eosinophilic pneumonia. A considerable number of patients with chronic eosinophilic pneumonia do not demonstrate characteristic x-ray findings.

Source Materials

1. Case records of the Massachusetts General Hospital. Case 39-1981. N Engl J Med 305:749, 1981.
2. Citro LA, Gordon ME, Miller WT. Eosinophilic lung disease (or how to slice P.I.E.). AJR 117:787, 1973.
3. Fox B, Seed WA. Chronic eosinophilic pneumonia. Thorax 35:570, 1980.
4. Gaensler EA, Carrington CB. Peripheral opacities in chronic eosinophilic pneumonia: The photographic negative of pulmonary edema. AJR 128:1, 1977.

Case 13

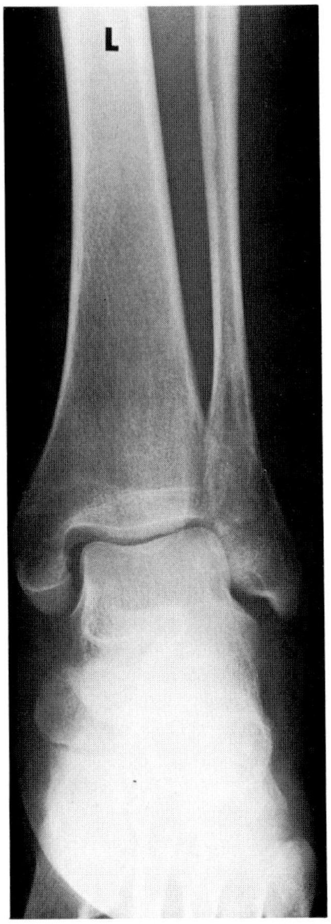

A

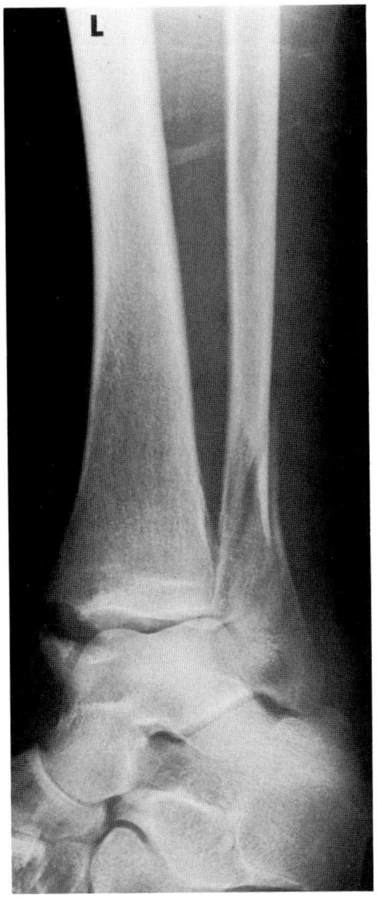

B

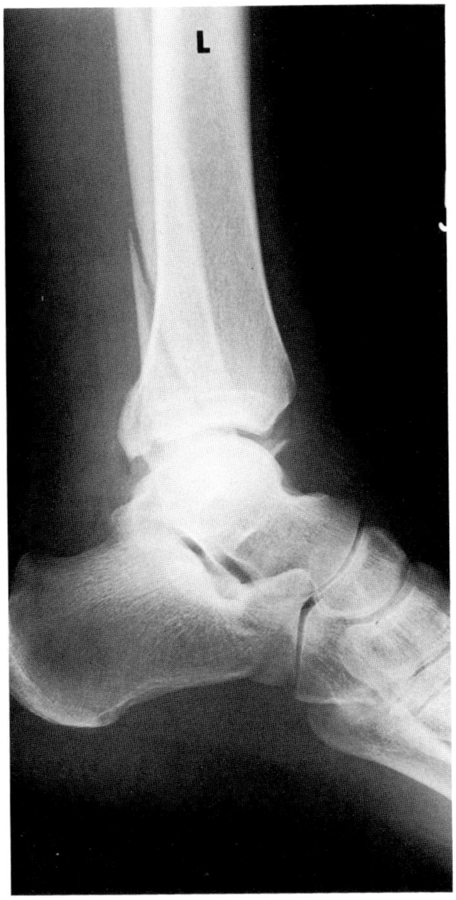

C

Ankle Fracture

Clinical Information

This 30-year-old male severely everted his left ankle while playing baseball. The fractures were treated with pin fixation. Healing was uneventful.

Roentgen Findings

Anteroposterior (A), oblique (B), and lateral (C) radiographs of the left ankle show a horizontal avulsion fracture of the medial malleolus at the level of the tibial plafond. There is also a small fracture through the lateral aspect of the posterior lip of the tibia. In addition, an oblique fracture of the distal fibula is seen to run proximally from near the level of the articular surface of the tibia at the ankle joint. The ankle mortice is mildly disturbed by medial widening from lateral slippage of the talus and foot. These changes are typical of an eversion injury with a tear in the tibiofibular ligament (2, 3).

Comments

Ankle injury is very frequent. This relatively small joint bears all of the body weight. Ankle injuries vary in severity from a mild strain to gross fracture and dislocation. Although the ankle joint can be injured from direct violence or vertical compression, most instances of trauma to this joint can result from inversion (supination) or eversion (pronation) (2, 3). This admitted oversimplification is useful in understanding the mechanics of these injuries. Other classifications of varying completeness and complexity exist (1).

Eversion injuries are very common. Minor trauma of this type causes at least a sprain of the medial collateral ligament. Additional force may rupture this ligament or (if the ligament remains intact) avulse the medial malleolus, which is seen radiologically as a transverse fracture near the level of the ankle joint. Still more force impacts the talus against the lateral aspect of the ankle joint. This may lead to an oblique fracture of the lateral malleolus below the tibial plafond. In general, avulsive forces lead to transverse fractures, whereas impactive forces cause oblique or spiral fractures. The fibular fracture may relieve the strain from the tibiofibular ligament, which can remain intact. Disruption of the distal portion of the tibiofibular ligament occurs in some patients. This permits separation of the tibia and fibula, with resultant widening of the ankle mortice. Such a separation can occur in the absence of a fracture. An eversion injury with a fracture of the fibula above the tibiofibular joint is invariably associated with a tear in the tibiofibular ligament. There may also be a fracture of the posterolateral tibial lip. The fibular fracture may be far above the ankle, even near the knee (Maisonneuve fracture). Consequently, x-ray evidence of a posterior lip tibial fracture demands a search for a fibular fracture, which may require films of its entire extent. It is important in the reduction and fixation of eversion fractures that the posterior lip be properly reduced and a normal length of the fibula restored.

In inversion injuries an avulsive stress is placed upon the lateral aspect of the joint. This can lead to rupture of the lateral collateral ligament or a transverse fracture of the lateral malleolus at the level of the ankle mortice. Further force may cause an oblique fracture of the distal medial malleolus. An inversion injury does not rupture the tibiofibular ligament. A consideration of the mechanics of ankle fractures in terms of inversion or eversion and the injuries that may result is important, because severe ligamentous injury may be sustained in the absence of an obvious fracture. Stress films are indicated in this circumstance, since patients with an extensive ligamentous tear should be treated by immobilization until healing occurs to prevent future degenerative joint changes (2).

Source Materials

1. Arimoto HK, Forrester DM. Classification of ankle fractures. An algorithm. AJR 135:1057, 1980.
2. Edeiken J, Cotler JM. Ankle injury. The need for stress films. JAMA 240:1182, 1978.
3. Edeiken J, Cotler JM. Ankle trauma. Semin Roentgenol 13:145, 1978.

Case 14

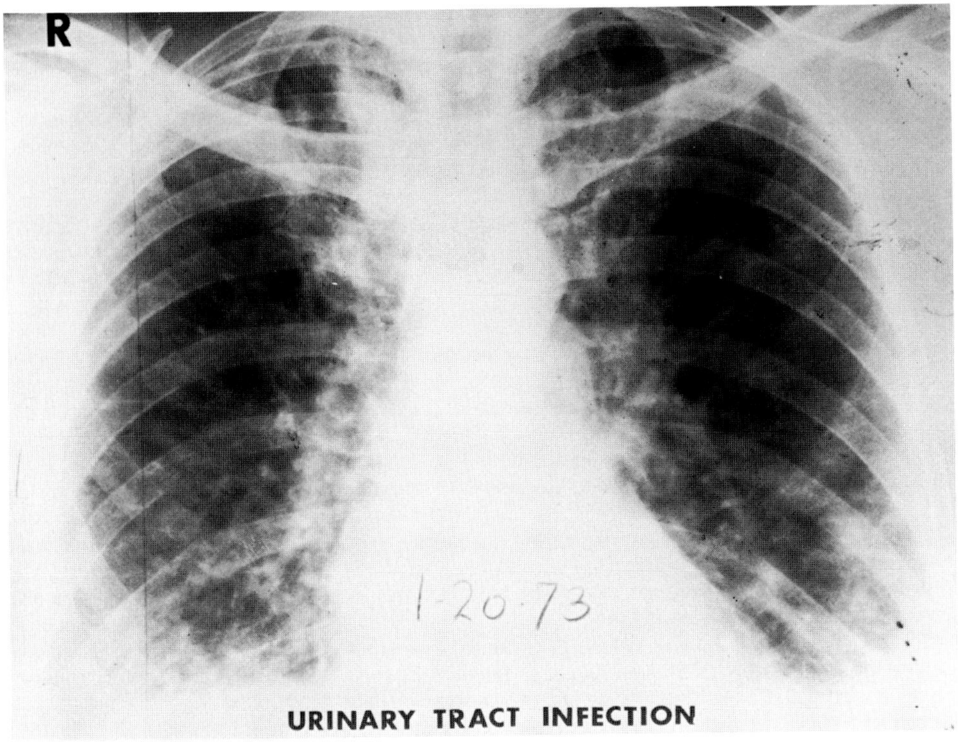

A

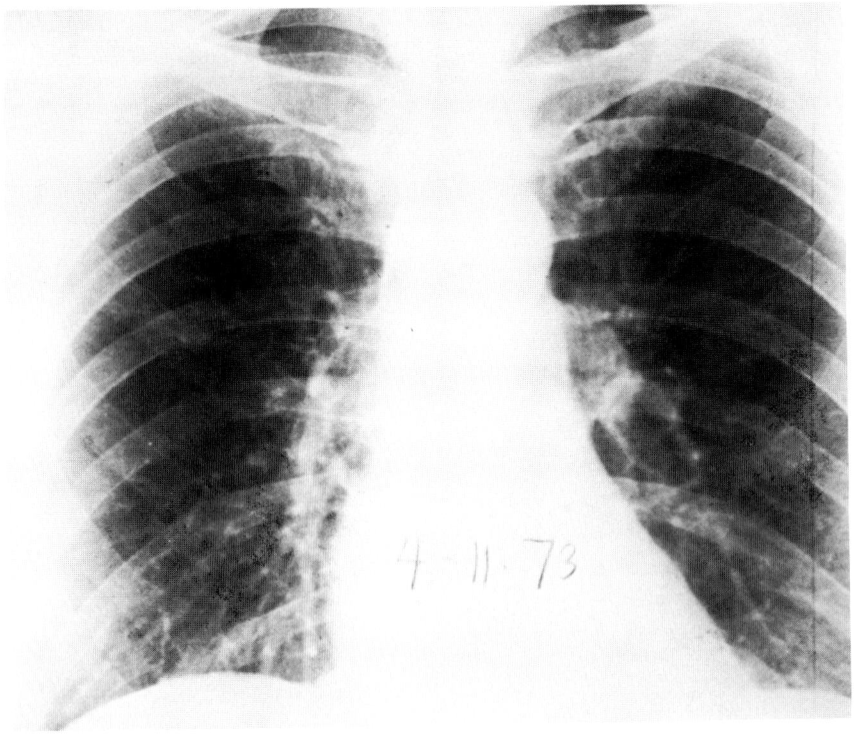

B

Nitrofurantoin Lung Disease

Clinical Information

This 60-year-old man with prostatism and urinary tract infection had been taking nitrofurantoin (Furadantin) for 1 week before he developed fever, cough, and shortness of breath. Laboratory studies revealed a peripheral blood eosinophilia. Furadantin therapy was continued for another week. His complaints worsened and the chest film dated 1-20-73 (A) was obtained. Furadantin was stopped and his symptoms and radiologic abnormalities cleared completely over the next several days.

Roentgen Findings

The film of the chest dated 1-20-73 shows abundant fluffy infiltrates distributed throughout both lung fields but most marked at the bases. There are small bilateral pleural effusions. A linear vertical artifact is evident along the right side of the radiograph. The chest film dated 4-11-73 (B) was obtained about 2½ months after cessation of therapy and reveals complete clearing of the infiltrates.

Comments

The administration of nitrofurantoin (trade name Furadantin) for a urinary tract infection has been recognized for many years as a very common etiology of drug-related pulmonary disease. Only oxygen and corticosteroids are more frequent causes. Aspiration of mineral oil does not often lead to permanent changes in the pulmonary parenchyma. The etiology of Furadantin lung disease, which can be either acute or chronic, is unknown, although the acute changes presumably represent an abnormal immunologic response. Pulmonary reaction can develop within hours after exposure, although many days or even weeks may elapse before symptoms and infiltrates appear. The pulmonary changes are seen as patches of soft infiltration that are often associated with pleural effusion. These radiologic abnormalities can simulate noncardiogenic pulmonary edema. They frequently are accompanied by fever and eosinophilia. Bronchospasm may be present. Some patients have chest pain. Such acute changes usually disappear promptly with cessation of the drug.

The chronic x-ray changes that can occur after Furadantin administration take the form of a diffuse, chronic interstitial pneumonitis characterized by reticulonodular densities and/or localized areas of consolidation. The chronic form is usually at least partially reversible following cessation of the drug. Although evidence of the acute manifestations of Furadantin lung disease disappears in a few days after the drug is stopped, weeks or months can be required for whatever measure of recovery may occur from the chronic form. Corticosteroids may be used. They are especially helpful in the chronic form of the disease, but discontinuance of Furadantin is essential. There is very little overlap between the acute and chronic forms of Furadantin lung disease.

Films of the chest are normal throughout the course of the disease in approximately 10% of patients with symptoms that abate following cessation of Furadantin therapy. Parenchymal changes are almost always bilateral in both acute and chronic Furadantin lung disease. Pleural effusion, on the other hand, is usually seen on only one side and is always accompanied by parenchymal disease. The diagnosis of Furadantin lung disease is made from a careful drug history, characteristic x-ray findings, and (if necessary) a drug challenge.

Source Materials

1. Glueck MA, Janower ML. Nitrofurantoin lung disease. Clues to pathogenesis. AJR 107:818, 1969.
2. Heap TR, Rebuck AS. Chronic nitrofurantoin (Furadantin) pulmonary reaction. Australas Radiol 16:236, 1972.
3. Morrison DA, Goldman AL. Radiographic patterns of drug-induced lung disease. Radiology 131:299, 1979.
4. Rosenow EC III. Drug-induced pulmonary disease. Clin Notes Respir Dis 16:3, 1977.

Case 15

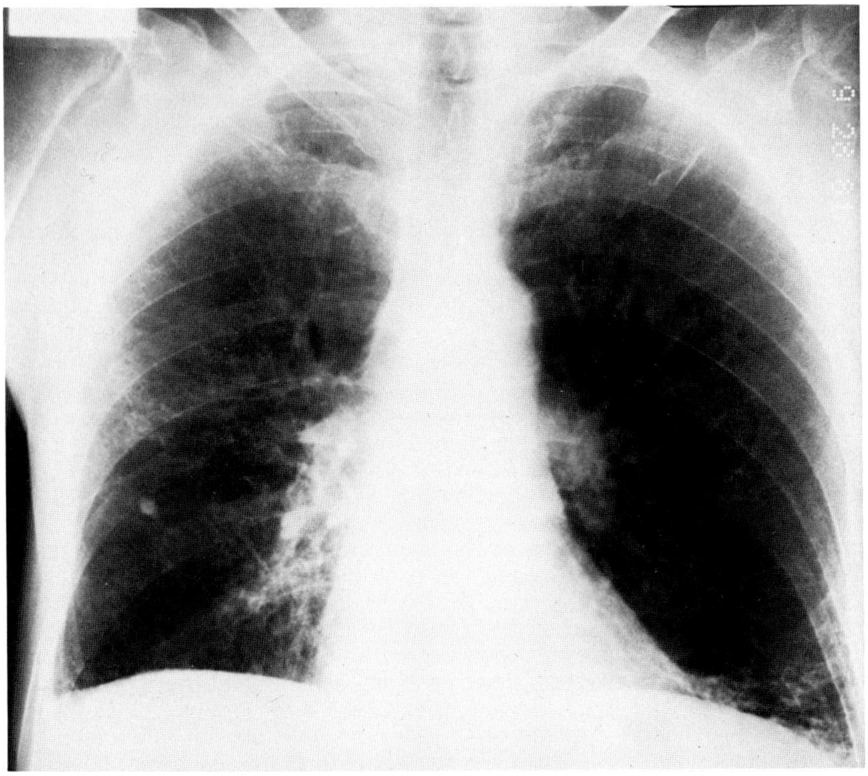

A

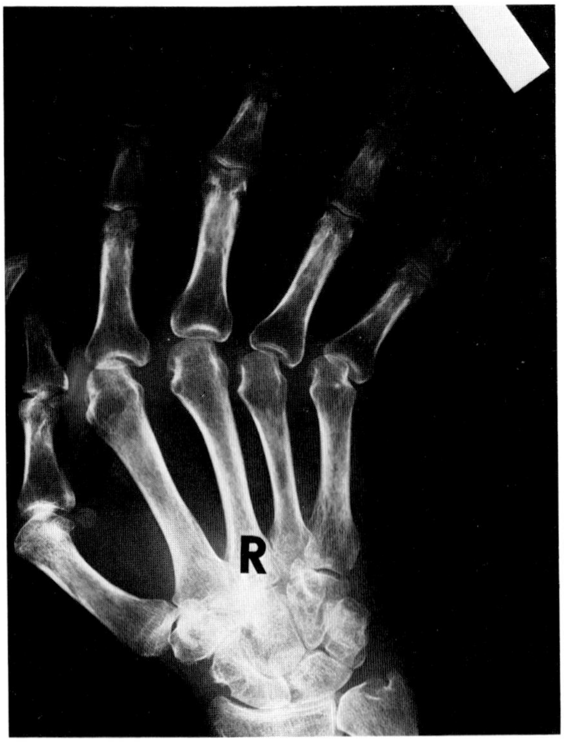

B

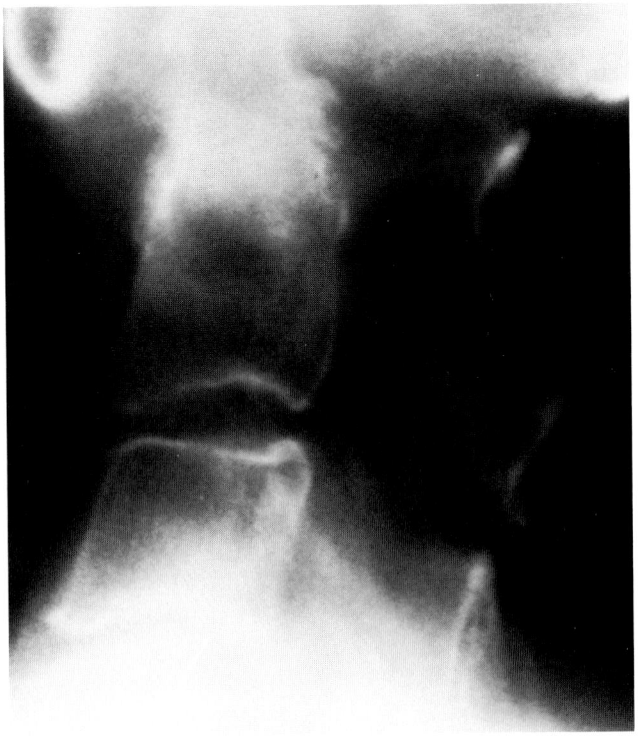

C

Rheumatoid Lung Disease

Clinical Information

This 50-year-old male with long-standing rheumatoid arthritis (RA) had no pulmonary complaints.

Roentgen Findings

A posteroanterior film of the chest (A) shows widespread reticulonodular densities. They are particularly prominent at the lung bases, where there is some loss of volume on the left. The right costophrenic angle is blunted. In addition, both shoulder joints are narrowed and somewhat irregular, a finding consistent with RA. An anteroposterior film of the right hand (B) and a lateral tomogram of the cervical spine (C) show typical changes of RA.

Comments

About 20% of patients affected with RA have extra-articular disease, most commonly subcutaneous nodules and/or rheumatoid lung disease (RLD). Pulmonary changes can be manifested as pleural effusion, pleural thickening, interstitial pneumonitis and fibrosis, pulmonary arteritis, microbiotic nodules, or rheumatoid nodules associated with pneumoconiosis (Caplan's syndrome). The last mentioned may be no more than a chance association. RLD usually follows long-standing severe RA but can precede the joint abnormalities. Patients with RLD commonly have an elevated rheumatoid factor, subcutaneous nodules, and severe joint involvement. RLD is more frequent in males by a ratio of 2:1 despite a striking predilection of RA for females. Respiratory symptoms are usually less severe than the radiographic abnormalities, which may be extensive in the absence of symptoms. This contrasts sharply with other causes of interstitial lung disease.

Pleural effusion is seen in males with RA more often than in females in a ratio of about 25:1. The effusion is usually small to moderate in size. There is a slight right-sided predominance, although the effusion is often bilateral. These effusions may remain unchanged for months or years. The pleura eventually becomes thickened. Pleural effusions of RLD exhibit the features of an exudate with a low glucose level, which, in contrast to a tuberculous pleural effusion, does not become elevated following intravenous glucose loading.

It is said that about 20% of all patients with interstitial pulmonary fibrosis have RLD, which is approximately the same percentage of patients with RA that develop RLD. The interstitial fibrosis of RLD is slowly progressive and irreversible. It may progress to an end-stage fibrotic lung. The most frequent radiologic change in the parenchyma is a reticulonodular pattern that usually is more marked at the bases. B lines of Kerley may be present in severe cases. The pulmonary nodules occasionally seen in RLD are usually small, multiple, and subpleural in location, and tend to cavitate. They are histologically identical to the subcutaneous nodules of RA. These nodules, in contrast to other manifestations of RLD, may wax and wane. The x-ray changes of RLD are not distinctive in themselves, but the diagnosis is justified when they are associated with joint changes that are consistent with RA.

Source Materials

1. Case records of the Massachusetts General Hospital. Case 3-1982. N Engl J Med 306:157, 1982.
2. Cervantes-Perez P, Toro-Perez AH, Rodriguez-Jurado P. Pulmonary involvement in rheumatoid arthritis. JAMA 242:1715, 1980.
3. Martel W, Abell MR, Mikkelsen WM, Whitehouse WM. Pulmonary and pleural lesions in rheumatoid disease. Radiology 90:641, 1968.
4. Reeder MM. RPC of the Month from AFIP. Radiology 92:1106, 1969.

Case 16

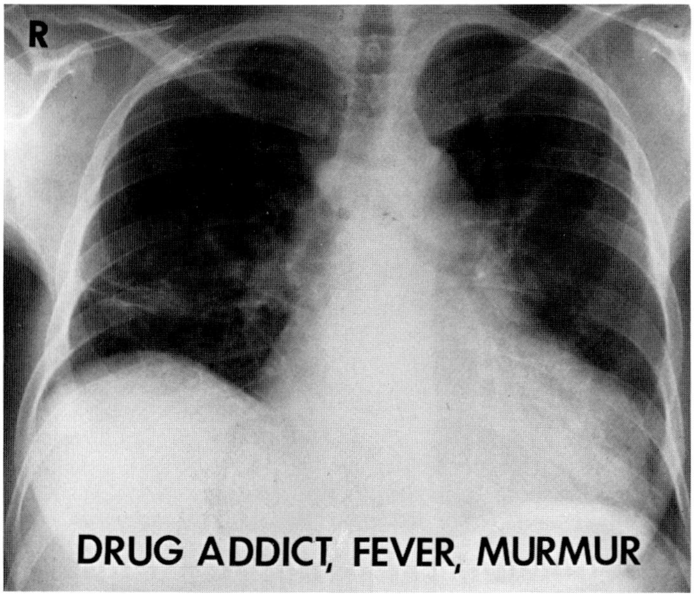

A

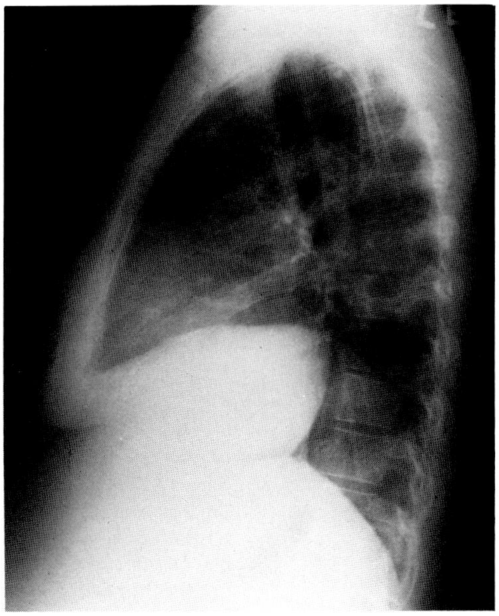

B

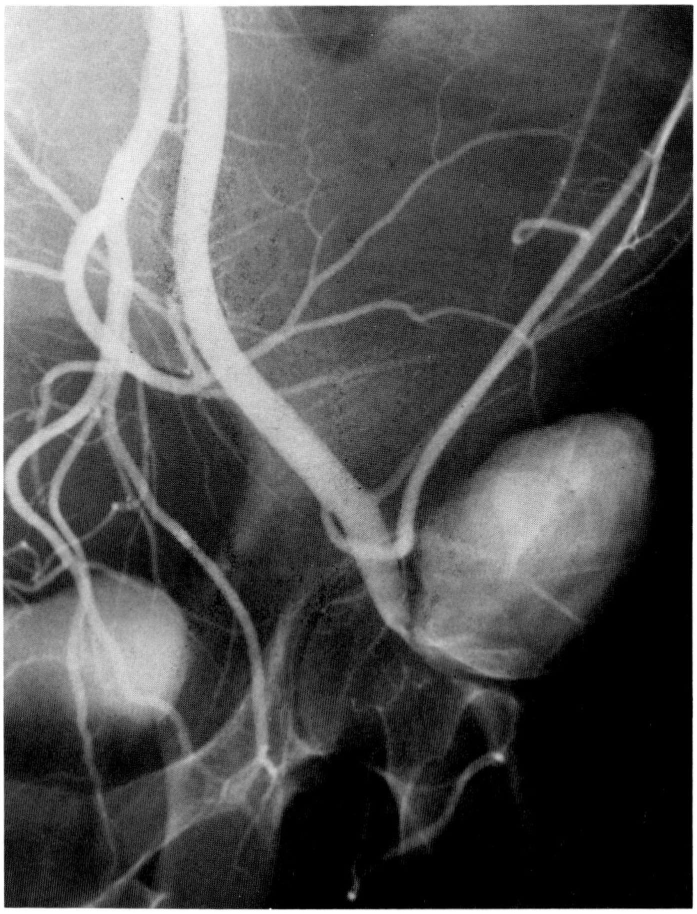

C

Tricuspid Endocarditis in a Drug Addict

Clinical Information

This 31-year-old white female heroin addict had suffered from increasing fever, cough, and evidence of congestive failure for several weeks. Ultrasonic evidence of tricuspid vegetations and multiple blood cultures positive for *Staphylococcus aureus* led to extensive chemotherapy and eventual replacement of the tricuspid valve. She also demonstrated a mycotic aneurysm of the left external iliac artery (see film C), which was also resected. The patient made a satisfactory recovery.

Roentgen Findings

Posteroanterior (A) and lateral (B) chest films show an enlarged heart and elevation of the right diaphragm. There are densities in both midlung fields, more marked on the right. The lateral film reveals an abscess with a fluid level in the superior segment of the right lower lobe. A portion of a needle can be seen in the soft tissues of the right axilla.

Comments

Narcotic addiction can lead to two types of radiologic findings (2). One represents reaction to the drug. This may take the form of pulmonary edema. Foreign material such as talcum can cause numerous pulmonary emboli, which appear as small, irregular densities. These emboli can lead to cor pulmonale. Severe gastrointestinal ileus and necrotizing angitis, particularly in the kidneys, have been reported. The other type of x-ray change is due to infection. Septic pulmonary emboli are particularly common. They usually are rounded or wedge-shaped, peripherally located, and can excavate rapidly, leaving a thin-walled cavity. Mycotic aneurysms can occur. Osteomyelitis, especially in the spine, has been reported frequently. Tetanus is seen quite often, as is hepatitis. These infections result from contamination of the injected material and lack of aseptic precautions. Drug addicts tend to be immunologically deficient and generally in poor health; these factors also make them liable.

Infective endocarditis is seen 30 times more frequently in addicts than in the normal population and four times more often than in patients with rheumatic heart disease. In some institutions 15% of the patients with infective endocarditis are addicts. The valves of the right heart, especially the tricuspid valve, are infected more often than the left-sided valves. Preexistent heart disease is not a necessary contributing factor. The infecting organism is *Staphylococcus aureus* in about 80% of these patients. Tricuspid insufficiency is usually present. Emboli from infected vegetations on the tricuspid valve can lead to septic pulmonary emboli, or they can progress beyond the lungs and involve the brain, kidney, liver, and spleen as well as other locations. Appropriate treatment involves 4–6 weeks of intravenous antibiotic therapy. A prosthetic valve is needed if the tricuspid valve is severely damaged. The prognosis of tricuspid endocarditis is better than with involvement of a left-sided heart valve. Death usually results from pulmonary infection rather than heart failure.

The diagnosis of endocarditis in an addict can be made from the history, evidence of infection, heart failure, pulmonary complaints, and x-ray evidence of septic emboli (1, 2). The presence of a needle or a portion thereof in the soft tissues is highly suggestive of this condition. Echocardiography can be useful. Septic emboli are usually multiple and peripheral in location. They tend to coalesce and frequently cavitate. A so-called "target lesion" has been said to be a specific sign (3). This sign consists of a thin-walled, rounded hyperlucency containing a central nodular density that is unaffected by gravity. The central density is presumed to be a nidus of suppuration surrounded by a small pneumatocele.

Source Materials

1. Davies W. Tricuspid endocarditis and embolic pneumonia in heroin addicts. Australas Radiol 24:27, 1980.
2. Stern WZ. Roentgenographic aspects of narcotic addiction. JAMA 236:963, 1976.
3. Zelefsky MN, Lutzker LG. The target sign: A new radiologic sign of septic pulmonary emboli. AJR 129:453, 1977.

Case 17

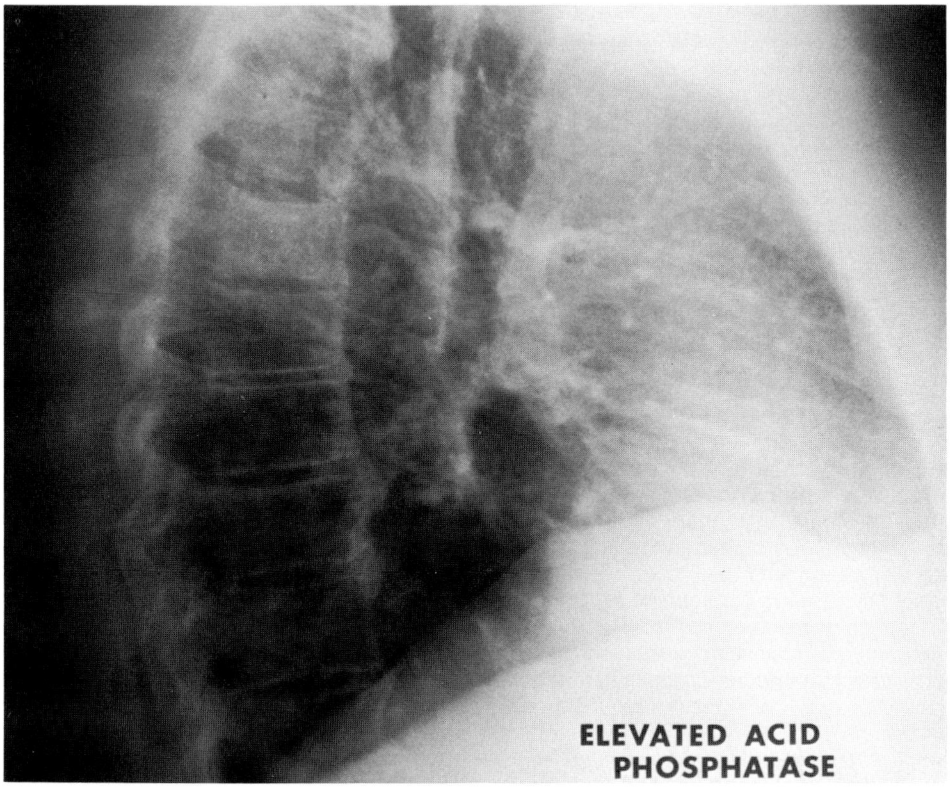

A

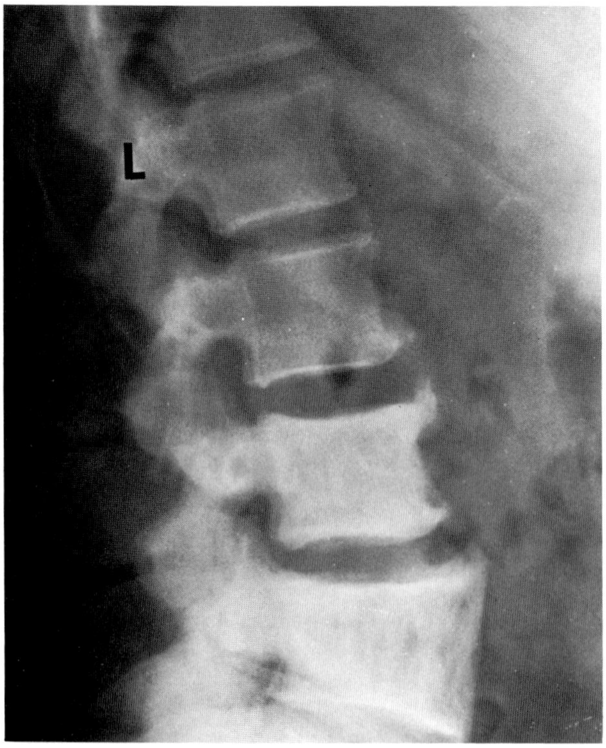

B (another patient)

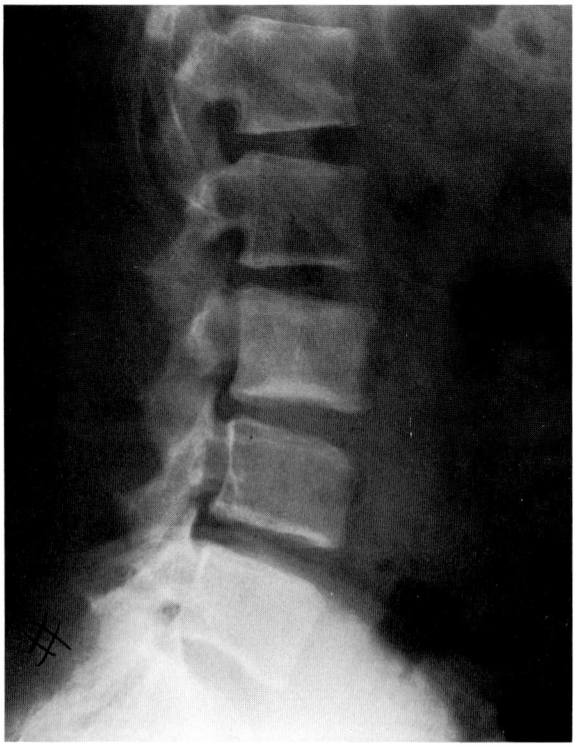

C (another patient)

Ivory Vertebra

Clinical Information

This 62-year-old plumber had complained of widespread bone pain for a few months. He was proved to have metastatic carcinoma of the prostate.

Roentgen Findings

A lateral film of the dorsal spine (A) shows a striking density of the body of T5, which is of normal size. The affected vertebral body has a smudged appearance but is not completely homogeneous. This appearance is typical of an ivory vertebra.

Comments

The term ivory vertebra was first used in 1925 in reference to metastatic carcinoma of the colon to a single vertebral body. Although this designation has been employed to describe multiple dense vertebral bodies, it most commonly refers to a single bone. Despite the fact that many conditions (osteomyelitis, fluorosis, healing fractures, osteopetrosis, etc.) can very uncommonly lead to this x-ray finding, the three most frequent causes by far are metastatic carcinoma (as seen in this case), Paget's disease (B, another patient), and lymphoma (C, a third patient) (1–4). There almost never is involvement of the adjacent intervertebral discs.

It is possible in most patients to distinguish among these three entities from their radiologic manifestations. Paget's disease usually can be identified by a coarsened trabecular pattern and/or an increase in the size of the vertebral body. The vertebral body enlargement is more evident in its anteroposterior and transverse dimensions than superoinferiorly, because Paget's disease softens bone and can lead to an element of collapse. The three lowest lumbar vertebral bodies show increased density and a coarsened trabecular pattern in the patient shown in B, but only L4 is enlarged. Paget's disease may also affect hypertrophic spurs and the posterior spinal elements. An ivory vertebra caused by lymphoma (C) or Hodgkin's disease is characteristically very homogeneous, more so than either Paget's disease or metastatic carcinoma. There uncommonly is erosion of the anterior surface of the vertebral body from adjacent enlarged lymph nodes. Sometimes the density occasioned by Hodgkin's disease or lymphoma will return to normal following radiation therapy or chemotherapy (3). An ivory vertebra caused by either lymphoma or metastatic carcinoma is more likely to be symptomatic than one that results from Paget's disease.

An ivory vertebra that represents metastatic disease is less likely to be so completely and homogeneously dense as is often seen with Hodgkin's disease or lymphoma. Also, metastatic deposits are frequently present in other bones. Metastases affect the vertebral pedicles more frequently than does lymphoma or Hodgkin's disease. The most common source of an ivory vertebra due to metastatic disease in a male is carcinoma of the prostate; in a female, carcinoma of the breast. The much less frequent causes of a dense vertebral body can usually be identified by abnormalities in other bones or other portions of the body. Only rarely is an isolated dense vertebra proved to be idiopathic. Consequently, the radiologic finding of an ivory vertebra nearly always represents significant disease.

Source Materials

1. Dennis JM. The solitary dense vertebral body. Radiology 77:618, 1961.
2. Harris DJ, Fornasier VL. An ivory vertebra. Monostotic Paget's disease of bone. Clin Orthop 136:173, 1978.
3. Mandell GA. Resolution of Hodgkin's induced ivory vertebrae. Pediatr Radiol 7:178, 1978.
4. Resnick D. The sclerotic vertebral body. JAMA 249:1761, 1983.

Case 18

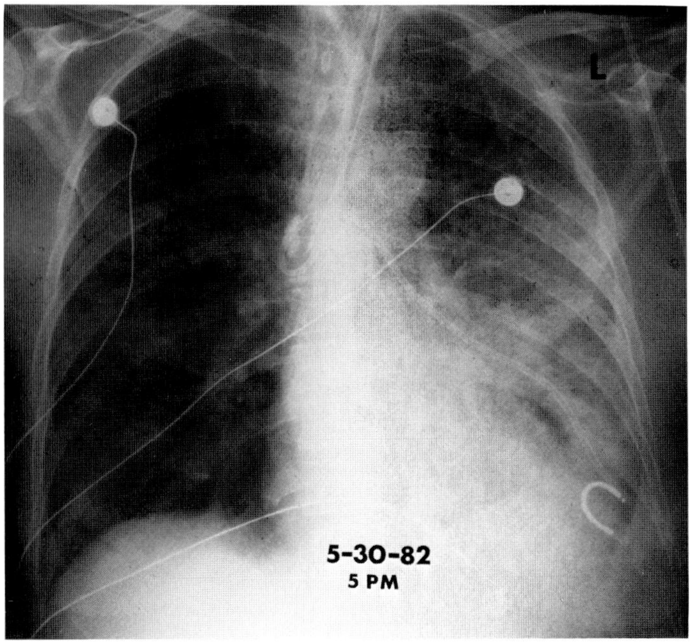

A

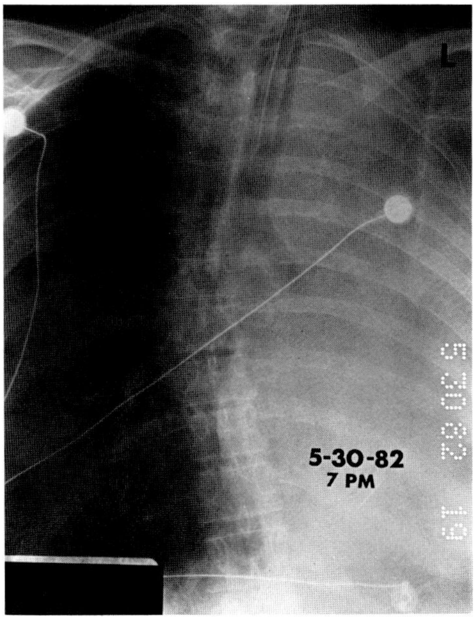

B

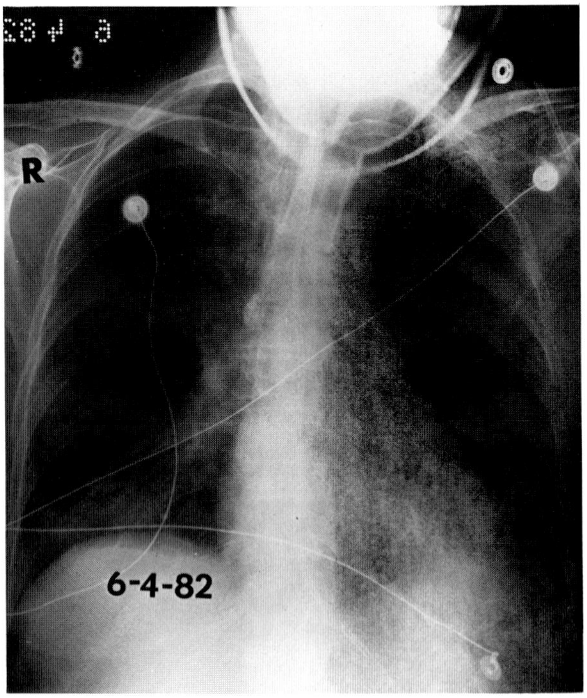

C

Nasogastric Tube in the Tracheobronchial Tree

Clinical Information

This 52-year-old female alcoholic, admitted for dysphagia, had been treated previously with surgery and radiation therapy for laryngeal carcinoma. Fifty milliters of Osmolite was injected through her inlying nasogastric tube at 4:30 PM on 5-30-82. The patient became very dyspneic and coughed repeatedly. Films were obtained at 5 PM (A) and 7 PM (B). The nasogastric tube was removed after the 5 PM radiograph was viewed. She was treated successfully (C) with suction, oxygen, and postural drainage.

Roentgen Findings

The film exposed at 5 PM on 5-30-82 shows a nasogastric tube with its tip lying far within the left lower lobe. The lower half of the left lung exhibits an abundance of patchy densities. The limited portable radiograph exposed at 7 PM on the same day shows all of the left hemithorax to be opaque. These densities are no longer visible on the film obtained on 6-4-82 (C).

Comments

A nasogastric tube is utilized frequently for alimentation or suction. Instillation of fluids through a tube that has been inadvertently placed within the tracheobronchial tree creates a serious situation, although most of the reported patients have survived. Promptly instituted postural drainage and percussion are usually effective. Bronchoscopy is rarely needed. A nasogastric tube can reach this location without provoking spasms of coughing if the patient is sufficiently depressed, particularly when there have been many previous aspirations into the tracheobronchial tree.

Several complications can be associated with a nasogastric tube. These include irritation of the esophagus and other problems due to pressure such as bleeding or perforation. Feeding tubes can perforate the esophagus to lie within the mediastinum or the pleural space (2). Such an event is especially likely in the pediatric age group or when used to establish a feeding pathway in the presence of esophageal malignancy (3). An abnormal position of the tube is particularly frequent after vomiting, especially with the narrow tubes currently in use (1). A nasogastric tube may reach the tracheobronchial tree, even though there is an inflated low-pressure, high-residual volume intratracheal tube cuff in place (4). This type of endotracheal tube cuff does not fit so tightly against the entire tracheal wall as a high-pressure cuff. Although it is much less likely to cause tracheal stenosis, the loose fit does not preclude the passage of a nasogastric tube between its outer margin and the tracheal wall.

Assurance must be obtained that the end of a feeding nasogastric tube is in the desired location, usually the stomach, before fluids are introduced. This can best be determined with radiographs, which are especially indicated following initial insertion of the tube or after repeated vomiting, which can regurgitate the tube to a more proximal location. Information concerning the position of the tube can sometimes be obtained by aspirating gastric juice, but only a radiograph will reveal many common problems such as location of a coiled tube within the esophagus or the pharynx.

Source Materials

1. Harvey PB, Bull PT, Harris DL. Accidental intrapulmonary Clinifeed. Anaesthesia 36:518, 1981.
2. Kassner EG, Baumstark A, Balsam D, Haller JO. Passage of feeding catheters into the pleural space: A radiographic sign of trauma to the pharynx and esophagus in the newborn. AJR 128:19, 1977.
3. Lipinski JK, Conway SS, Kottler RE, Werner DI. The radiology of oesophageal tubes for malignant strictures. Clin Radiol 33:453, 1982.
4. Stark P. Inadvertent nasogastric tube insertion into the tracheobronchial tree. A hazard of new high-residual volume cuffs. Radiology 142:239, 1982.

Case 19

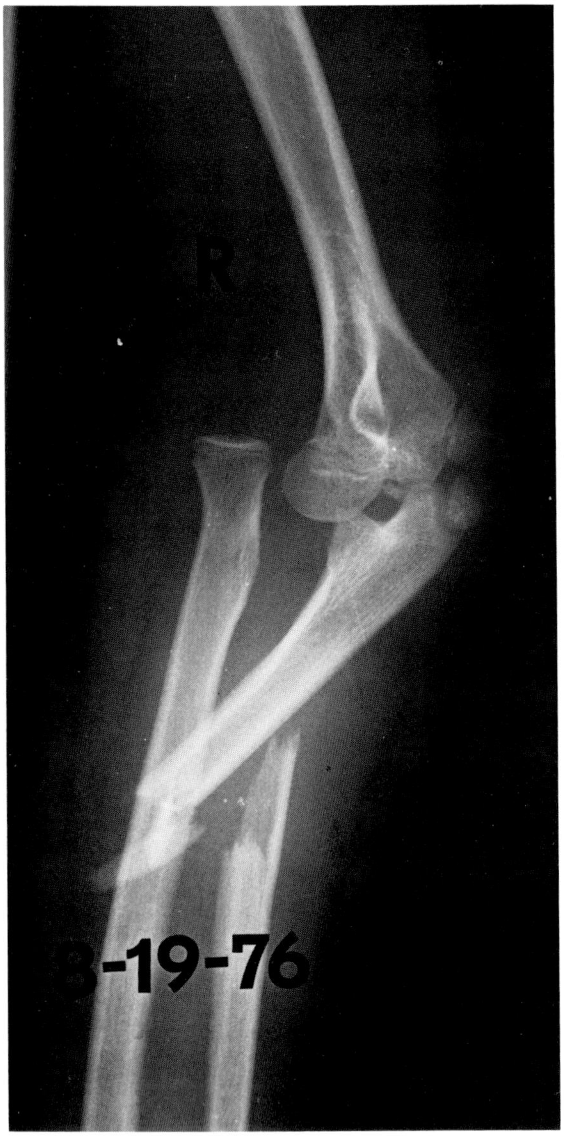

A

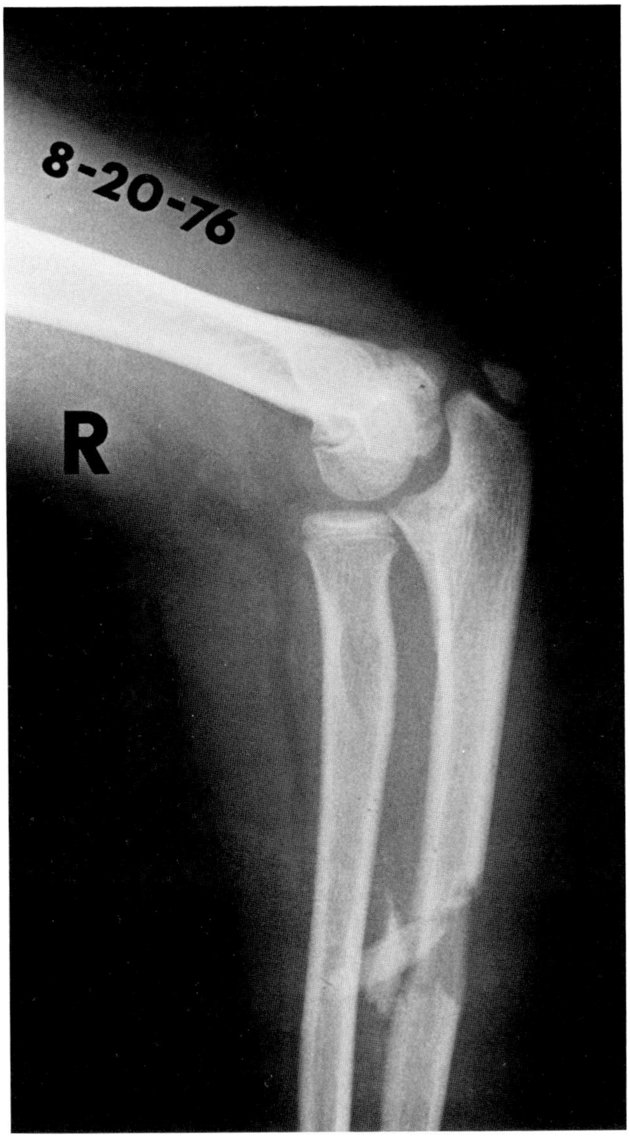

B

Monteggia's Fracture

Clinical Information

A severe blow was delivered to the dorsum of the right forearm of this young boy, creating an immediate deformity. The injury healed following reduction and casting.

Roentgen Findings

Film A shows a comminuted fracture of the proximal third of the right ulna with anterior angulation. The radial head is dislocated anteriorly. Film B reveals excellent reduction of both the fracture and the dislocation.

Comments

A classical Monteggia's injury is characterized by a fracture in the proximal third of the ulna with anterior angulation and anterior dislocation of the radial head. The associated radial head dislocation may not be diagnosed immediately. It was, in fact, missed by Monteggia on his first patient with this condition. There was a reasonable excuse for Monteggia's error, since it occurred in the early portion of the 19th century, well before the discovery of x rays. There are many variations or types of Monteggia's injury. Although anterior radial head dislocation and anterior angulation of the ulnar fracture occur in the majority of these patients, the dislocation and angulation may be directed posteriorly or laterally. Posterior dislocation of the radial head is often called a reverse Monteggia's fracture. The radial head always dislocates in the same direction as the fracture angulates. Fracture with angulation of either bone of the forearm leads to dislocation of the other at the elbow or wrist, because the radius and the ulna are held firmly together throughout their entire lengths by a very strong interosseous membrane. A fracture with angulation of the distal radius is almost invariably associated with dislocation of the ulna at the wrist. This injury is called a Galeazzi's fracture-dislocation (see Case 47).

Monteggia's fractures usually result from direct trauma, although some evidence indicates that forced pronation, particularly at the time of injury, may promote anterior radial head dislocation. These patients often present with the forearm in pronation. Supination may effect a successful reduction. By the same token, posterior dislocations are more likely if the forearm is injured in supination. Monteggia's fractures can usually be treated successfully in children with closed reduction, but adults often require open reduction.

Failure to note a radial head dislocation can lead to very significant complications, the most common of which is loss of adequate supination and pronation. Nerve palsies can appear early or late (2). Monteggia's fractures are frequently missed because the injury is relatively rare, there often is abundant soft tissue swelling, and the joints at both ends of the injured forearm are not always evaluated (1). At least two radiographs, preferably perpendicular views, must be evaluated before one can be sure the radial head is not dislocated, since the appearance may be entirely normal in the presence of dislocation on any single projection. Normal location of the radial head, even in children, can be confirmed by use of the radiocapitellar line. This line is drawn through the center of the radial shaft and extended upward. It will intersect the center of the capitellum in all projections in the absence of dislocation. A Monteggia's injury in children must not be confused with separation of the entire distal humeral epiphysis, in which the radiocapitellar line remains normal. Dislocation of the entire distal humeral epiphysis can simulate complete dislocation at the elbow joint. The radius and the ulna move laterally in elbow joint dislocation. They are displaced medially when there is separation of the entire distal humeral epiphysis (3).

Source Materials

1. Giustra PE, Killoran PJ, Furman RS, Rott JA. The missed Monteggia fracture. Radiology 110:45, 1974.
2. Morris AH. Irreducible Monteggia lesion with radial-nerve entrapment. A case report. J Bone Joint Surg 56A:1744, 1974.
3. Rogers LF. Fractures and dislocations of the elbow. Semin Roentgenol 13:97, 1978.
4. Tompkins DG. The anterior Monteggia fracture. Observations on etiology and treatment. J Bone Joint Surg 53A:1109, 1971.

Case 20

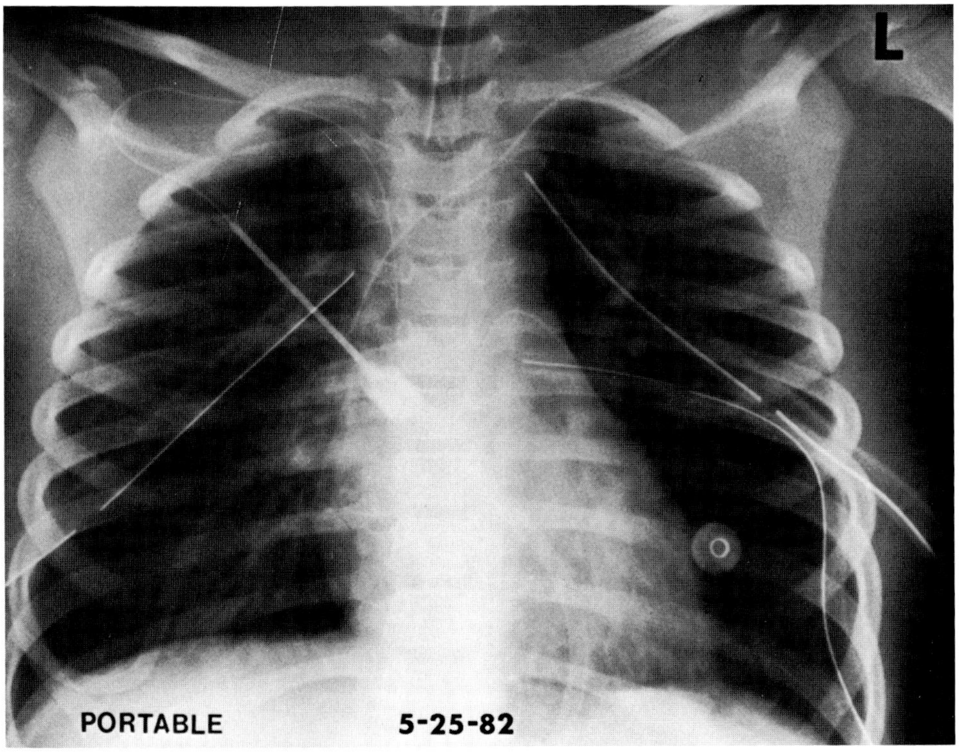
L
PORTABLE
5-25-82

A

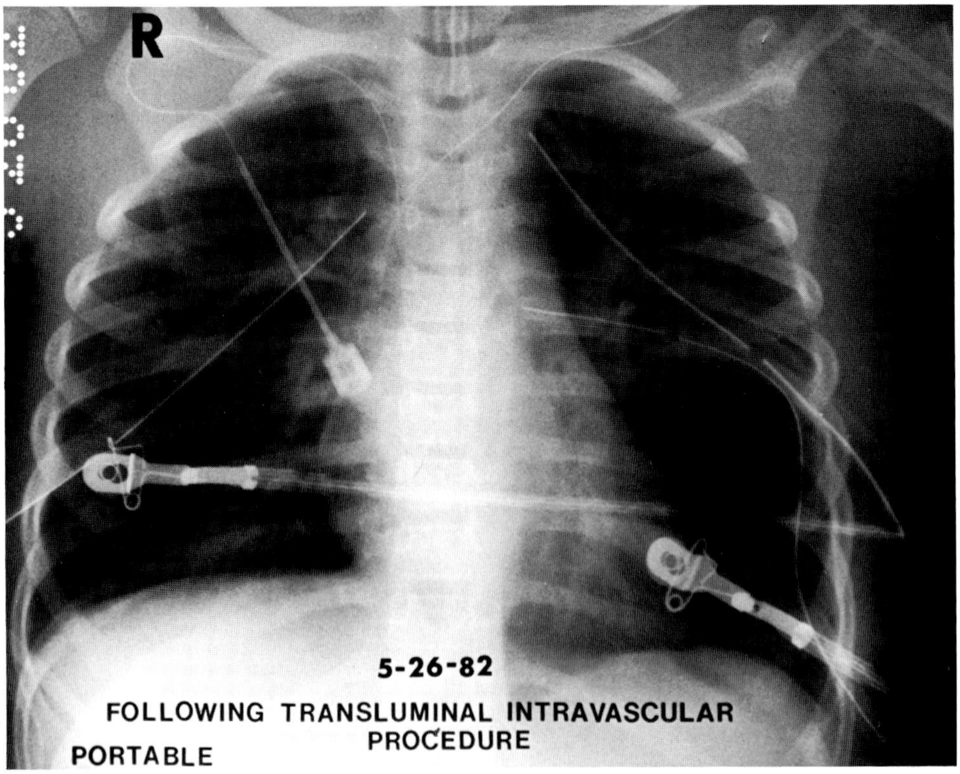
R
5-26-82
FOLLOWING TRANSLUMINAL INTRAVASCULAR PROCEDURE
PORTABLE

B

Intravascular Foreign Body

Clinical Information

A central venous catheter that was used in the treatment of this severely burned child was severed. The severed portion lodged in the main pulmonary artery. It was removed using a loop snare.

Roentgen Findings

A portable anteroposterior chest film (A) shows a nasogastric tube, bilateral chest tubes, an intratracheal tube, and a central venous catheter in place. Another tube overlies the patient's lower right chest, and a fragment of a central venous catheter is visible in the main pulmonary artery. Film B shows the fragment to have been removed.

Comments

Many types of tubing and other devices are used with benefit for the administration of fluids, to obtain pressure measurements, for cardiac pacing, and so forth. Most iatrogenic intravascular foreign bodies consist of a segment of tubing that is inadvertently cut off during its use. The most commonly severed tubing is a polyethylene central venous catheter. The needle used in the introduction of tubing should be dull, and the catheter should not be withdrawn through an inlying needle. Both of these precautions will reduce the incidence of this complication. All catheters used should be radiopaque. It is important to measure the length of a catheter before its insertion so one can determine whether all is removed when it is withdrawn.

Intra-arterial foreign bodies embolize blood vessels in the peripheral vascular bed of the extremities, abdomen, or central nervous system. Foreign bodies in the venous side of the circulation tend to lodge within the right atrium near the tricuspid annulus, but they can migrate into or beyond the right ventricle. Long pieces of tubing usually arrest within the superior vena cava. All foreign bodies can penetrate the vascular wall and excite a foreign body reaction. Perforation of the heart can lead to tamponade. There may be recurrent pericardial effusion. Superimposed infection may cause an abscess or endocarditis. A thrombus can develop, with subsequent embolic episodes. Myocarditis or arrhythmias may also occur. Cardiac complications increase in direct proportion to the length of time a foreign body is within the heart. It has been said that failure to remove an intracardiac catheter fragment will lead to death in about 75% of patients with this complication (2).

Various transluminal techniques have been used since about 1950 to successfully remove intravascular foreign bodies such as segments of tubing (1–4). Such foreign bodies were previously removed surgically. Among the various maneuvers is a loop snare when the end of the tubing can be engaged. A hooked catheter can be utilized when it is impossible to reach the end of the severed tubing (4). A basket or grasping forceps can be successfully employed at times. Percutaneous transluminal extraction is usually possible. Complications are uncommon. The vascular structures are rarely torn, lacerated, or perforated. Transluminal removal is not possible, indeed is contraindicated, after a large thrombus develops near the foreign body. Consequently, angiographic studies often are justified for exact localization or to reveal a nonopaque catheter or a surrounding thrombus. Fluoroscopy is obviously required during the procedure. Extraction should not be attempted if the foreign body has been within the heart for a long period of time because fibrosis will have developed. Removal of the foreign body under such circumstances may seriously damage intracardiac structures.

Source Materials

1. Dotter CT, Rösch J, Bilbao MK. Transluminal extraction of catheter and guide fragments from the heart and great vessels: 29 collected cases. AJR 111:467, 1971.
2. Fisher RG, Ferreyro R. Evaluation of current techniques for nonsurgical removal of intravascular iatrogenic foreign bodies. AJR 130:541, 1978.
3. Fisher RG, Romero JR. Extraction of embolized central venous catheter using percutaneous technique. Radiology 116:735, 1975.
4. Maxwell DD, Anderson RE. Transfemoral retrieval of an intracardiac catheter fragment using a simple hook-shaped catheter. Radiology 103:213, 1972.

Case 21

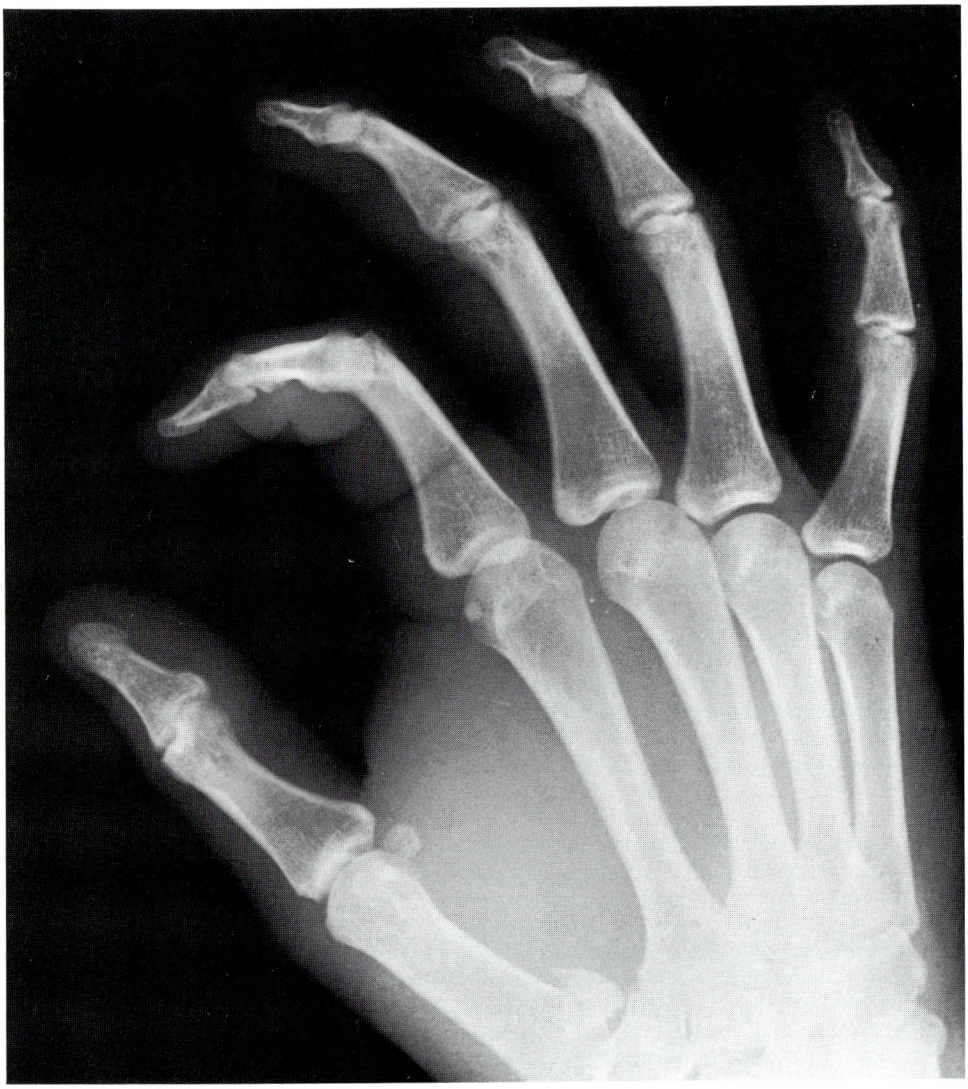

Bennett's Fracture

Clinical Information

This 30-year-old male fell on his opened left hand, impacting his weight upon his abducted thumb. The resulting Bennett's fracture was reduced and fixed in good position with an internal pin, which ran from the main portion of the first metacarpal into the trapezium. Healing occurred without sequelae.

Roentgen Findings

An oblique film of the left hand shows an intra-articular oblique fracture line extending from the medial and volar aspect of the first metacarpal into the joint between this bone and the trapezium (greater multangular). There is dorsolateral and proximal displacement of the first metacarpal.

Comments

Bennett's fracture was first described in 1882. It is characterized by an oblique fracture at the base of the first metacarpal, which extends into the joint between this bone and the trapezium. This is an unusual fracture that is more common in adults, particularly males. The dominant hand is involved in 90% of cases. A Bennett's fracture is virtually always associated with displacement of the major portion of the first metacarpal. The smaller, triangular fractured medial fragment maintains a normal position because it is held in place by the relatively strong ulnar volar ligament. The major portion of the fractured first metacarpal has no remaining strong attachments to the capsule of the affected joint. It becomes displaced laterally and proximally from the pull of the abductor pollicis longus muscle, which is attached to its base beyond the capsular attachments. The amount of dislocation varies from case to case.

A Bennett's fracture can be incapacitating because the thumb has numerous and very valuable functions. Improper reduction will lead to a weak thumb, poor grasping, inability to make a strong fist, and, in general, weak "thumb" power. Workmen's compensation in Sweden allows 25% disability for a Bennett's fracture that heals in poor position (1). This is similar to the amount of disability allowed for a fractured femur that heals in poor position. Motions of the thumb include flexion, extension, abduction, apposition, rotation, and circumduction. The thumb is especially important in grasping. Stability of the joint between the trapezium and the first metacarpal is maintained by ligaments and by the shape of the bony surfaces. The bony relationships at the base of the first metacarpal have been likened to a rider sitting in the "saddle" of the trapezium. The extensive use of the thumb in daily activities accounts for the osteoarthritic changes frequently seen around the margins of this joint.

Bennett's fractures result from direct trauma, which usually is secondary to falls. The thumb is usually extended and abducted at the time of impact. The injury can also be sustained when the first is clenched with the thumb abducted. In this situation the causative blow impacts directly against the first metacarpal. Such an event may occur during a fist fight. It is said to result from a hook but not a jab.

Accurate reduction is essential and relatively easy. Proper reduction is best gauged by a truly lateral projection (1). Maintenance of the reduction may be difficult because of the abductor pollicis longus. Good reduction can be maintained by rigid internal fixation. Fixation pins may extend through the smaller fractured fragment but often run directly from the first metacarpal into the trapezium. The small triangular piece of bone has little tendency to change its position. The thumb is usually casted in abduction. Healing can be expected to occur in 4–8 weeks.

Source Materials

1. Billing L, Gedda K-O. Roentgen examination of Bennett's fracture. Acta Radiol 38:471, 1952.
2. Dial WB, Berg E. Bennett's fracture. Hand 4:229, 1972.
3. Fisher E. Bennett's fracture in general practice. Med J Aust 1:434, 1976.
4. Hambury HJ. Bennett's fracture. Hand 4:224, 1972.

Case 22

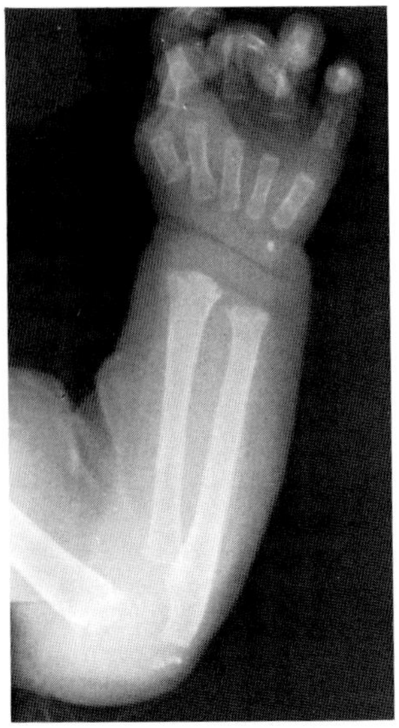

A

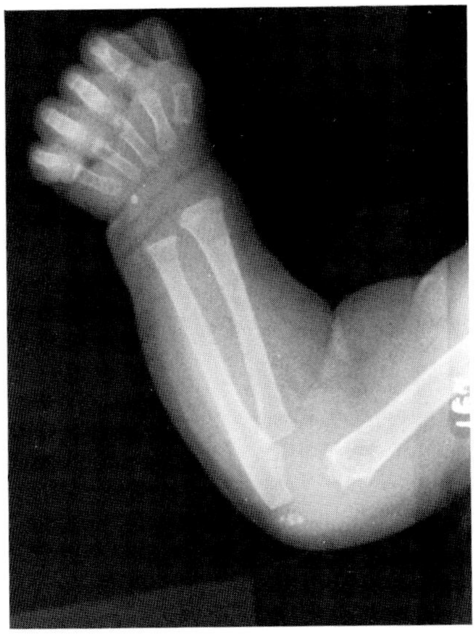

B

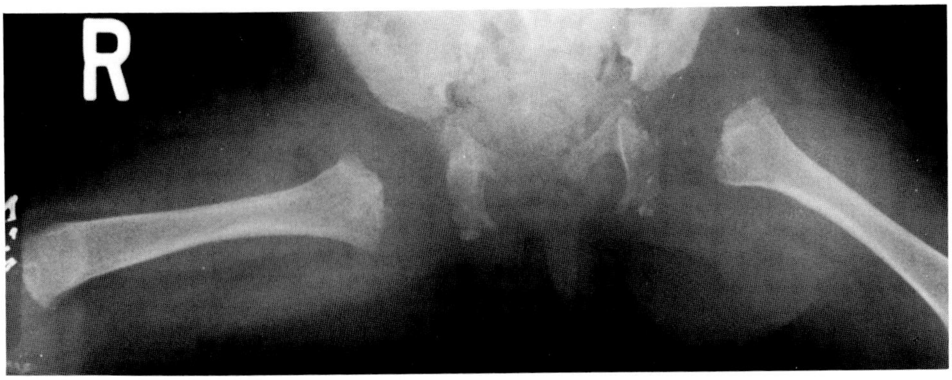

C

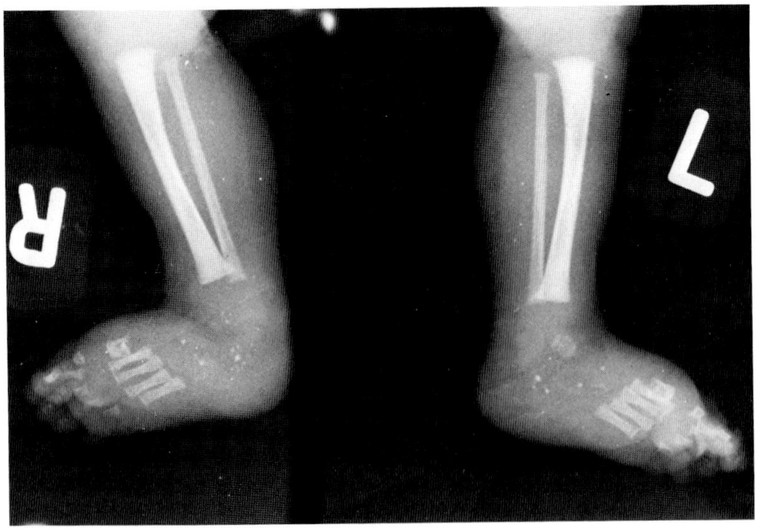

D

Chondrodysplasia Punctata

Clinical Information

This newborn infant with short, stubby fingers progressed satisfactorily after birth. No follow-up is available. The patient's mother is said to have had small hands and presented a similar general appearance. Her radiographs were alleged to show shortened metacarpals and deformities of one radius and of the carpal bones.

Roentgen Findings

Films of the extremities (A–D) show multiple punctate calcifications in many epiphyses. The stippling is especially prominent in the tarsal bones and olecranon cartilages.

Comments

Many names have been used to designate chondrodysplasia punctata (CP). These include chondrodystrophia calcificans congenita, stippled epiphyses, and Conradi's disease. CP is a form of multiple epiphyseal dysplasia characterized by punctate calcifications in cartilaginous epiphyseal centers and other nonskeletal cartilage. These calcifications are radiologically evident at birth but disappear by 5 years of age if the patient survives. Survivors may be entirely normal, or there may be various levels of disability. The end result often depends upon commonly associated anomalies, which include a saddle nose, cataracts, contractures, shortened limbs, short stature, spinal anomalies, scoliosis, and skin abnormalities.

There are at least two types of CP. The rhizomelic form, an autosomal recessive trait, almost invariably leads to death very early in life. Bilaterally symmetrical shortened extremities are common. Cataracts are seen in about 75% of these individuals, who often show coronal vertebral clefts and psychomotor retardation. The less severe Conradi-Hünermann form demonstrates dominant inheritance and may be associated with a normal life span (4). These patients usually have normal intelligence. Spinal anomalies and scoliosis are fairly common. Cataracts are less frequent in the Conradi-Hünermann form, and extremity shortening tends to be asymmetrical. It is held by some that a third, X-linked dominant type exists that is universally fatal in utero in males (1). These patients present characteristic icthyosiform skin changes and otherwise are much like the Conradi-Hünermann form of CP. It has been suggested that the three types of CP may, in fact, represent three different diseases rather than variations of one process, although all show similar epiphyseal calcifications.

The fine stippling in the epiphyses coalesces with time, leaving either a normal or a deformed epiphysis. Stippled calcifications may also be seen in synovial membranes and in cartilage outside the skeletal system, such as the trachea. The vertebrae, ribs, sternum, scapulae, ilia, and ischiae are especially likely to be affected. The stippling tends to be small, regular, and punctate but can be irregular. Similar bony changes can occur following the administration of warfarin during pregnancy (3). The shortened extremities of CP develop in bones associated with epiphyses that have demonstrated stippled calcification (2). Differential diagnostic possibilities include cretinoid epiphyseal dysplasia, in which the epiphyseal fragments are larger and tend to conform to the expected shape of the epiphysis. Osteopoikilosis can be differentiated by denser and larger sclerotic areas, which are located both within and outside the epiphyses. The stippled calcifications of CP are much finer than those in either of these disorders. Stippled calcification can occur about the hips, especially in the Y-cartilages and the patellae, in Zellwegger's (cerebrohepatorenal) syndrome. Zellwegger's calcification is typically located in the medial and inferior aspect of the patella but usually spares the tarsal and carpal bones, a common location of the CP stippling.

Source Materials

1. Manzke H, Christophers E, Wiedmann HR. Dominant sex-linked inherited chondrodysplasia punctata. A distinct type of chondrodysplasia punctata. Clin Genet 17:97, 1980.
2. Theander G, Pettersson H. Calcification in chondrodysplasia punctata. Relation to ossification and skeletal growth. Acta Radiol 19:205, 1978.
3. Whitfield MF. Chondrodysplasia punctata after warfarin in early pregnancy. Case report and summary of the literature. Arch Dis Child 55:139, 1980.
4. Young LW. Radiological case of the month. (Chondrodysplasia punctata, Conradi-Hünermann form). Am J Dis Child 133:1191, 1979.

Case 23

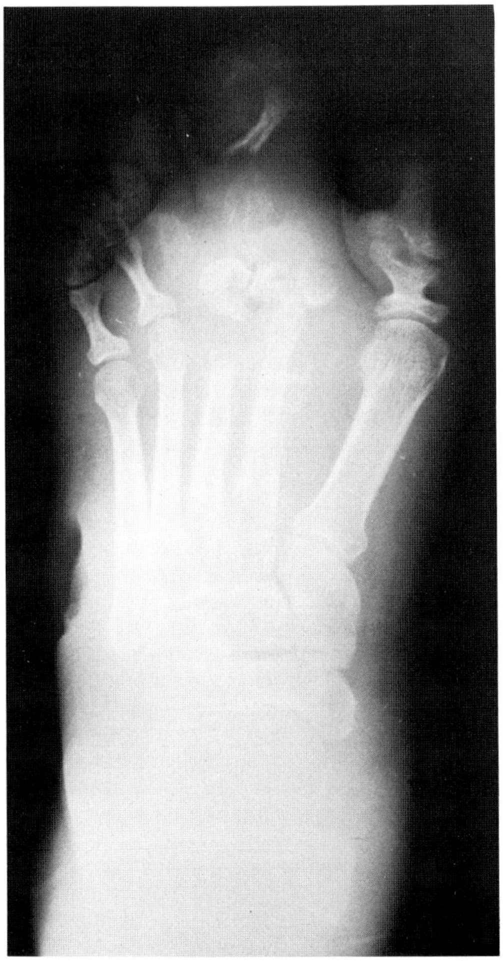

A

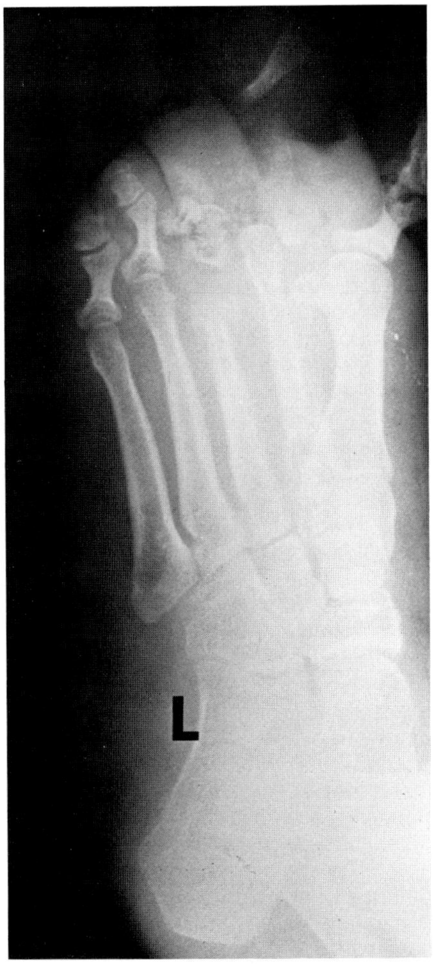

B

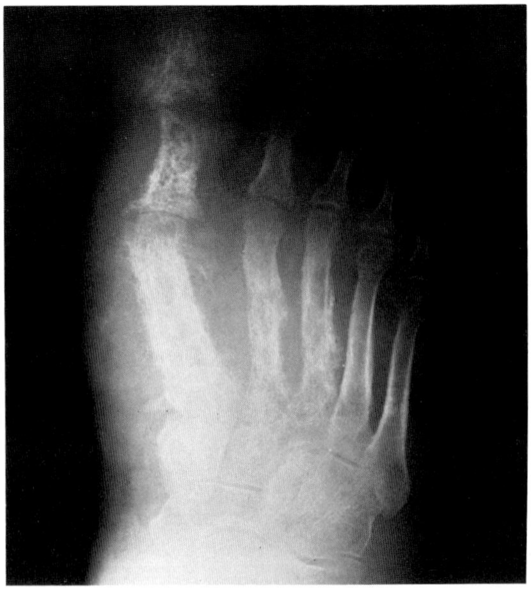

C (another patient)

Madura Foot

Clinical Information

This Nicaraguan farm laborer had noted painless sinus tracts and extensive left foot swelling for years. White granules discharged from the sinuses.

Roentgen Findings

Anteroposterior (A) and oblique (B) radiographs of the left foot show marked and slightly irregular soft tissue swelling as well as extensive bony destruction in the second and third toes on both sides of their metacarpophalangeal joints. Periosteal reaction is evident along their metatarsal shafts. There is considerable destruction on opposing bony surfaces of the interphalangeal joint of the great toe. Another patient from Africa (C) reveals medial soft tissue swelling and irregular periosteal reaction, with somewhat moth-eaten bony destruction.

Comments

Madura foot is a generic name for chronic infection of the foot with fungi or fungus-like organisms. The condition is most commonly seen in India, Africa, southern Arabia, South and Central America, and Mexico. Occasional cases have been reported in the United States (4). This type of foot mycetoma was first described in 1840 in Madura, India, thus accounting for its name. The infection is contracted through the bare feet. A preceding thorn injury is frequent. Fissures can provide a portal of entry. Usually only one extremity, most commonly the foot, is affected. Fever and associated lymphadenopathy are rare. The condition is not painful, since the organisms do not attack nerves.

Spread of the infection depends upon its site of implantation, the virulence of the organism, the presence of secondary infection, and, very importantly, the duration of the disease. A prolonged period of time is required before the infection extends beyond the soft tissues. Involvement of the bone can proceed once the plantar aponeurosis is breached. Many different fungi and fungus-like organisms can cause a Madura foot. Some information concerning the offending organism can be obtained from the radiologic findings and from the color and consistency of the granules that often pour from the sinus tracts. Some granules are hard; others are soft. Treatment can be effective but it must be very prolonged.

X-ray examinations show only swelling and alterations in the external contours of the foot when the infection is localized to the soft tissues. Normal fat lines are often distorted or obscured. Many abnormalities are seen once the infection attacks the bones. The earliest change is loss of a definite cortical outline. This is followed by adjacent sclerosis. Nocardia infection is particularly likely to lead to sclerosis. The bones in the second row of tarsals and their adjacent metatarsals are said to be the most frequent sites of initial involvement. There may be numerous erosions and periosteal new bone formation. Bony expansion may be seen due to the periosteal proliferation. Endosteal cavitation is common. Cavitation results from bony destruction caused by growth of the fungal granules. A honeycombed appearance may develop. Sequestra are not usually seen. Some bones may be completely destroyed. At times the tarsal bones present a "melting snow" appearance from an admixture of demineralization and destruction, which blurs the bony outlines. Joints are usually preserved much longer than in other types of infection because the fungal grains are not proteolytic. Cartilage destruction does not occur in the absence of secondary infection. The diagnosis of a Madura foot is not difficult in the presence of a painless extremity with severe bony involvement and numerous sinus tracts that discharge fungal granules. Abundant periosteal reaction helps differentiate Madura foot from tuberculosis.

Source Materials

1. Reeder MM. Tropical diseases of the foot. Semin Roentgenol 5:378, 1970.
2. Reeder MM, Palmer PES. The Radiology of Tropical Diseases with Epidemiological, Pathological and Clinical Correlation. Williams & Wilkins, Baltimore, 1981, pp 365–377.
3. Subbarao K, Lubetsky H. Massive swelling of the foot in a 63-year-old man. JAMA 248:3173, 1982.
4. Warintarawej A, Winter WG Jr, Goodman NL. Maduromycosis (Madura foot) in Kentucky. South Med J 68:1570, 1975.

Case 24

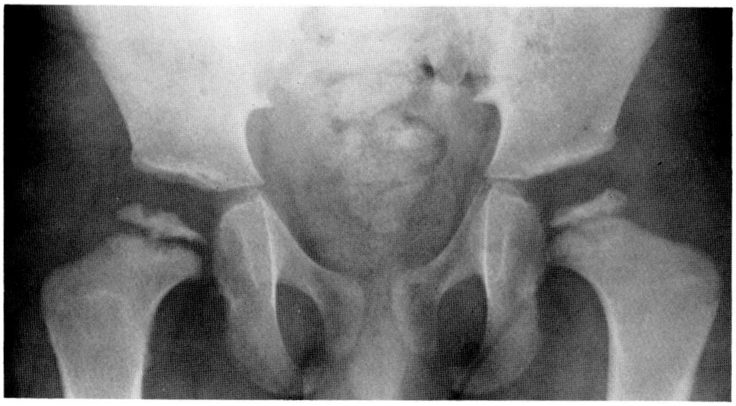

A

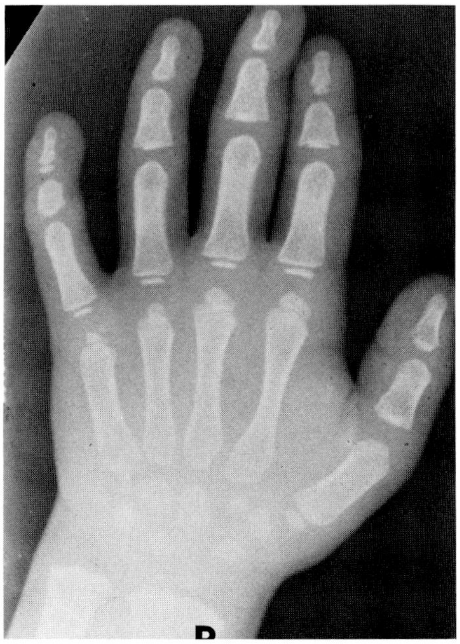

B

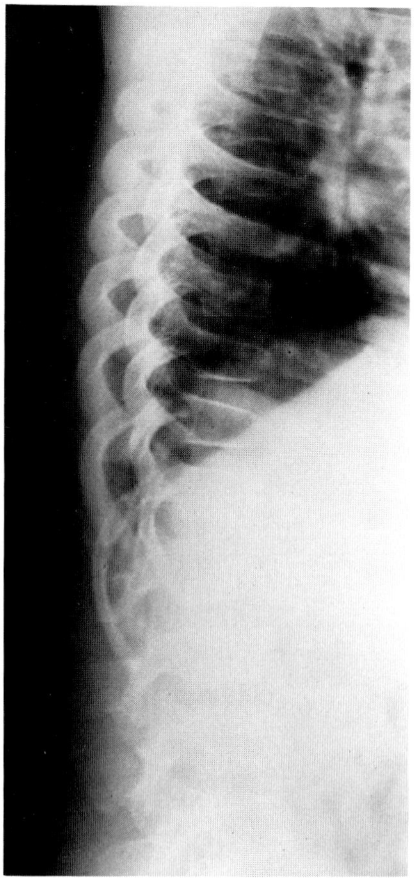

C

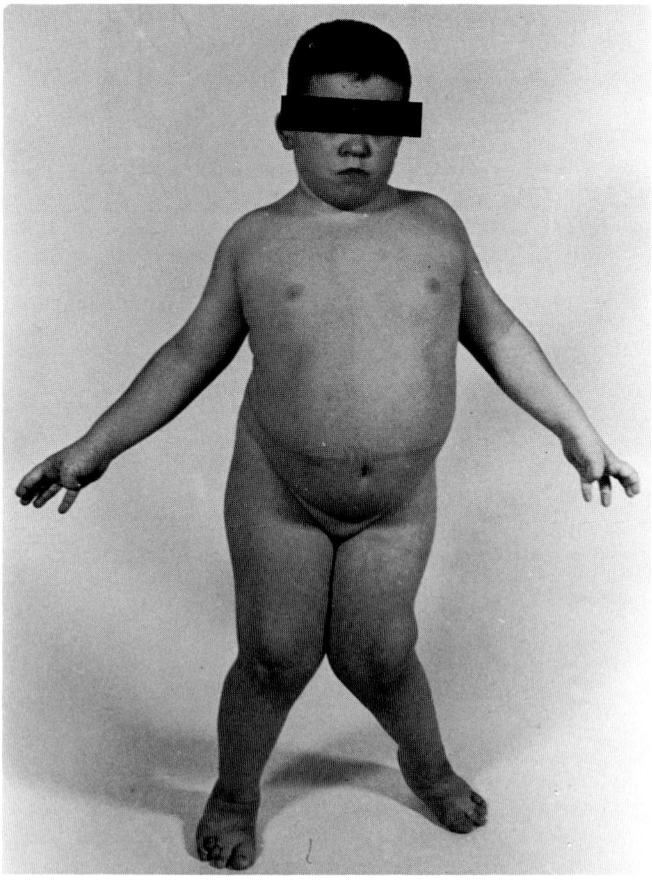

D

Multiple Epiphyseal Dysplasia

Clinical Information

This 10-year-old, moderately retarded boy was admitted for a diagnostic workup. Previous diagnoses had included Legg-Perthes disease and Hurler's syndrome. He was 44 inches tall (below the 3rd percentile), overweight, and knock-kneed (see D).

Roentgen Findings

The femoral capital epiphyses are small, flat, and irregular (A). Similar changes were present in many peripheral epiphyses (B). The fingers are short and stubby with both ivory and cupped epiphyses. Similar findings are present in the toes. Only minimal spinal abnormalities are evident (C). These x-ray findings are characteristic of multiple epiphyseal dysplasia.

Comments

Multiple epiphyseal dysplasia (MED), also know as dysplasia epiphysialis multiplex and Fairbank's disease, is characterized by bilateral and symmetrical irregular development of the epiphyseal ossification centers of the peripheral bones. Most patients show dominant inheritance, although some have demonstrated recessive characteristics (2). Individuals with MED are short (rarely more than 60 inches tall) and have stubby hands and feet. Intelligence is usually normal. Histologic studies show abnormalities of the epiphyseal chondrocytes. They are reduced in number and demonstrate deranged organization, which eventually leads to structural abnormalities. Symptoms concern ambulation, usually appear at about 4 years of age, and include such things as pain and a waddling gait. Knock-knees are common. There is a tendency for the symptoms to improve after puberty at the time radiologic studies show consolidation of the epiphyses. The amount of final deformity varies, even in the same family. The bones may become almost normal, although some flattening and irregularities usually persist. Such changes can lead to secondary degenerative joint disease. Many individuals are minimally affected and may not seek medical advice. Chondrodysplasia punctata is a specific type of MED.

The x-ray changes of MED include late appearance of the epiphyses, which are small, irregular, and sometimes fragmented. They often present a mulberry appearance. The x-ray findings are often more marked than the patient's symptoms. The epiphyses in an adult with MED are somewhat irregular and flattened. There may be associated premature degenerative changes. Epiphyseal abnormalities are widespread, bilateral, and symmetrical, being particularly pronounced in the hips, knees, and shoulders. The distal tibia may develop abnormally and lead to a talar tilt with deformity of the ankle joint. The tarsal and carpal bones are often hypoplastic and somewhat irregular. Coxa vara is relatively common. A double-layered patella has been reported to be characteristic of MED. Spinal epiphyses show minimal, variable, or even no abnormalities (1). This characteristic distinguishes MED from spondyloepiphyseal dysplasia.

It is not difficult to reach a confident diagnosis of MED when the history, clinical findings, and x-ray manifestations are considered in concert. Other diseases can similarly affect a single bone or a very few bones. These include Legg-Perthes disease and other osteochondroses. Clinical findings will identify cretinism, juvenile rheumatoid arthritis, and achondroplasia. Patients with Stickler syndrome have many similarities to MED, but these patients also exhibit marfanoid bony changes and dislocated lens. More spinal abnormalities are present with Morquio's disease and spondyloepiphyseal dysplasia. It has been said that individuals in families known to have MED are more likely to show diagnostic x-ray abnormalities if they have hand deformities than are those who either are short of stature or have symptoms (3).

Source Materials

1. Hulvey JT, Keats T. Multiple epiphyseal dysplasia. A contribution to the problem of spinal involvement. AJR 106:170, 1969.
2. Juberg RC, Holt JF. Inheritance of multiple epiphyseal dysplasia tarda. Am J Hum Gen 20:549, 1968.
3. Mena HR, Pearson EO. Multiple epiphyseal dysplasia. A family case report. JAMA 236:2629, 1976.
4. Short LA, Hume RL, Gudas CJ. Multiple epiphyseal dysplasia. A review of the literature and case report. J Am Podiatry Ass 69:695, 1979.

Case 25

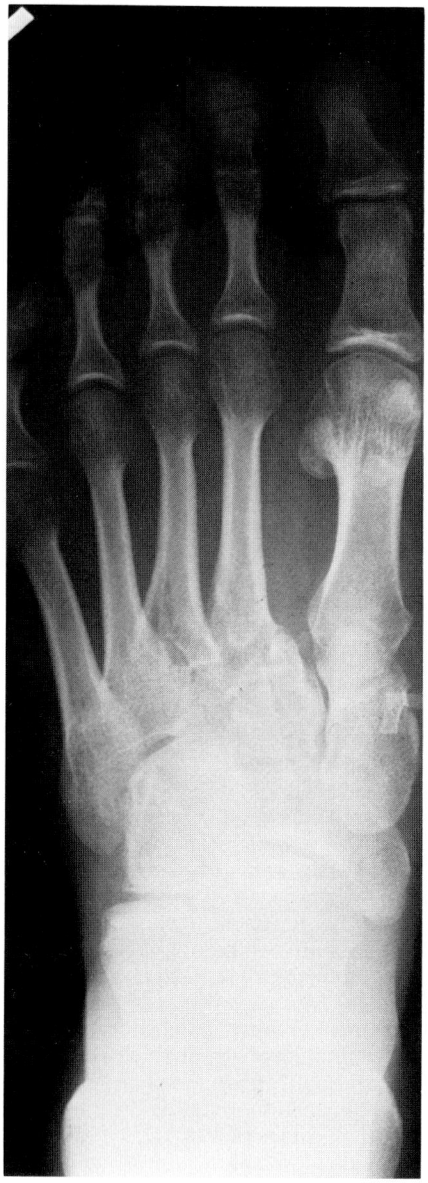

A

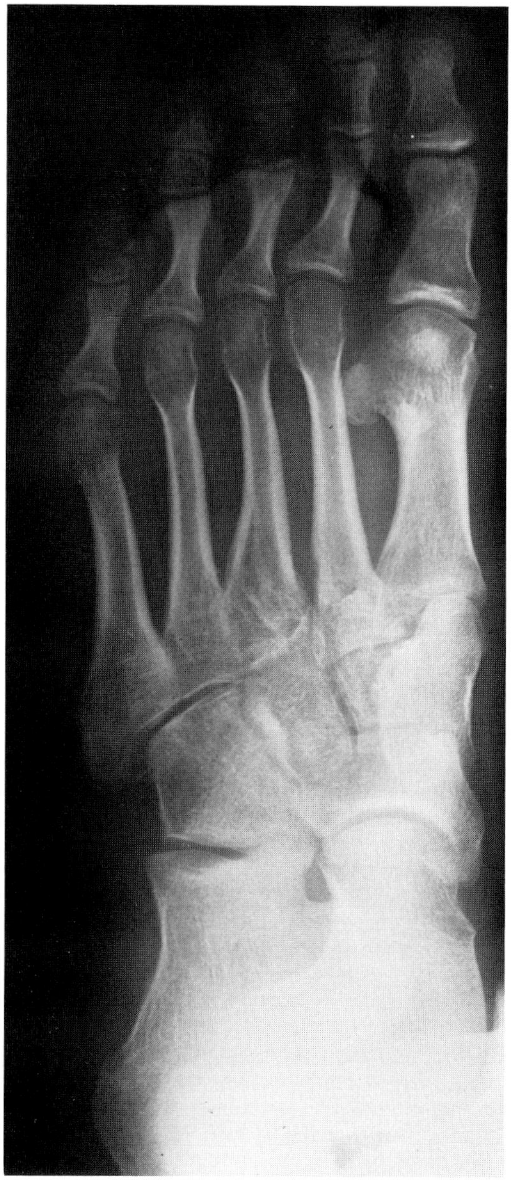

B

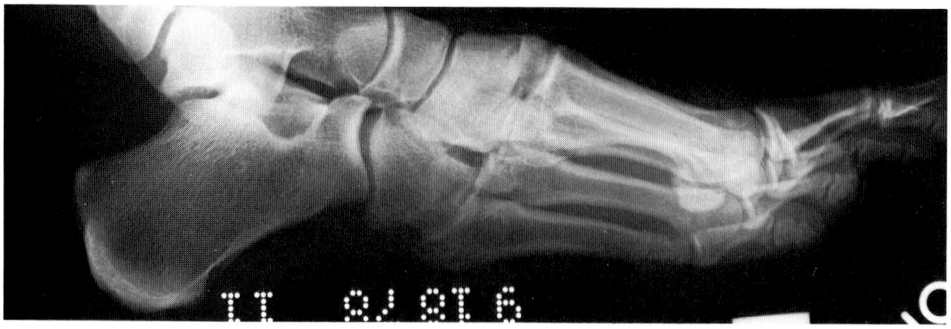

C

Lisfranc Injury

Clinical Information

This 30-year-old male injured his left foot in a motor vehicle accident.

Roentgen Findings

Anteroposterior (A), oblique (B), and lateral (C) radiographs of the left foot show an abnormally increased width of the space between the bases of the first and second metatarsals. The medial edge of the proximal end of the second metatarsal does not align with the middle (second) cuneiform, confirming the presence of a Lisfranc injury. There is lateral and dorsal subluxation of the second and third toes and lateral subluxation of the fourth toe at their tarsometatarsal (TMT) joints. The proximal portion of the first metatarsal may be slightly subluxed dorsally. The calcaneus is also subluxed dorsally on the cuboid. Fractures are seen at the base of the second and third metatarsals, the cuboid, and the medial (first) cuneiform.

Comments

A Lisfranc injury involves dislocation, or at least subluxation, of one or more of the TMT joints, most commonly the second. There frequently are associated fractures. Although this type of trauma is named for Jacques Lisfranc, a French Army surgeon who described a method of amputation of the forefoot through the joint that bears his name, he did not describe the injury. The bones that form the five TMT joints constitute a transverse arch that is maintained by the wedged shape of some of the bones and by dorsal, plantar, and interosseous ligaments. A strong Lisfranc ligament connects the base of the second metatarsal to the medial cuneiform. The joint between the middle cuneiform and the second metatarsal is situated at the summit of the arch and is slightly recessed. It is the keystone that locks the transverse arch in place.

Most Lisfranc injuries occur in automobile accidents, jumping from a height, or stepping into a hole. Children are often injured jumping from the top of a bunk bed (2). The impact is always impressed upon a markedly plantarflexed foot. The wedge shape of the second cuneiform abets the dislocation, which generally is in a dorsal and lateral direction. Wedging of the obliquely oriented medial cuneiform and first metatarsal epiphysis between the bases of the first and second metatarsal bones is common. This type of injury in children can lead to a minimal deformity of the proximal portion of the first metatarsal, which may be the only indication of a severe Lisfranc injury, since the cuneiforms and metatarsal epiphyses are not calcified before 18–24 months of age. Although dislocation of all five metatarsals may occur, malalignment most frequently involves the second metatarsal. The posterior tibial artery may be avulsed. Most Lisfranc subluxations are treated with closed reduction, but many require surgery with internal fracture. Inadequate reduction leads to a painful, crippled foot with early degenerative changes. Arthrodesis eventually may be required.

The radiologic diagnosis of a Lisfranc injury is usually easy but at times is difficult, especially in children. Nonweightbearing anteroposterior, oblique, and lateral films are usually sufficient. Malalignment may be visible on only one of these views. Because limited motion is possible at the TMT joints, offsets of up to 3 mm may be normal. Alignment of the first three metatarsals with the three cuneiforms and the fourth or fifth metatarsals with cuboid is seen in 80–100% of normal individuals (3). Parallelism is most constant between the middle cuneiform and the second metatarsal. The lateral radiograph permits identification of the first TMT joint, because the great toe is large and lies at the top of the foot. The second TMT joint is the most proximal, and the third lies between and below the first and second. The tarsal bones are normally situated at the same level or slightly dorsal to the metatarsals.

Source Materials

1. Foster SC, Foster RR. Lisfranc's tarsometatarsal fracture-dislocation. Radiology 120:79, 1976.
2. Johnson GF. Pediatric Lisfranc injury: "Bunk bed" fracture. AJR 137:1041, 1981.
3. Norfray JF, Geline RA, Steinberg RI, et al. Subtleties of Lisfranc fracture-dislocations. AJR 137:1151, 1981.

Case 26

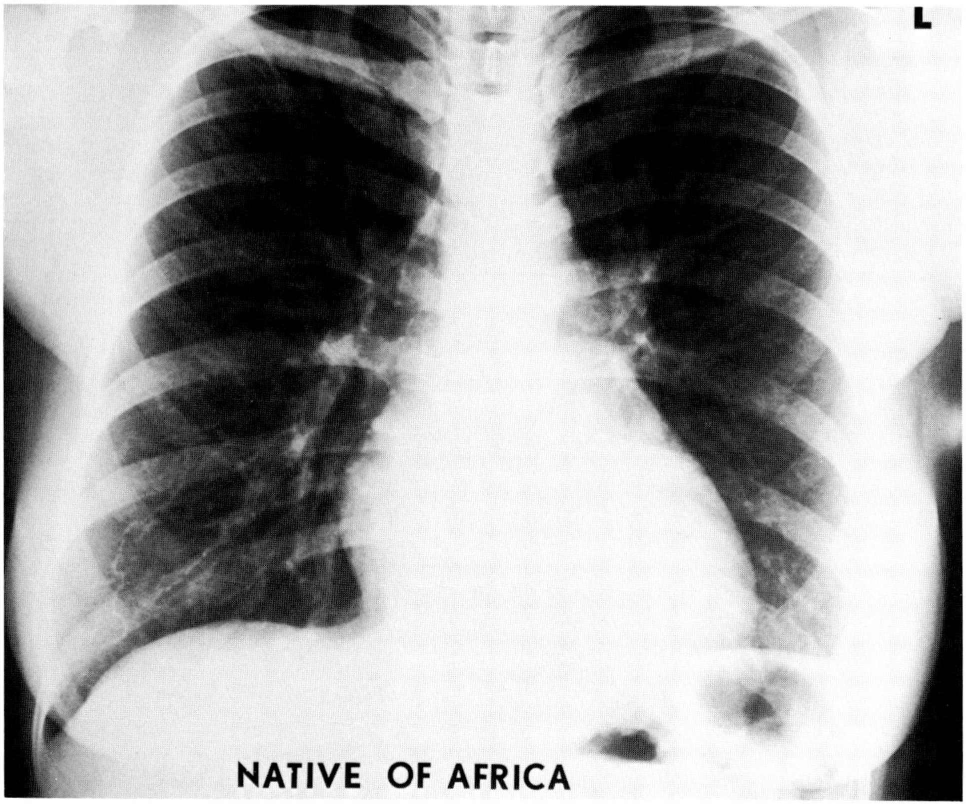

A

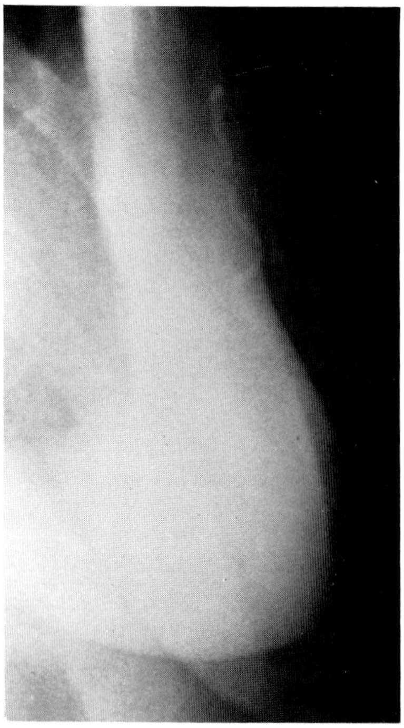

B

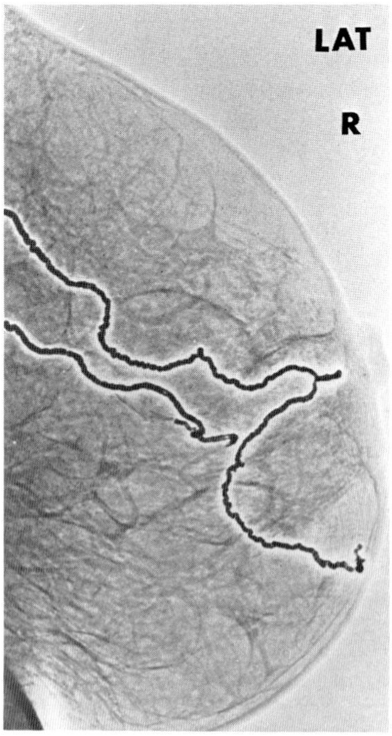

C

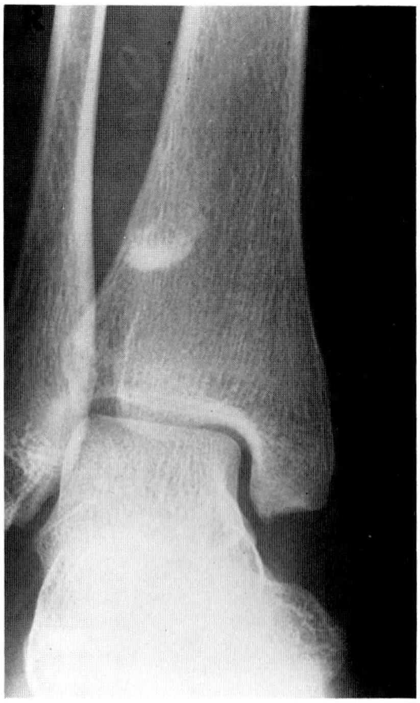

D

Dracunculiasis

Clinical Information

This patient, previously reported, immigrated from Ghana (2). She developed a right ankle effusion associated with a sterile abscess in the posterior portion of her lower right leg. A guinea worm could be palpated beneath the skin of her right breast.

Roentgen Findings

Films of the chest (A,B) are negative except for a stringlike, curved, and beaded ("chain mail") calcification within the right breast. This appearance is better shown on the xeromammograms (C). An anteroposterior film of the right ankle (D) shows whorled calcification, also characteristic of a guinea worm, situated between the tibia and the fibula. It lies just above a collection of amorphous calcification.

Comments

The offending parasite that causes dracunculiasis is the guinea worm, *Dracunculus medinensis.* This condition was called the "plague of the fiery serpents" in the Book of Numbers. The guinea worm is so named because of its prevalence in Guinea. "Medinensis" derives from the frequency of human guinea worm infestation near the city of Medina in Saudi Arabia. Dracunculiasis is widespread in many parts of the Middle East, Asia, and Africa. It previously existed in South America but has died out in the Western Hemisphere. Over 50 million people in the world are affected. As many as 85% of the young adult and middle-aged individuals in some communities have the condition.

A tiny crustacean (cyclops) ingests the dracunculus larvae in contaminated water. Human beings become infested from drinking water containing these cyclops. Acid in the stomach destroys the cyclops, which releases the dracunculus larvae. The larvae burrow into the retroperitoneal tissues where the females become fertilized by the males, who apparently subsequently die. Male guinea worms are very small and are absorbed. The female larvae burrow into the deep connective tissues, usually of dependent areas of the body. Uncommon sites of involvement are the extradural space, with possible compression of the spinal cord, or even the pericardium. The pregnant female worm moves toward the skin surface, where in due time vesicles will form through which she will discharge her developing larvae. The entire process takes about a year following ingestion of the contaminated water. If the female worm does not reach the skin surface she will discharge the products of conception within the tissues. This excites a severe reaction and usually leads to a sterile abscess.

The manifestations of guinea worm infestation, besides skin blisters and a sterile abscess, include an acute aseptic arthritis and asymptomatic calcification. More than 50% of infested individuals show two or more areas of involvement. The most common clinical effect of dracunculiasis is a skin vesicle, which often is associated with an allergic reaction. The vesicle can become secondarily infected. The mortality of dracunculiasis is extremely low but morbidity is high. An individual can be incapacitated for up to 3 months, and a few are permanently disabled. The best treatment is prevention, although appropriate medication can kill the adult guinea worm, which also can be slowly extracted over a period of several days if it is wound around a twig.

The female worm eventually dies and can become calcified. The dead worm may disintegrate, become coiled, and occupy a rather localized area, or it may remain elongated. The radiologic appearance of the intact calcified worm is absolutely diagnostic. No other parasite or condition simulates the elongated linear or coiled beaded appearance of a dead, calcified guinea worm. It can measure up to 100 cm in length. Although there is a tendency for the guinea worm to migrate to the lower extremities, the breast, scrotum, and other tissues may be affected. Guinea worms rarely invade the viscera. At times the worm disintegrates and leads to a localized area of amorphous mottled calcification. This appearance is not diagnostic and, when it is located on the chest wall, can simulate the chest film manifestations of a granuloma or even calcified lymph nodes.

Source Materials

1. Reeder MM, Palmer PES. The Radiology of Tropical Diseases with Epidemiological, Pathological and Clinical Correlation. Williams & Wilkins, Baltimore, 1981, pp 687–705.
2. Stelling CB. Dracunculiasis presenting as sterile abscess. AJR 138:1159, 1982.

Illustrations C and D courtesy of Carol B. Stelling. Reprinted with permission from AJR 138:1159, 1982 (Ref. 2).

Case 27

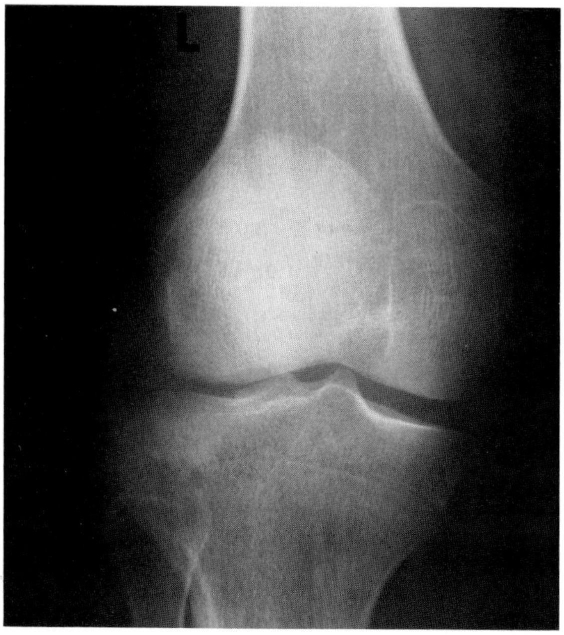

A

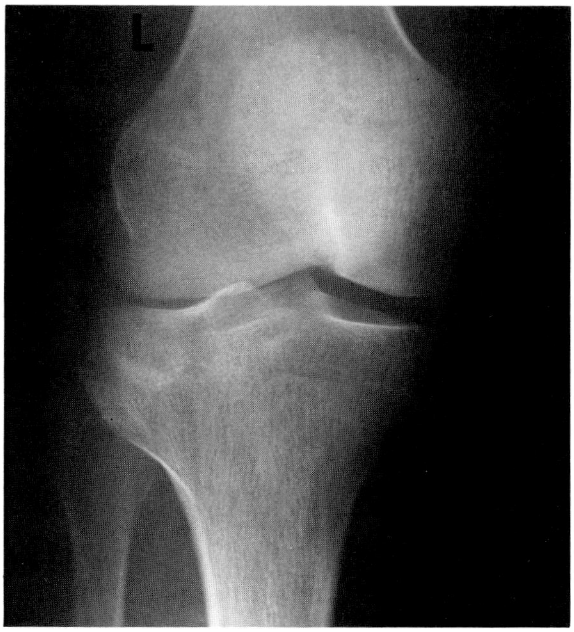

B

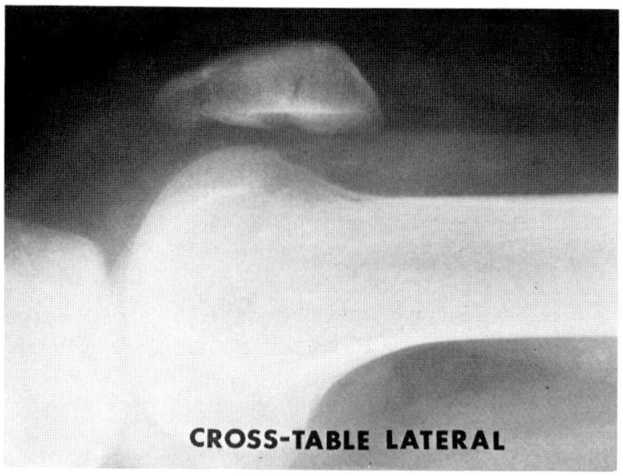

C

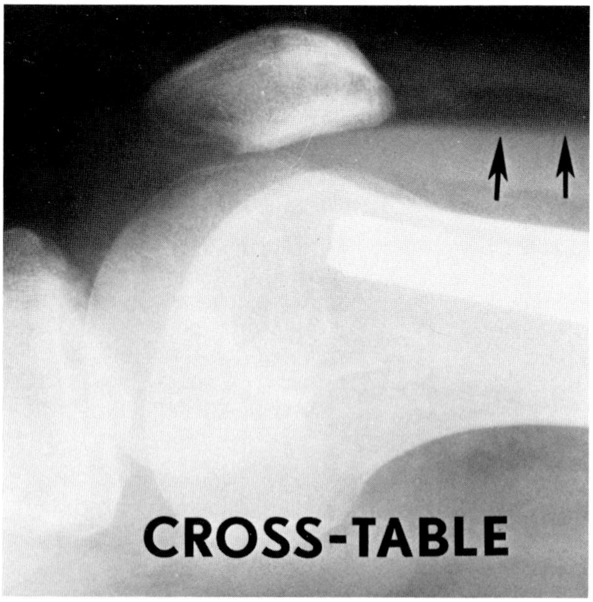

D (another patient)

Lipohemarthrosis

Clinical Information

This 39-year-old black male injured his left knee in an automobile accident.

Roentgen Findings

Anteroposterior (A) and oblique (B) views of the left knee indistinctly reveal a fracture of the lateral tibial plateau and a mildly comminuted patellar fracture. The cross-table lateral projection of this knee (C) shows a blood-fat fluid level in the suprapatellar portion of the knee joint. Film D shows a similar blood-fat fluid level in the knee joint of a patient who previously had an intramedullary rod inserted to stabilize a broken femur but recently had fractured his lateral tibial plateau (not visible on this projection).

Comments

The presence of blood and fat in a joint space following trauma is indicative of an intracapsular fracture. The fracture permits both bone marrow, with its contained fat, and blood to escape into the joint. Lipohemarthrosis may be the only evidence of an occult fracture—an especially frequent circumstance in fracture of a tibial plateau. This x-ray finding was first demonstrated about 40 years ago. A horizontal beam is required to demonstrate a blood-fat fluid level. The fat is seen as a zone of radiolucency layered above the denser blood. It was proved more than 50 years ago by aspiration that fat can accumulate in a joint space after an intracapsular fracture (2). It has been said that 10–20 ml of fat and 80–100 ml of blood are required to produce a radiologically visible blood-fat level, although the sign has been demonstrated in cadavers with as little as 5 ml of cooking oil and 10 ml of water (3, 4). Lipohemarthrosis has been most frequently visualized in the knee, but the condition has been noted in other locations, particularly in large joints such as the shoulder. This finding has been observed in up to 50% of intracapsular knee fractures.

If a fracture is never demonstrated, the fat probably is released from the synovium or else represents periarticular fat that enters the joint space through a tear in the capsule (1). Lipohemarthrosis in the absence of a fracture is particularly common with shoulder dislocations. A blood-fat fluid level should not be confused with an air-fluid level after joint aspiration or following a compound fracture that tears the joint capsule. It is said that lipohemarthrosis can also be simulated by fat beneath the lateral half of the acromion secondary to a torn supraspinatus tendon. On some occasions a small triangular suprapatellar fat pad may somewhat resemble a blood-fat fluid level, but this radiolucency will not change its orientation when the patient is placed in the upright position as occurs with a true blood-fat fluid level.

Although fat and blood within the joint space are best demonstrated by a horizontal beam, a relatively large quantity of fat in the knee joint can be seen with a vertical beam (3). Both sides of the joint capsule become visible. The outer surface of the capsule is seen because fat is normally present in this location. The inner surface of the capsule is outlined by the intracapsular fat. This situation is very similar to visualization of both walls of a bowel loop in a patient with pneumoperitoneum. The radiologic appearance of the capsule depends upon the amount of fat within the joint. The discovery of a blood-fat fluid level in the knee is equally as valuable in the diagnosis of a fracture as are displaced fat lines in a fracture of the elbow.

Source Materials

1. Arger PH, Oberkircher PE, Miller WT. Lipohemarthrosis. AJR 121:97, 1974.
2. Kling DH. Fat in traumatic effusions of knee joint. Am J Surg 6:71, 1929.
3. Sacks BA, Rosenthal DI, Hall FM. Capsular visualization in lipohemarthrosis of the knee. Radiology 122:31, 1977.
4. Saxton HM. Lipohaemarthrosis. Br J Radiol 35:122, 1962.

Case 28

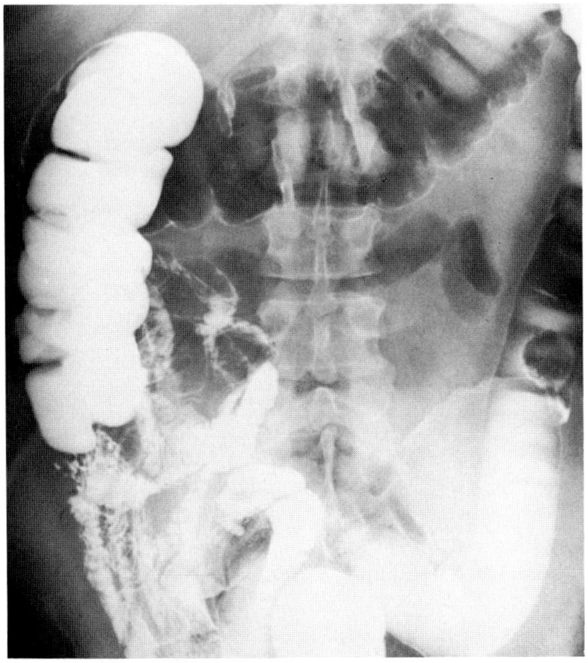

A

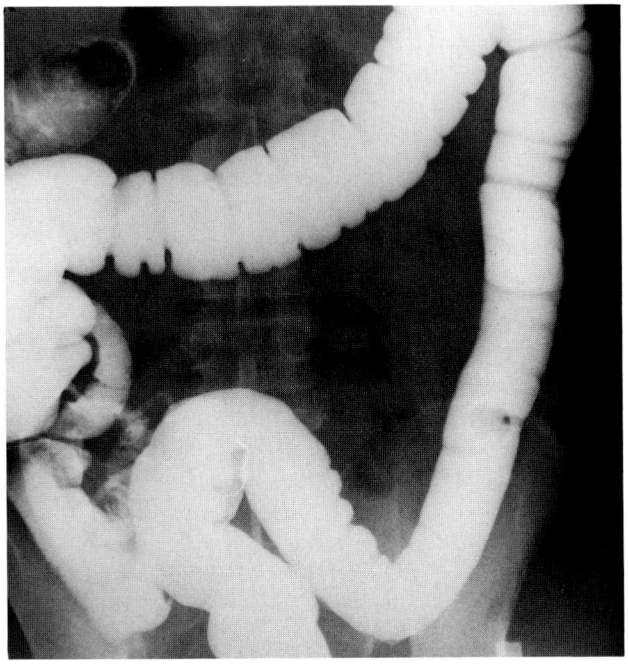

B

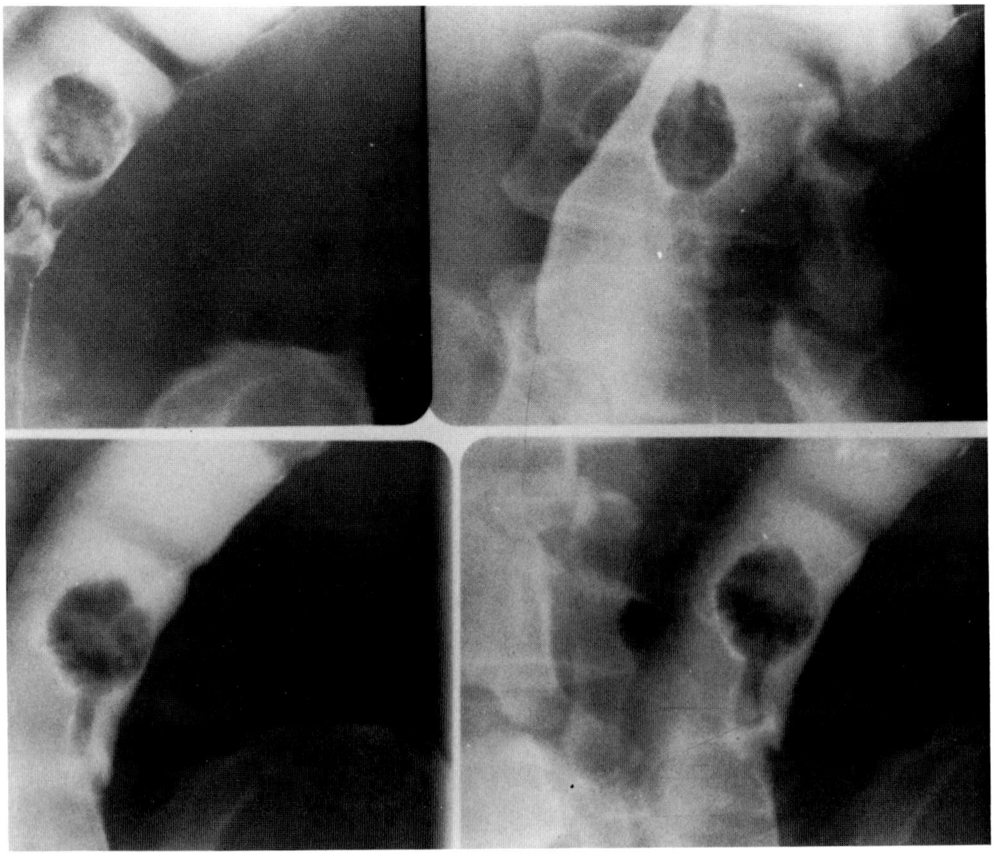

C

Colonic Polyp

Clinical Information

This anemic 39-year-old white male complained of passing bright red blood by rectum. A benign adenomatous polyp was subsequently resected.

Roentgen Findings

A barium enema (A, B) reveals a smooth, rounded filling defect measuring 2.5 cm in the distal portion of the descending colon. It is attached to the colonic wall by a slender stalk. The appearance is confirmed on multiple spot films (C).

Comments

Colonic polyps are very common. Their exact incidence is unknown, but perhaps 15% of adults harbor one or more of these lesions. About 60% are adenomatous polyps, another 10–15% are villous adenomas, and the remainder represent a variety of other lesions. An adenomatous polyp is generally thought to be an important precursor of colorectal carcinoma, which accounts for approximately 50,000 deaths in the United States each year (2). About 100,000 new cases are discovered annually. The survival rate of colonic cancer has not improved substantially over the past 40 years, although removal of asymptomatic lesions will cure about 80%. The majority of investigators believe colorectal cancer develops slowly over several years, most often from an adenomatous polyp. Some maintain a polypoid colonic lesion is either malignant or benign from onset. Such is true in some instances, since polypoid lesions as small as 0.5 cm have been shown to be malignant (3). All easily accessible polyps probably should be removed. Careful follow-up with repeated barium enemas or a colonoscopic examination is certainly indicated. The likelihood of malignancy increases with the size of the polyp. Polyps that exceed 3 cm in diameter most certainly should be removed. The most common symptom of a colonic polyp is rectal bleeding.

Colonic polyps are a manifestation of many syndromes. These include familial polyposis and Gardner's syndrome, both of which have a very high incidence of malignancy in the colonic lesions. Other conditions associated with colonic polyps include Peutz-Jeghers syndrome, Turcot syndrome, Cronkhite-Canada syndrome, juvenile polyposis, and Cowden's disease.

A double-contrast barium enema is considerably more sensitive in the detection of colonic polyps than a single-contrast study. About 90% of colonic polyps can be discovered with a double-contrast examination. A colonoscopy is probably somewhat more sensitive. This is particularly true of lesions located in the left side of the colon, although barium studies are more likely to reveal polyps in the right colon (4). The two modalities are complementary. There are many descriptions of the usual and unusual x-ray appearances (figure eight sign, bowler hat sign, etc.) of colonic polyps. Uncommon presentations can be explained by the disposition of the barium-coated polyp in the air-filled colon and the direction of the x-ray beam (1). Several x-ray findings are said to be associated with an increased incidence of malignancy. These include ulceration, broad-based irregular margins, retraction of the colonic wall at the base of the lesion, and an increase in size on subsequent examinations. Benignity is favored by smooth margins and pedunculation. The x-ray characteristics of malignancy are much more likely to be evident when a polyp reaches 3 cm in diameter. The single most important factor is size. Polyps below 1 cm in diameter are rarely malignant. Those larger than 2 cm have a 20% likelihood of being malignant.

Source Materials

1. Ament AE, Alfidi RJ. Sessile polyps: Analysis of radiographic projections with the aid of a double-contrast phantom. AJR 139:111, 1982.
2. Munyer TP, Margulis AR. Detection and management of polypoid lesions of large bowel. Rev Interam Radiol 7:79, 1982.
3. Skucas J, Spataro RF, Cannucciari DP. The radiographic features of small colon cancers. Radiology 143:335, 1982.
4. Thoeni RF, Petras A. Double-contrast barium-enema examination and endoscopy in the detection of polypoid lesions in the cecum and ascending colon. Radiology 144:257, 1982.

Case 29

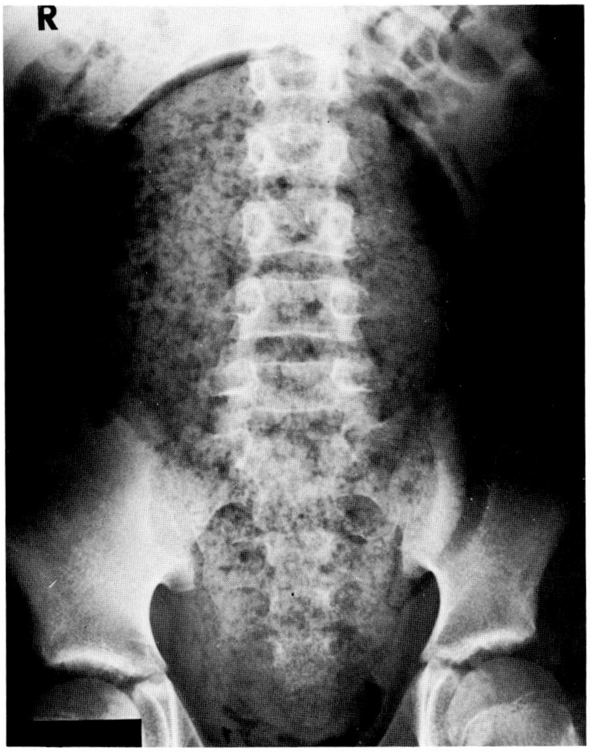

A

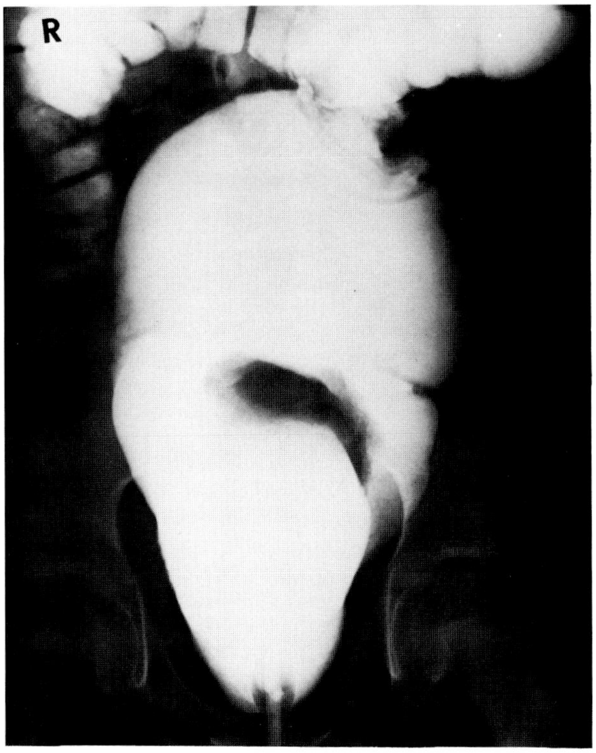

B

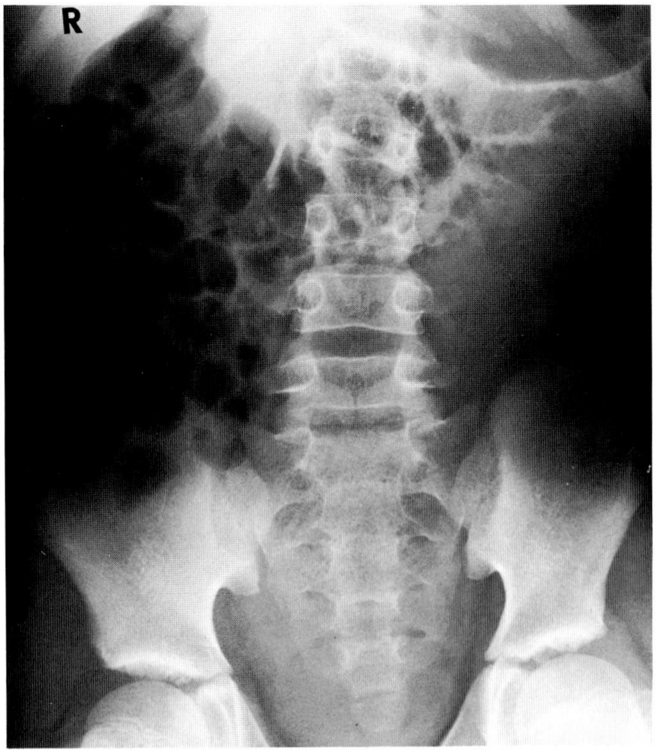

C

Functional Megacolon

Clinical Information

This 13-year-old boy was admitted for fecal impaction. He had been constipated since the first year of life and had passed very large stools every 4–5 days with intervening fecal soiling. The patient's parents were recently divorced and his father suffered from manic-depressive episodes. Many family members had various intestinal diseases or complaints, especially chronic constipation. Rectal biopsy showed abundant ganglion cells. Medical management relieved his immediate problem (film C).

Roentgen Findings

A supine abdominal film (A) shows massive amounts of feces in the colon, especially the sigmoid and the rectum. Dilatation of the rectum extends to the anus. A barium enema (B) did not reveal a transition zone.

Comments

Functional megacolon is very common in children. It must be differentiated from Hirschsprung's disease and hypothyroidism. Hypothyroidism usually can be distinguished easily from clinical evidence. Clinical differences also exist between Hirschsprung's disease and functional megacolon. The former causes symptoms from birth, which usually are manifested by inability to pass formed stools. Bowel movements tend to be small and relatively liquid. Children with Hirschsprung's disease do not show evidence of attempting to withhold stooling (leg crossing, etc.). They rarely experience fecal soiling. Although the majority of patients with functional megacolon develop complaints within the first year of life, the condition usually worsens with time. Bowel movements are voluminous and occur at long intervals. There frequently is fecal soiling. The abdomen is continuously distended in Hirschsprung's disease and the rectum is of normal size and empty. This contrasts with functional megacolon, in which the abdomen is of variable size and the rectum is very large and filled with feces. There often are strong psychological overlays in functional megacolon. The children frequently come from families with disturbed social relationships. There usually is a family obsession with toilet training and constipation. Appropriate treatment, following symptomatic therapy for the chronic constipation, is directed toward resolving parental-child conflicts.

The x-ray differentiation between Hirschsprung's disease and functional megacolon can be very difficult, particularly early in life (3). Plain films in Hirschsprung's disease reveal the rectal diameter to be smaller than the diameter of the sigmoid, which is the opposite of findings in normal individuals or those with functional megacolon (2). A diagnostic narrowed transition zone is not always clearly evident in Hirschsprung's disease. The colon proximal to the narrowing (usually located in the high rectum or low sigmoid) is characteristically dilated. In functional megacolon the colon is dilated to the anus. Evacuation films in functional megacolon usually show better emptying than with Hirschsprung's disease. Functional megacolon may lead to marked elongation and redundancy of the rectosigmoid. Manometry may show lack of relaxation of the internal sphincter in Hirschsprung's disease but not in functional megacolon or normal individuals (1). An indubitable diagnosis of Hirschsprung's disease requires absence of the ganglion cells in Auerbach's myenteric plexus on a deep rectal muscle biopsy.

Source Materials

1. Mahboubi S, Schnaufer L. The barium-enema examination and rectal manometry in Hirschsprung disease. Radiology 130:643, 1979.
2. Pochaczevesky R, Leonidas JC. The "rectosigmoid index": A measurement for the early diagnosis of Hirschsprung's disease. AJR 123:770, 1975.
3. Schey WL, White H. Hirschsprung's disease. Problems in the roentgen interpretation. AJR 112:105, 1971.

Case 30

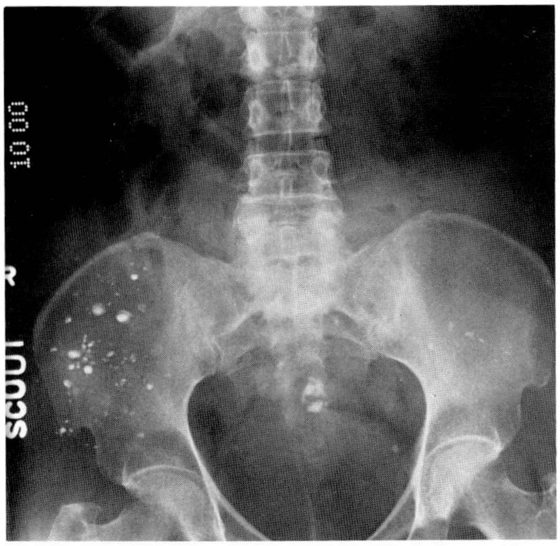

A

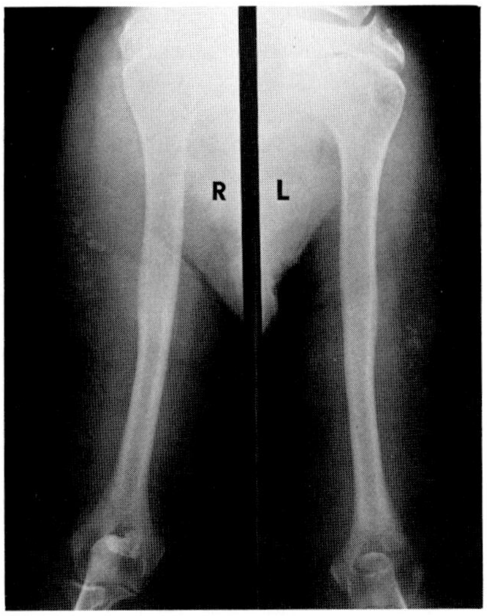

B

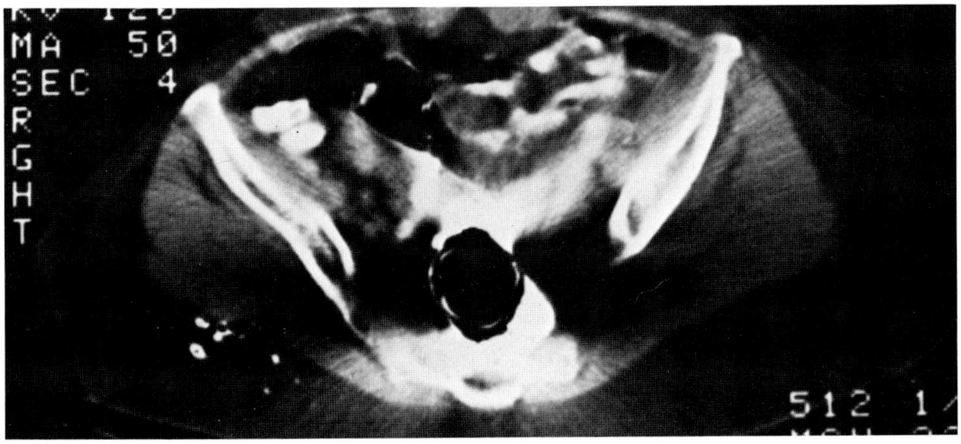

C

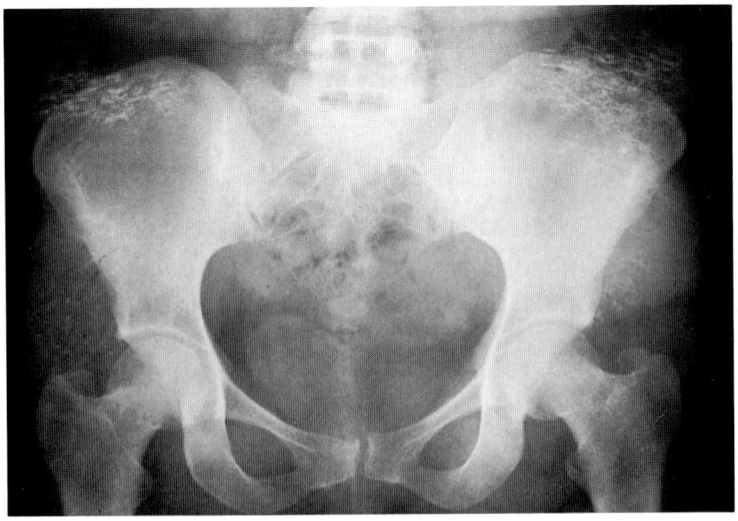

D (another patient)

Postinjectional Fat Necrosis

Clinical Information

This 74-year-old female with chronic renal failure and multiple myeloma had received numerous injections into her buttocks and shoulders. She did not complain of distress in either area, nor did she give a history of unusual soreness or pain following the injections. There was no evidence of alcoholism or pancreatitis.

Roentgen Findings

Anteroposterior films of the pelvis (A) and both arms (B) show numerous rounded soft tissue calcifications. Some of the densities are speckled or dotlike in appearance; some exhibit a circle of peripheral calcification; others are more homogeneously calcified. These calcifications are located within the subcutaneous fat rather than the underlying muscles (C). There is a single small, calcified uterine fibroid in the pelvis.

Comments

Although fat necrosis in the subcutaneous tissues can follow many types of trauma, the radiologic findings in this patient are most commonly seen after so-called intramuscular injections. Recent studies have shown that most parenteral injections are subcutaneous rather than intramuscular (1). The needles commonly employed are not long enough to reach the gluteal muscles, particularly in females. Such was the circumstance in this patient. Figure C is a computed tomogram of this patient's pelvic region. The shoulder injections were also subcutaneous.

Other types of trauma can lead to subcutaneous fat necrosis. The patient shown in D is a Nicaraguan female with abundant subcutaneous fat necrosis in her buttocks. This appearance is not an uncommon x-ray finding in Nicaragua and presumably represents the end result of chronic trauma from sleeping on the ground. The subcutaneous fat necrosis sometimes seen in pendulous breasts and the scrotum is presumably due to chronic trauma. Rather extensive subcutaneous fat necrosis may be seen in a newborn infant who has experienced perinatal distress. It usually is widespread, appears within the first and second months, and gradually clears without sequelae. Although the etiology is unknown, there may be a relationship to neonatal anoxia or prolonged hypothermia. The subcutaneous fat necrosis occasionally seen in pancreatic disease may be associated with lytic bony lesions (2).

Parenteral injections can cause a local inflammatory reaction, a sterile abscess of sorts. Secondary fat necrosis may result and appears as yellowish-white necrotic foci within the adipose tissue. Chemical analysis reveals an increased quantity of calcium and free fatty acids. The fatty acids are released by hydrolysis of neutral fat. These fatty acids combine with calcium to form calcium soaps. An elevation of serum calcium frequently is present in patients with multiple myeloma. An elevated calcium in this patient, along with the chronic renal failure, probably abetted the development of subcutaneous calcification.

It is important to differentiate postinjectional subcutaneous fat necrosis in the buttocks from the streaky metallic densities of bismuth deposits that are still occasionally seen in older patients who received this type of treatment for syphilis. Calcification in the soft tissues is sometimes evident in Weber-Christian syndrome (nonsuppurative nodular panniculitis), but it is not so circumscribed or rounded as the calcification that can develop secondary to injections. On rare occasions, calcified abdominal lymph nodes or ureteral calculus can be confused with postinjectional calcification.

Source Materials

1. Cockshott WP, Thompson GR, Howlett LJ, Seeley ET. Intramuscular or intralipomatous injections? N Engl J Med 307:356, 1982.
2. Hollingworth P, Isaacs D, Bydder G. Recurrent osteolytic lesions and subcutaneous fat necrosis in association with a developmental pancreatic cyst. Arch Dis Child 54:790, 1979.

Case 31

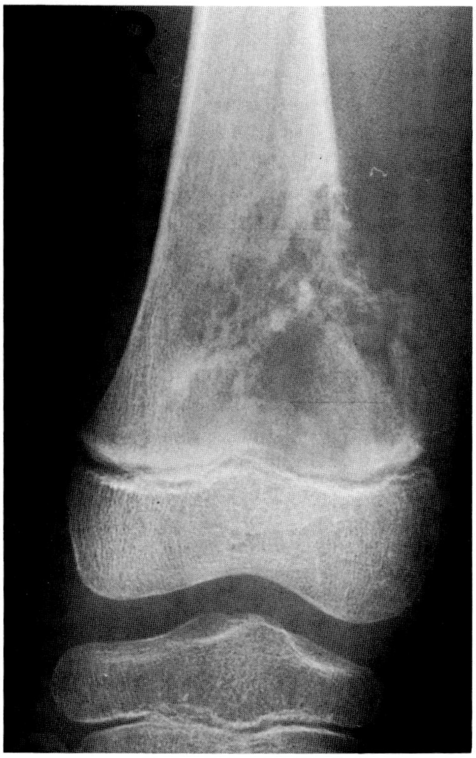

A

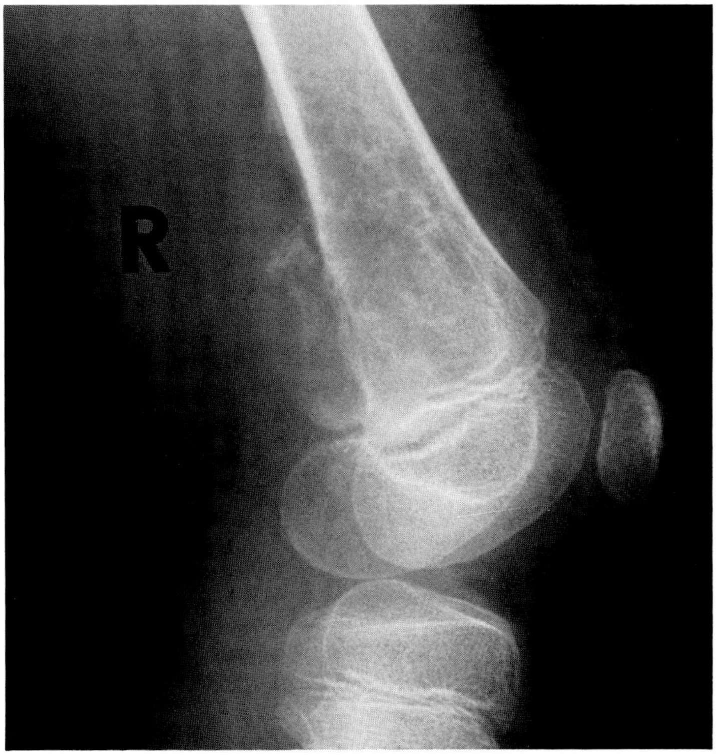

B

Osteosarcoma

Clinical Information

This 11-year-old boy complained of pain and swelling in his right knee. A diagnosis of osteosarcoma was made and his leg amputated. He died 9 months later.

Roentgen Findings

Anteroposterior (A) and lateral (B) films of the right knee show an extensive, predominantly destructive lesion in the distal metaphysis of the femur. The cortex is disrupted. Tumor calcification is seen in a soft tissue extension of the tumor, which protrudes posteriorly and medially. A Codman's triangle is evident on both radiographs.

Comments

Although osteosarcoma is the second most frequently encountered primary bone tumor (after plasma cell myeloma) and comprises almost a quarter of all primary malignant bone neoplasms, it represents only 0.2% of all malignancies. Patients with osteosarcoma usually complain of localized swelling or pain. Laboratory findings are negative except for an elevated alkaline phosphatase. The disease is usually seen in individuals between the ages of 10 and 25 years, but there also is another peak of increased prevalence beyond 50 years. Osteosarcoma in older individuals is frequently a complication of Paget's disease or radiation, but there often is no known predisposing factor (3). Younger patients show a 2:1 male predominance. This sex ratio is reversed in older patients. About 75% of osteosarcomas occur around the knee, most commonly in the distal femur, but almost any bone can be affected. Metastases are usually hematogenous and most commonly involve the lungs. The favored treatment is amputation, which should be far proximal to the lesion, since skip areas of marrow involvement are well known and can account for a local recurrence. Chemotherapy seems to improve survival rates. Radiation therapy is used primarily for palliation. The 5-year survival rate is less than 20%.

Fibrous, cartilaginous, or malignant osseous tissue may be present in various proportions in osteosarcomatous lesions. The usual form of osteosarcoma must be differentiated from multiple sclerotic osteosarcoma that occurs in early childhood, is apparently multifocal in origin, is seen predominantly in females below the age of 10 years, and is invariably fatal. Parosteal (juxtacortical) and periosteal osteosarcoma are variant forms that primarily affect cortical bone and only uncommonly extend into the medullary canal. Both have a better prognosis than the usual form of osteosarcoma. Patients with parosteal osteosarcoma tend to be in the third decade of life (4). Periosteal osteosarcomas comprise about 2% of all osteosarcomas (2). Primary soft tissue osteogenic sarcoma is very rare.

An osteosarcoma appears radiologically as predominantly osteosclerotic, osteolytic, or a mixture of bone destruction and bone formation. Some cortical bone destruction is always present. Intramedullary extension is indicated by an increase in radiodensity. This may not be evident on plain radiographs. It is always better seen on CT scans, which also can show skip areas (1). Skip areas, said to occur in approximately 20% of osteosarcomas, may be missed on plain films or nuclear scans. CT scanning can identify extraosseous extensions, which may contain abnormal bone formed by the osteogenic tumor tissue. A Codman's triangle is visible in about half of these patients. Some osteosarcomas are telangiectatic and present an x-ray appearance suggestive of an aneurysmal bone cyst. An area of the tumor that is not mineralized should be identified by either plain films or CT to mark a preferred site for needle biopsy.

Source Materials

1. de Santos LA, Bernardino ME, Murray JA. Computed tomography in the evaluation of osteosarcoma: Experience with 25 cases. AJR 132:535, 1979.
2. de Santos LA, Murray JA, Finklestein JB. The Radiographic spectrum of periosteal osteosarcoma. Radiology 127:123, 1978.
3. de Santos LA, Rosengren J-E, Wooten WB, Murray JA. Osteogenic sarcoma after age of 50: A radiographic evaluation. AJR 131:481, 1978.
4. Smith J, Ahuja SC, Huvos AG, Bullough PG. Parosteal (juxtacortical) osteogenic sarcoma—A roentgenological study of 30 patients. J Can Assoc Radiol 29:167, 1978.

Case 32

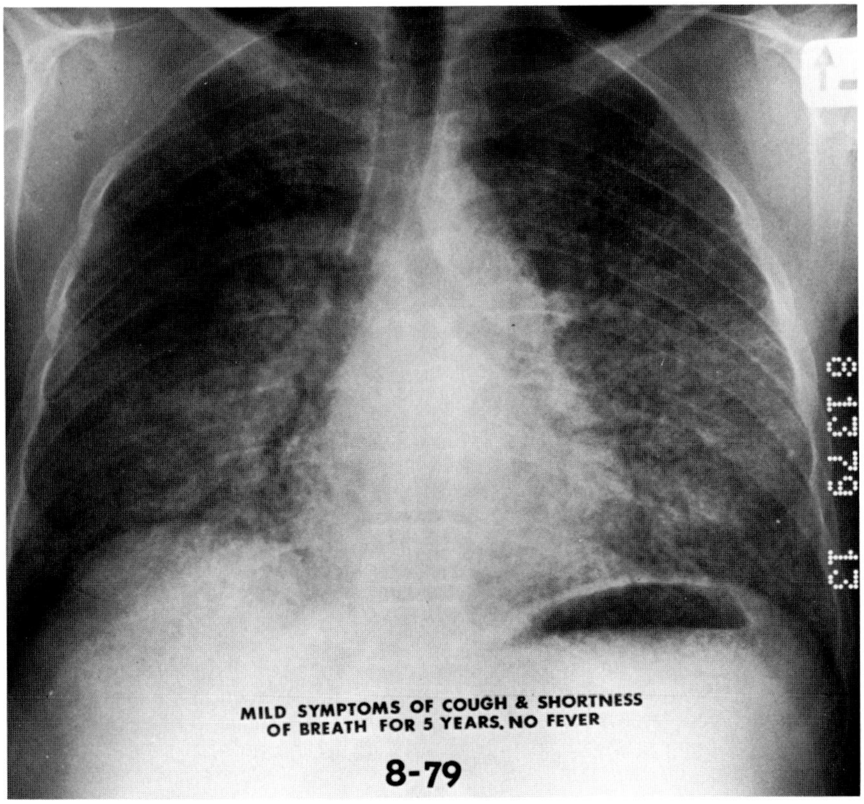
MILD SYMPTOMS OF COUGH & SHORTNESS
OF BREATH FOR 5 YEARS, NO FEVER
8-79

A

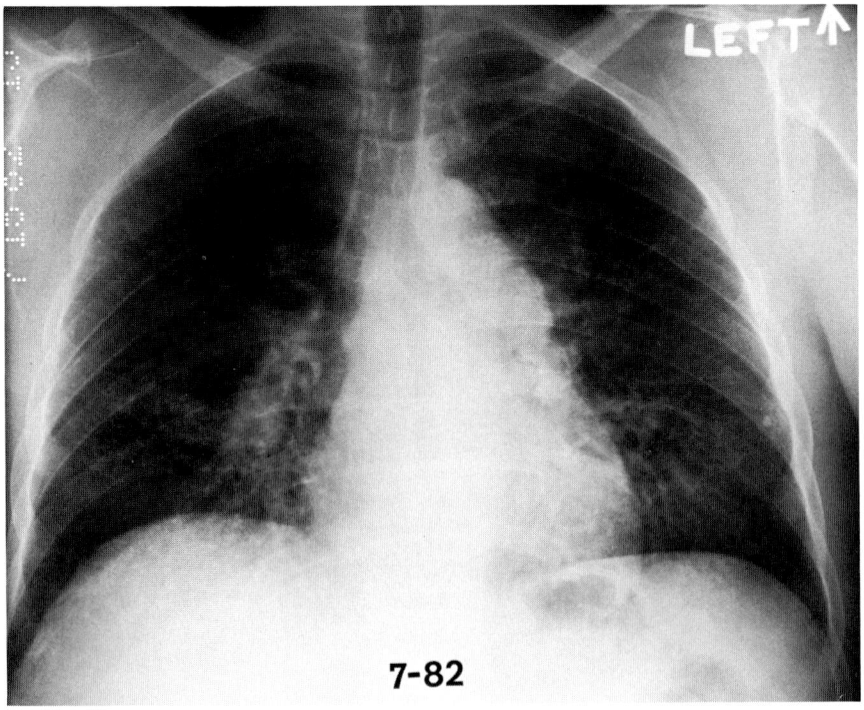
LEFT
7-82

B

Pulmonary Alveolar Proteinosis

Clinical Information

This 49-year-old white male had noted mild shortness of breath and a minimal cough for many years. He was known for at least 8 years to have biopsy-proved pulmonary alveolar proteinosis (PAP). There was no clinical or electrocardiographic evidence of pulmonary arteriolar hypertension. His symptoms improved following multiple pulmonary saline lavages.

Roentgen Findings

A posteroanterior chest film (A) shows abundant bilateral alveolar infiltrates. They are more marked in the perihilar regions and lower lung fields. No pleural effusion or mediastinal lymphadenopathy is seen. The pulmonary artery segment is prominent. Film B, taken after repeated pulmonary saline lavages, shows marked improvement.

Comments

PAP is a rare condition characterized by periodic-acid-Schiff-positive lipoproteinaceous material within the pulmonary alveoli. This material, chemically similar to the surfactants, probably originates from sloughed septal lining cells and can interfere with gaseous exchange. PAP is occasionally associated with silicosis, infections, or lymphoma; this association suggests the condition is basically a response of the lung to a variety of insults. There may be associated impairment of the defense mechanisms against microorganisms (1). The cause of PAP is unknown. It possibly is an overproduction of surfactants by the granular pneumocytes (type II cells). Another theory holds the fundamental abnormality to be defective clearance of surfactant by the alveolar macrophages. Defective macrophage function of the alveolar cells could be either a primary defect or secondary to overingestion of the surfactant-like material (2).

This disease occurs most often in individuals between 20 and 50 years of age. There is a 2:1 male ratio. Children with the condition frequently have an immunologic deficient state (3). A third of patients with PAP are asymptomatic, and most of the remainder have only mild complaints of cough, dyspnea, and/or weight loss. A low-grade fever may be present at its onset. The physical examination is usually negative. Pulmonary function tests are commonly normal but may show a reduction in diffusion capacity and vital capacity. The majority of patients with PAP eventually recover, but there occasionally is steady progress of the disease with eventual pulmonary insufficiency due to interstitial involvement (4). Death frequently results from infection by secondary invaders. The alveolar macrophages in patients with PAP have been shown by in vitro studies to have defective antibacterial activity. Treatment with bilateral tracheobronchial saline lavages and antibiotics is justified only in patients with distressing symptoms. Steroids are contraindicated.

The x-ray findings of PAP are characteristically more striking than the patient's symptoms. In a typical case the densities are bilateral, fluffy, and alveolar (2). They often are more prominent in the perihilar regions with radiation toward the bases, creating a "butterfly" pattern. This appearance closely simulates pulmonary edema but tends to remain unchanged for long periods of time. There is no associated cardiac enlargement or other x-ray findings of cardiac decompensation. Many patients with PAP do not have a characteristic x-ray appearance. There may be coalescence of the acinar densities, which can simulate a dense mass. Atypical x-ray findings can include almost any appearance. Unusual radiologic findings are particularly likely to be seen as the densities clear.

Source Materials

1. Case records of the Massachusetts General Hospital. Case 19-1983. N Engl J Med 308:1147, 1983.
2. Corsello BF, Varkey B. Central bilateral pulmonary infiltrates in an asymptomatic man. JAMA 248:2499, 1982.
3. McCook TA, Kirks DR, Merten DF, et al. Pulmonary alveolar proteinosis in children. AJR 137:1023, 1981.
4. Miller PA, Ravin CE, Smith GJ, Osborne DR. Pulmonary alveolar proteinosis with interstitial involvement. AJR 137:1069, 1981.

Case 33

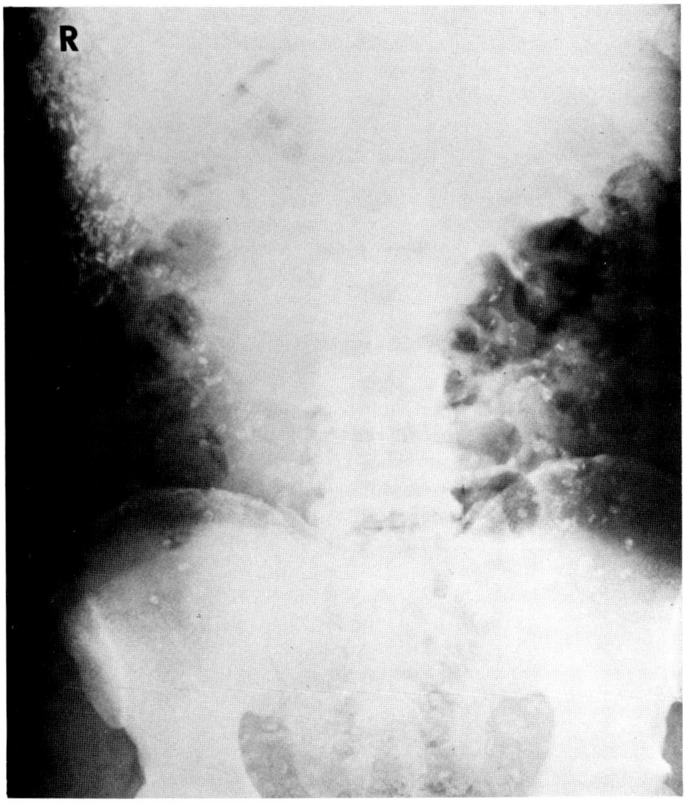

A

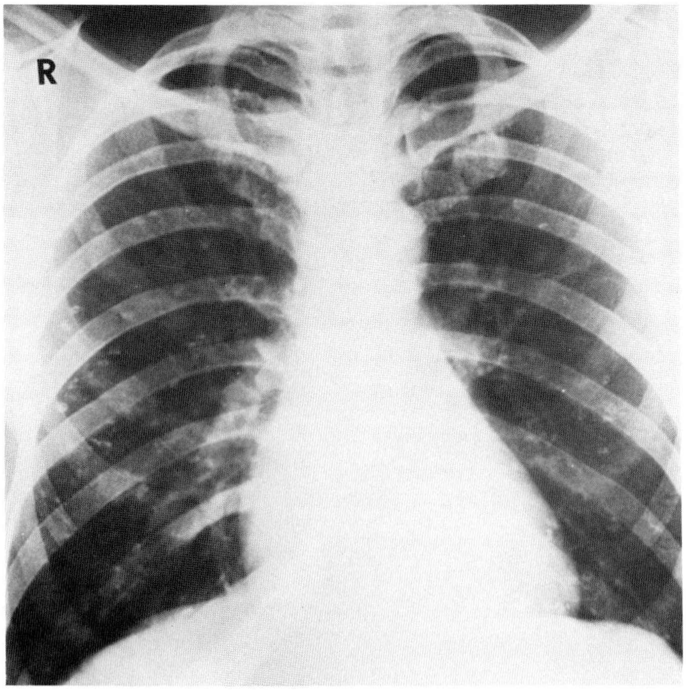

B

Porocephalosis (Armillifer Infestation)

Clinical Information

This 46-year-old male Ghanian immigrant was undergoing a complete physical examination for mild hypertension. He had no symptoms that could be related to his porocephalosis.

Roentgen Findings

A supine film of the abdomen (A) shows discrete, smoothly marginated calcifications dispersed throughout the peritoneal cavity. They are especially numerous in the right upper quadrant. Similar, although less marked, calcifications are seen on the pleural surfaces (B). Some of these calcific densities are rounded, others comma-shaped. This radiologic appearance and the distribution of the calcifications are diagnostic of porocephalosis.

Comments

Porocephalosis is a tongue worm infestation that is rarely seen outside West Africa and portions of Southeast Asia. This pentastomid infestation is caused by two varieties of tongue worms. Infestation with *Armillifer armillatus* occurs in Africa, whereas *Armillifer multiformis* is usually encountered in Malaysia. Up to 50% of the population in endemic areas can be affected. The adult parasite lives in the tracheobronchial tree of some snakes. Puff adders, cobras, and royal pythons are particularly likely to be infested. The male tongue worm is about 4 cm in length, the female 12 cm.

An adult female worm deposits her eggs within the snake's tracheobronchial tree. These eggs are passed in the reptile's excreta or bronchial secretions, which can contaminate the food or water that is ingested by the intermediate hosts, which include rats, mice, hedgehogs, hyenas, lions, and human beings. The duodenal juices of the intermediate host release the developing larvae. These larval nymphs migrate through the bowel wall and mesentery to become implanted upon peritoneal or pleural surfaces, more abundantly upon the former. The life cycle of the parasite is completed when a snake eats the smaller varieties of these intermediate hosts and the nymphs become adults. In human beings the larvae become encysted and calcified after reaching the peritoneal and pleural surfaces, where they usually cause little reaction. Vital structures such as the bile ducts, bronchi, ureters, and even the bowel lumen occasionally can be compressed. The parasites very rarely invade organs to cause pneumonitis, hepatitis, and so forth. Infestation within the abdominal cavity can be extremely abundant. It has been said that larvae may virtually cover the hands and arms of the pathologist during an autopsy.

The radiologic appearance of the dead calcified larvae is characteristic. They present as distinctive coiled calcifications that vary from 3 to 7 mm in size and are horseshoe, crescentic, or comma-shaped. If seen on end they may appear rectilinear or rounded. The calcifications are especially abundant within the abdomen, particularly over the liver. Calcifications have been seen within the scrotum. The location of the calcifications differentiates porocephalosis from cysticercosis. The calcifications of cysticercosis are characteristically located within the muscles of the extremities, a location virtually never reached by armillifer larvae.

Source Materials

1. Bretland PM. *Armillifer armillatus* infestation: Radiological diagnosis in two Ghanian soldiers. Br J Radiol 35:603, 1962.
2. Linder RR. Retrospective x-ray survey for porocephalosis. J Trop Med Hyg 68:155, 1965.
3. Reeder MM, Palmer PES. The Radiology of Tropical Diseases with Epidemiological, Pathological and Clinical Correlation. Williams & Wilkins, Baltimore, 1981, pp. 933–941.
4. Steinbach HL, Johnstone HG. The roentgen diagnosis of Armillifer infection (porocephalosis) in man. Radiology 68:234, 1967.

Case 34

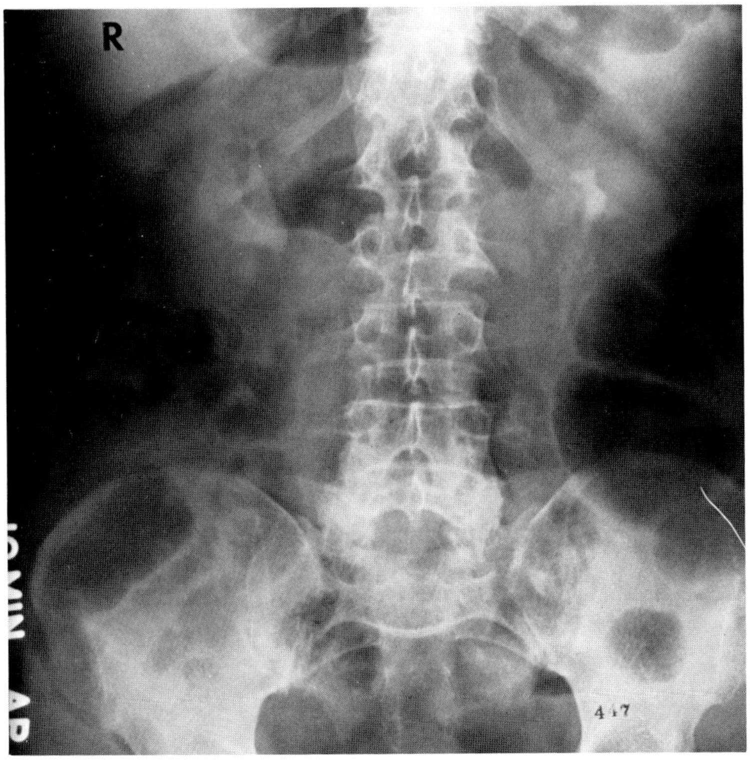

A

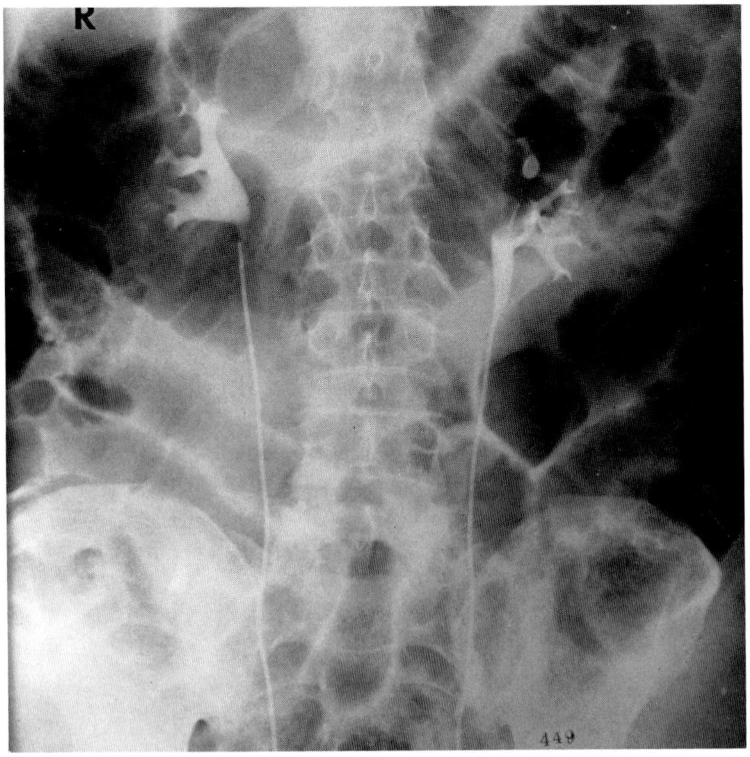

B

Transitional Cell Carcinoma of the Renal Pelvis

Clinical Information

This 75-year-old man had developed intermittent hematuria during the preceding several weeks. He was hospitalized for diagnosis and underwent resection of his left kidney and ureter for a polypoid transitional cell carcinoma of the renal pelvis. Recovery was uneventful.

Roentgen Findings

An intravenous urogram (A) shows extremely poor function bilaterally. A retrograde pyelogram (B) reveals a normal drainage system on the right. There is a lobulated, smoothly marginated filling defect within the central portion of the left renal pelvis. This lesion measures about 2.2 cm in diameter and has the radiologic characteristics of a transitional cell tumor.

Comments

Tumors of the renal pelvis, which most commonly are transitional cell carcinomas, comprise about 8% of all malignant lesions of the kidney. This cancer is three times more common in men than in women. Eighty percent of patients with this tumor are between the ages of 40 and 70 years. The pathogenesis of a renal pelvis transitional cell carcinoma is not known with certainty, but the etiology is very likely similar, if not identical, to like tumors of the urinary bladder. Simultaneous transitional cell tumors in both locations often occur.

An increased frequency of these lesions is noted following exposure to aniline dyes and possibly after prolonged ingestion of synthetic sweeteners, food coloring, coffee, or cyclophosphamides. Cigarette smoking has been associated with an increased incidence of this tumor. Transitional cell tumors are particulalry common in individuals who have suffered from Balkan nephropathy or analgesic nephropathy, both of which are interstitial nephritides characterized by destructive changes in the renal papillae (1).

Transitional cell carcinomas are frequently multiple. This may represent spread along the uroepithelium or possibly multicentric sites of origin. There is often simultaneous involvement of the ipsilateral ureter and the bladder. The bladder tumors are usually located near the related ureteral orifice. The tumor can spread by direct extension or by metastases. Frequent symptoms are hematuria and flank pain. The tumor can entirely replace an affected kidney. This usually occurs without evidence of renal enlargement. There may be considerable associated fibrosis. Appropriate treatment is surgical resection, usually with removal of the ureter and a cuff of bladder near the ureteral opening. The prognosis is worsened by an advanced stage or grade of the tumor. Survival rates vary between 5% and 80%.

The typical radiologic finding is a smooth filling defect in the renal pelvis, which usually is easily appreciated on an intravenous urogram. A retrograde study may be required if renal function is poor. The lesion can occupy any location within the pelvicalyceal system. It can be obstructive and cause hydronephrosis, although complete lack of renal function is more likely to result from replacement of the kidney by the tumor than from complete obstruction. Calcification is rare. The filling defect, if small, must be differentiated from a radiolucent stone, blood clot, or inflammatory polyp (4). These tumors have been said to be hypervascular at angiography, but such changes, if present at all, are very subtle. The lesion also may be evident on sonographic studies.

Source Materials

1. Burnett KR, Miller JB, Greenbaum EI. Transitional cell carcinoma: Rapid development in phenacetin abuse. AJR 134:1259, 1980.
2. Case records of the Massachusetts General Hospital. Case 11-1981. N. Engl J Med 304:657, 1981.
3. Lowe PP, Roylance J. Transitional cell carcinoma of the kidney. Clin Radiol 27:503, 1976.
4. Reuter KL, Krolikowski FJ, D'Orso CJ, et al. Inflammatory polyp of the renal pelvis simulating transitional cell carcinoma. Radiology 144:505, 1982.

Case 35

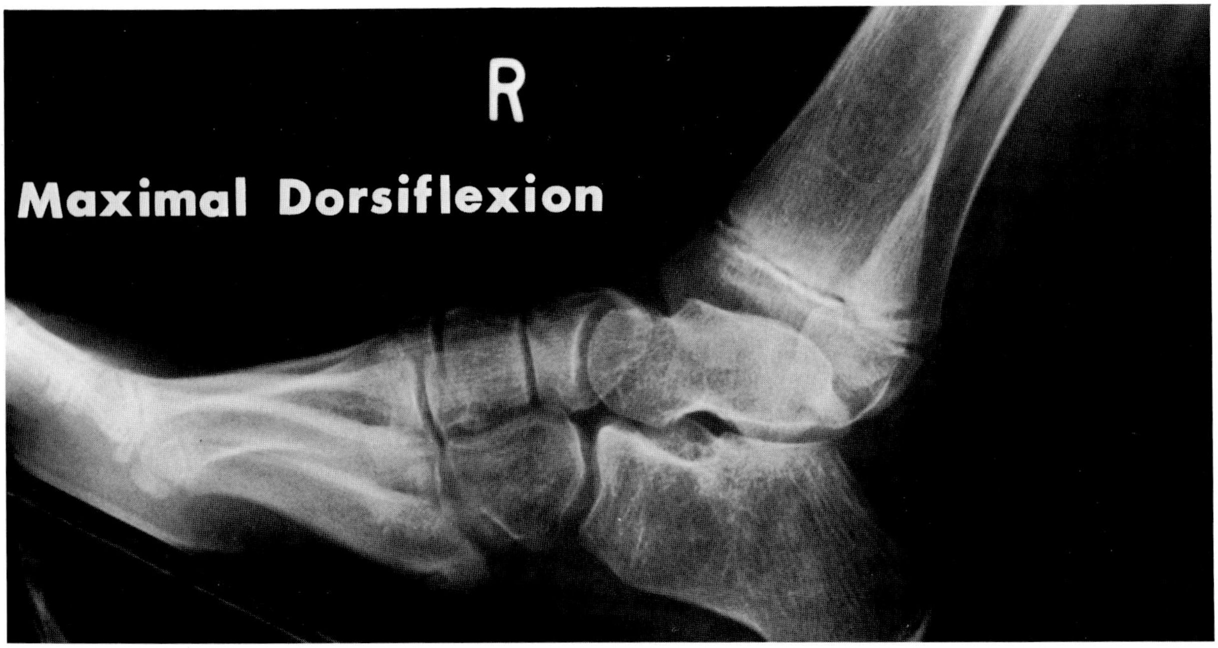

A

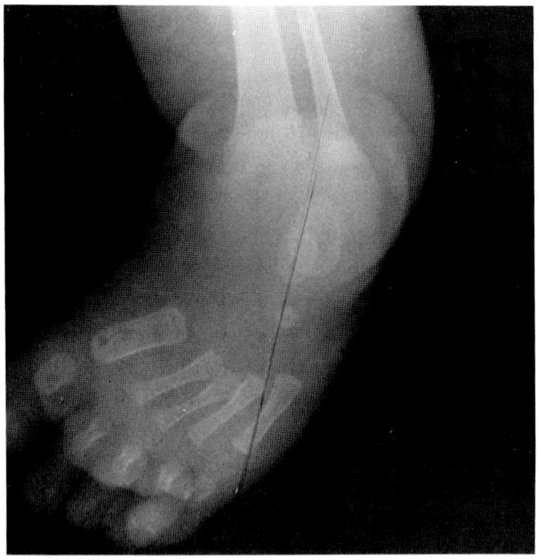

B

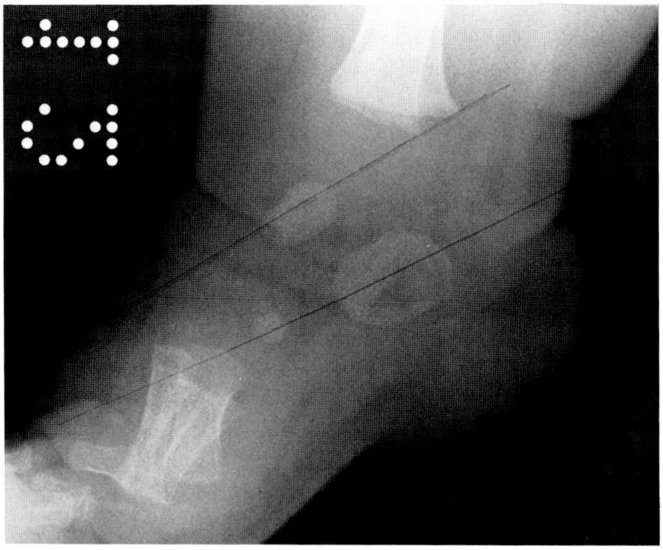

C

Flat-Top Talus

Clinical Information

This 13-year-old boy had been treated with bandages and splints during the first several years of his life for a right clubfoot. His foot thereafter functioned satisfactorily.

Roentgen Findings

A lateral film of the maximally dorsiflexed right foot (A) shows the angle between the foot and the tibia to be barely 90°, indicating a slight limitation of dorsiflexion. The talocalcaneal angle is somewhat less than normal, and the talus at its tibial articulation is flattened and reduced in height. This is the typical appearance of a flat-top talus, which is sometimes encountered after treatment of a clubfoot in early infancy.

Comments

Clubfoot (talipes equinovarus) is an ancient disease, evident in tomb paintings of ancient Egyptians and the Aztecs. Hippocrates recommended about 300 B.C. that clubfeet be treated with manipulation and bandages. The cause of this relatively common deformity is unknown. Half of affected individuals have bilateral clubfeet. When unilateral, the right foot is involved more often than the left. Associated congenital anomalies may exist (4).

Positioning of the extremity is very important in a radiologic examination of an infant for clubfeet (1) The anteroposterior radiograph should be exposed with the tibia in a normal anteroposterior position regardless of the resulting attitude of the abnormal foot (3). The lateral view should be taken in maximal dorsiflexion. In a normal individual, a line drawn through the longitudinal axis of the talus on the anteroposterior view, when extended, will pass near the longitudinal axis of the first metatarsal shaft. Likewise, a line drawn in a similar manner through the calcaneus will tend to pass near the longitudinal plane of the fourth metatarsal. In a clubfoot the talar line runs well lateral to the first metatarsal due to forefoot and heel varus. A normal foot on the lateral film reveals an angle between the midtalar and midcalcaneal lines of about 40°, whereas in a clubfoot these two lines become almost parallel. Films B and C show this patient's right foot in infancy. His left foot was normal.

Forced dorsiflexion of the foot in a plaster cast before the equinovarus deformity of the calcaneus is corrected, particularly when the ankle joint capsule and associated ligaments are tight, will lead to abnormal pressure between the superior surface of the talus and the tibia. This occurs because the calcaneus lies immediately beneath the talus. The usual result is a flat-top talus as seen in this patient (2). It is clear that the calcaneus must be moved laterally before flexion of the talus can occur. Extreme force in this situation can cause a "rocker bottom" deformity from midfoot extension. A "rocker bottom" deformity from forceful dorsiflexion of a clubfoot must be distinguished from the "rocker bottom" of a congenital vertical talus in which the talus is flexed and the tarsal scaphoid is dislocated. Patients with a flat-top talus are liable to early development of degenerative changes.

Source Materials

1. Davis LA, Hatt WS. Congenital abnormalities of the feet. Radiology 64:818, 1955.
2. Dunn HK, Samuelson KM. Flat-top talus. A long-term report of twenty club feet. J Bone Joint Surg 56A:67, 1974.
3. Freiberger RH, Hersh A, Harrison MO. Roentgen examination of the deformed foot. Semin Roentgenol 5:341, 1970.
4. Gilsanz V, Teitelbaum G, Condon VR. Clubfoot deformity and tibiofibular diastasis. AJR 140:759, 1983.

Case 36

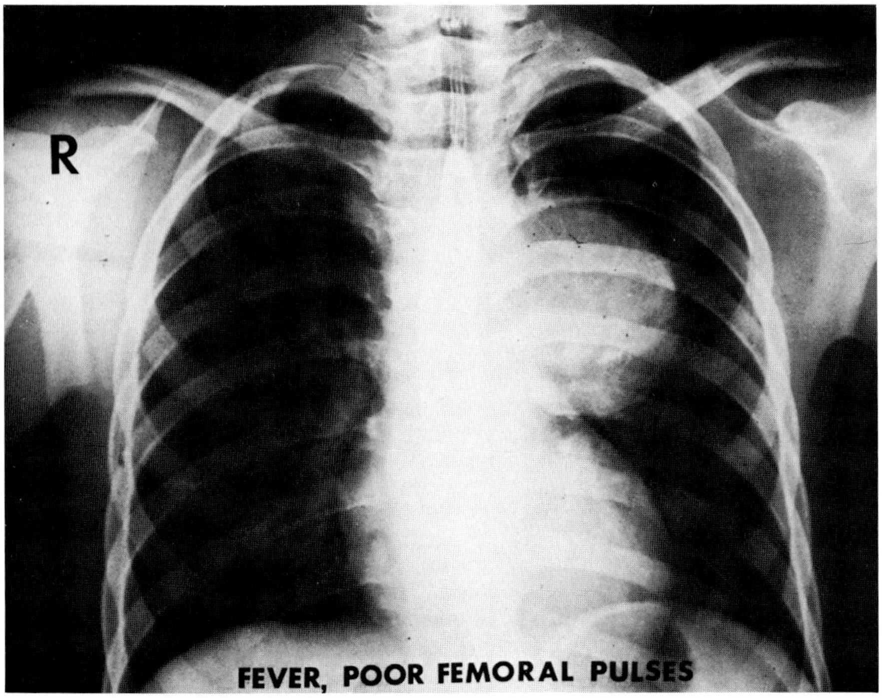

A

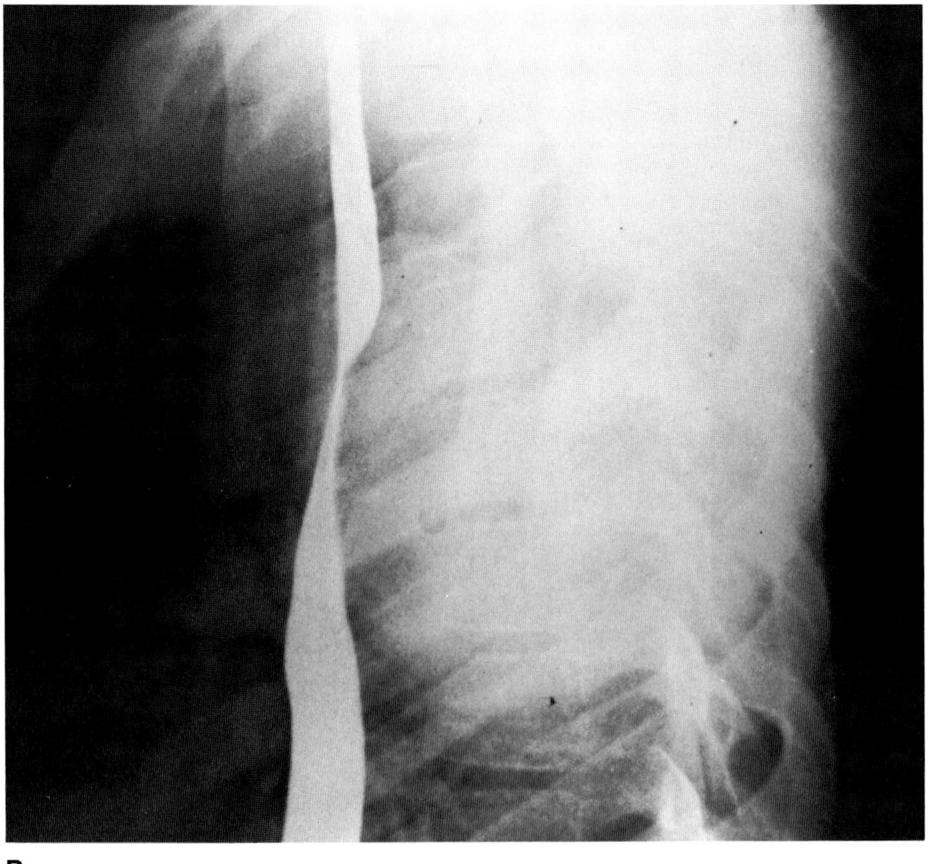

B

Mycotic Aortic Aneurysm

Clinical Information

This 4-year-old male had been febrile for the preceding 3 weeks. He collapsed and died shortly after it was noted that he had very poor femoral pulses bilaterally. Autopsy showed coarctation of the aorta near its isthmus and a ruptured mycotic aortic aneurysm. The aneurysm was situated immediately beyond the point of coarctation.

Roentgen Findings

Posteroanterior (A) and lateral (B) films of the chest with barium swallows show a smoothly outlined soft tissue mass that is rounded in configuration and measures about 6.5 cm in diameter. It is situated posteriorly in the central portion of the left hemithorax at the level of the aortic arch and indents the posterior aspect of the esophagus. Bilateral rib notching is present. It is most easily appreciated on the undersurface of the right fourth and fifth ribs.

Comments

The term mycotic aneurysm was first used by Osler about 100 years ago to refer to aneurysms caused by septic emboli in patients with bacterial endocarditis. The term now includes all types of infected aneurysms. A mycotic etiology is present in about 2.5% of aneurysms (4). These aneurysms can result from lymphatic spread or direct extension of an infection or from septic emboli (most often from bacterial endocarditis) that lodge either within the vasa vasorum or else upon damaged or abnormal portions of the vascular endothelium (2). Lymphatic spread is very uncommon. Drug abusers may develop these lesions, which actually are false aneurysms since there is destruction of most or all of the intima and media of an affected vessel. Mycotic aneurysms are very rare in children (1, 4). Trauma, particularly injury from an umbilical arterial catheter in premature infants, can lead to this lesion. Patients with congenital heart disease, especially those with coarctation of the aorta, can develop this type of aneurysm. A mycotic aneurysm is most commonly situated in the aorta and can cause a variety of symptoms (3). Fever is usually present. A palpable mass or a bruit may be appreciated in the region of the lesion.

Subclinical bacteremia, which occurs in a variety of circumstances, can lead to a so-called primary mycotic aneurysm. Infective organisms apparently lodge on a normal or near-normal aorta. Virtually all adults have small intimal plaques upon which bacteria might arrest. Such primary infections are most commonly caused by salmonella that apparently reach the bloodstream from the gut. Common pathogens such as streptococcus and staphylococcus are the usual offending organisms in other types of mycotic aneurysms. The prognosis of the condition is poor. These aneurysms rapidly increase in size and often rupture. Prompt surgical excision is the treatment of choice.

X-ray findings vary with the location of the aneurysm and its rate of progression. These lesions frequently are not recognized before they rupture, which usually is a fatal event. A correct diagnosis requires a high level of clinical suspicion. Mycotic aneurysms are usually saccular but without features that distinguish them from any other aneurysm. The presence of an appropriate predisposing condition, an enlarging mass, and fever should alert the radiologist to the possibility of this lesion. A definitive diagnosis can be obtained with an angiogram.

Source Materials

1. Faer MJ, Taybi H. Mycotic aortic aneurysm in premature infants. Radiology 125:177, 1977.
2. Felson B, Akers PV, Hall GS, et al. Mycotic tuberculous aneurysm of the thoracic aorta. JAMA 237:1104, 1977.
3. Kaufman SL, White RI Jr, Harrington DP, et al. Protean manifestations of mycotic aneurysms. AJR 131:1019, 1978.
4. Siegel MJ, McAlister WH. Aortic aneurysms in children. Radiology 132:615, 1979.

Case 37

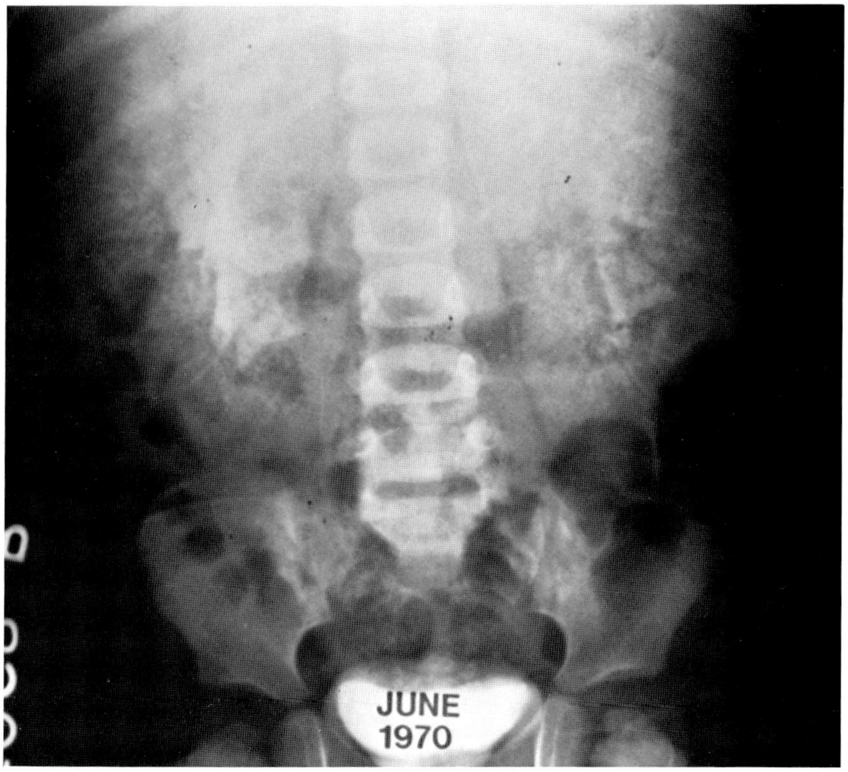

A

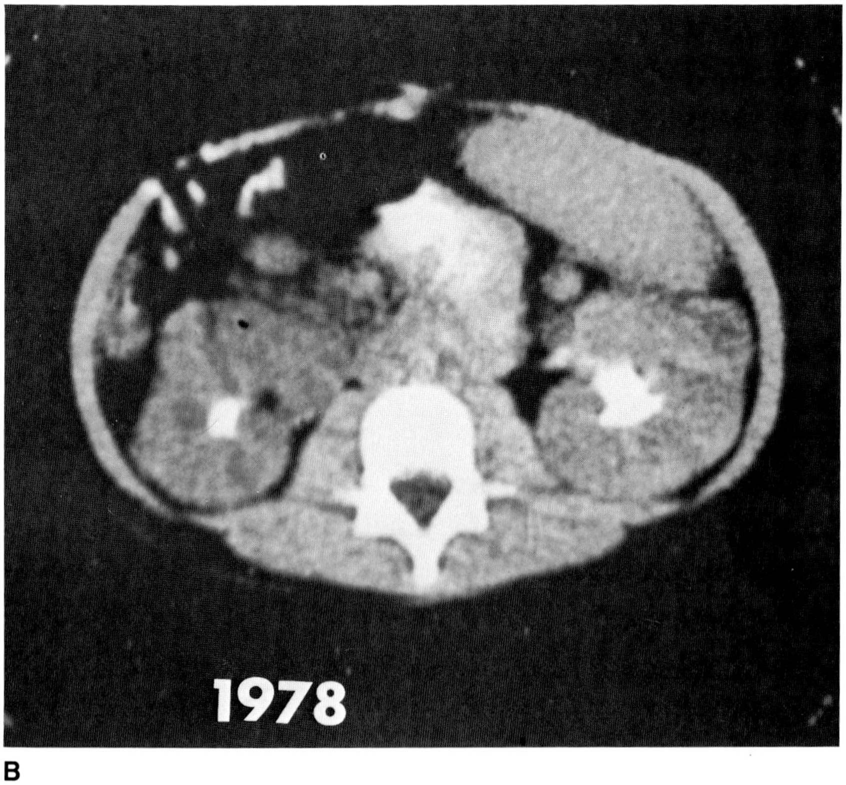

B

Infantile Polycystic Disease

Clinical Information

Flank masses became evident in this child at 2 years of age. Hypersplenism and esophageal varices developed at 10 years of age. Renal and hepatic function were relatively normal at the time of the last x-ray study. The patient's family history is unknown.

Roentgen Findings

The intravenous urogram at 2 years of age (A) shows good concentration of the excreted contrast medium. The kidneys are markedly and symmetrically enlarged. The renal parenchyma displays a radially striated appearance due to opaque medium within dilated ducts. The calyces and pelves are poorly seen. A computed tomographic examination 8 years later (B) shows both kidneys to be enlarged with somewhat nodular outlines and also demonstrates striated densities of opaque material within the parenchyma. The pelves are not enlarged. These x-ray findings are diagnostic of the childhood type or juvenile form of infantile polycystic disease.

Comments

Infantile polycystic disease (IPCD), by most accounts, represents a single disease process with a broad spectrum of clinical and pathologic manifestations (3). The condition has been known by many other names, including hamartomatous cystic disease, infantile sponge kidney, and microcystic kidneys. Although the adult form of polycystic disease may be seen in infants, the two processes have distinctive clinical manifestations, inheritance, and radiologic findings, as well as different ages of initial clinical presentation. IPCD is an autosomal recessive trait that affects both kidneys uniformly and symmetrically. Its etiology, although uncertain, is most likely developmental and dysplastic. Three or four forms of the condition have been described. These variations depend upon relative involvement of the renal and hepatobiliary systems. The most severe form affects almost all of the renal tubules and leads to perinatal death. There often is associated oligohydramnios and secondary pulmonary hypoplasia. Death may occur somewhat later, although still very early in life, if there is less extensive renal involvement. The fatal outcome in these patients results from kidney failure with azotemia and often hypertension. The mildest form of IPCD occurs when 10% or fewer of the renal tubules are affected. These patients have symptoms secondary to hepatic fibrosis and consequent portal hypertension. This condition, often called juvenile polycystic disease or congenital hepatic fibrosis, may be heralded by massive gastrointestinal bleeding from esophageal varices. Hepatosplenomegaly is frequent. Liver and renal function are usually normal or near normal.

In contrast to IPCD, the adult type of polycystic kidney disease is inherited as an autosomal dominant trait and does not usually cause symptoms until later in life. The kidneys, although markedly enlarged, are less uniform in contour. Adult polycystic disease also presents a different pathologic appearance characterized by nephronic dilatation and cyst formation, whereas the nephrons are not specifically involved in IPCD. The cysts of IPCD are smaller and more uniform in size and distribution than are the cysts seen with adult polycystic disease.

The radiologic findings caused by IPCD can be diagnostic. They are characterized by a prolonged nephrogram and a striated appearance of the renal parenchyma. The latter results from opaque medium within dilated ducts. Both kidneys are markedly and symmetrically enlarged with smooth or mildly nodular contours. The pelvicalyceal system, if visible, is normal, although a brush border along the margins of the calyces may be seen. Ultrasonic studies reveal increased echogenicity of the cortex and medulla due to the ectatic tubules, which create multiple tissue interfaces (1). CT examinations show linear striations, which represent the contrast medium within the dilated collecting tubules (2).

Source Materials

1. Habif DV Jr, Berdon WE, Yeh M-N. Infantile polycystic kidney disease: *In utero* sonographic diagnosis. Radiology 142:475, 1982.
2. Howie JL, Nicholson RL. CT evaluation of infantile polycystic disease. J Can Assoc Radiol 31:202, 1980.
3. Madewell JE, Hartman DS, Lichtenstein JE. Radiologic-pathologic correlations in cystic disease of kidney. Radiol Clin North Am 17:261, 1979.

Case 38

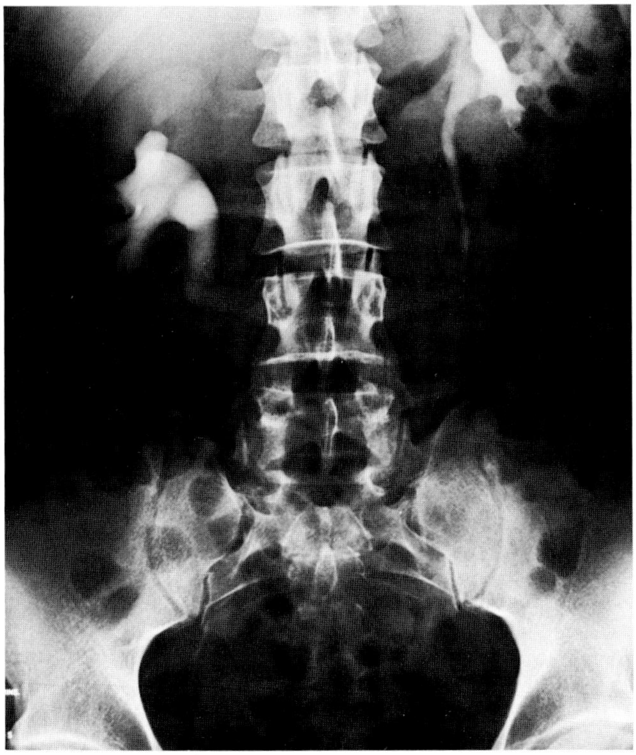

A

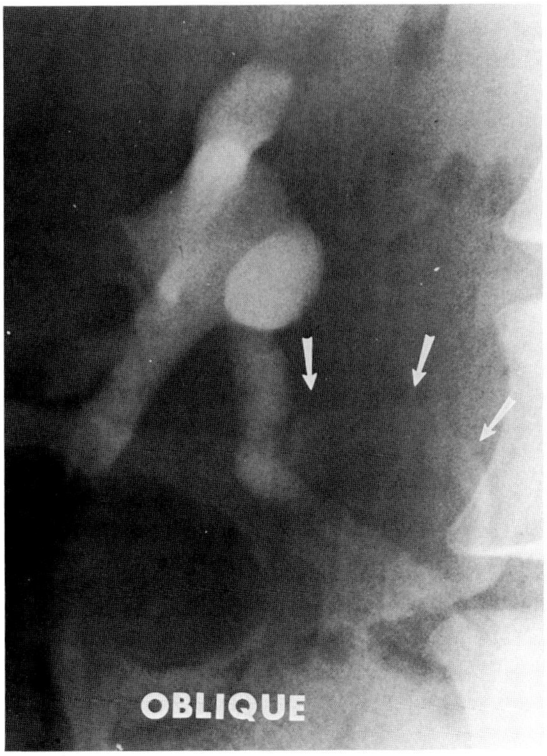

B

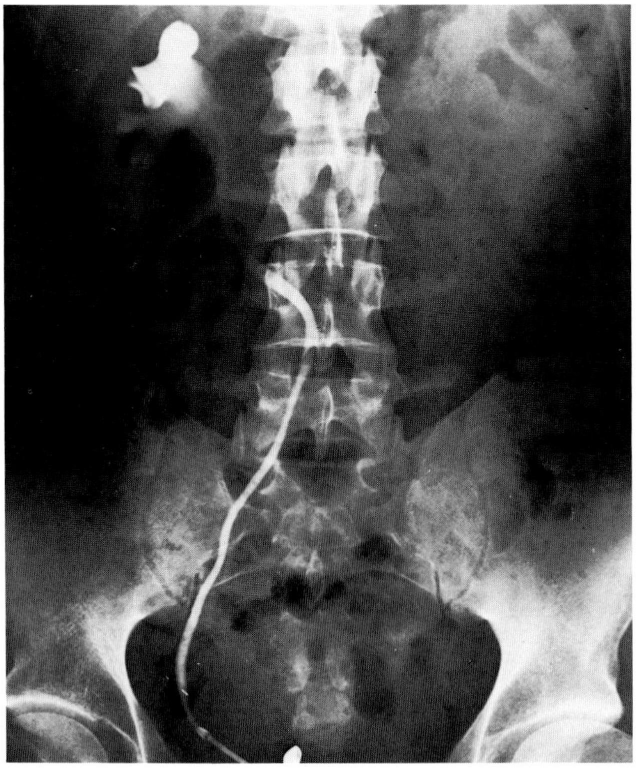

C

Retrocaval Ureter

Clinical Information

This 30-year-old man complained of intermittent right flank pain.

Roentgen Findings

An intravenous urogram (A) shows good function bilaterally. The left drainage system is normal. The calyces, pelvis, and upper portion of the right ureter are moderately dilated. The right ureter curves medially at the level of the fourth lumbar vertebra to reach a position slightly medial to the right pedicle of L4. At this location the ureter forms a hooklike configuration and progresses downwardly and laterally to reach its normal retroperitoneal location near the brim of the pelvis. The affected portion of the ureter is displaced both posteriorly and medially (B). The ureter beyond its displaced portion is not dilated. A right retrograde pyelogram (C) confirms the abnormal course of the ureter. This x-ray appearance is diagnostic of a retrocaval ureter.

Comments

A retrocaval ureter has also been called a postcaval ureter, circumcaval ureter, deflected ureter, and a preureteric vena cava (2). This condition occurs in approximately 0.1% of all individuals and predominates in males by a ratio of about 3:1. The anomalous ureter courses behind the inferior vena cava. The developmental aberration results from abnormal development of embryonic retroperitoneal venous structures. Failure of normal regression of ventrally situated embryonic right-sided venules leads to their incorporation into an inferior vena cava that is located anterior to the right ureter (1, 4).

Most patients with a retrocaval ureter are asymptomatic. This x-ray finding usually has no clinical significance. Some patients show dilatation of the drainage system proximal to the point where the ureter is located behind the inferior vena cava. This situation may lead to the symptoms and complications that can attend hydronephrosis. Such is unusual before the third or fourth decade of life. Relative ureteral obstruction can result from pressure created by the anteriorly situated inferior vena cava and the posterior vertebral column. Occasionally a stricture is present in the ureter at this location. Surgery is rarely indicated. Occasionally the symptoms are sufficiently severe to demand intervention for relief of the obstruction. Anastomosis of the ureter anterior to the inferior vena cava is the favored surgical procedure (3).

The x-ray findings of a retrocaval ureter are diagnostic. The characteristic medial and posterior displacement of the ureter, usually at the level of the fourth lumbar vertebra, is pathognomonic. The abnormally located ureter creates an "S", reversed "J", or hooked configuration, which usually extends slightly medial to the right-sided vertebral pedicle. There may or may not be associated dilatation of the ureter proximal to this point. The diagnosis is usually made by excretory urography. It can also be confirmed with computed tomography. Retrograde studies are rarely needed. There are no significant differential diagnostic possibilities. Although other diseases may cause medial ureteric displacement, nothing else leads to this configuration.

Source Materials

1. Chuang VP, Mena CE, Hoskins PA. Congenital anomalies of the inferior vena cava. Review of embryogenesis and presentation of a simplified classification. Br J Radiol 47:206, 1794.
2. Crosse JEW, Soderdall DW, Teplick SK, Clark RE. Nonobstructive circumcaval (retrocaval) ureter. Radiology 116:69, 1975.
3. Feldman SL, DiMarco ER, Tencer T, Ross LS. Retrocaval ureter: Radiographic techniques directing surgical management. Br J Urol 54:212, 1982.
4. Mayo J, Gray R, St. Louis E, et al. Anomalies of the inferior vena cava. AJR 140:339, 1983.

Case 39

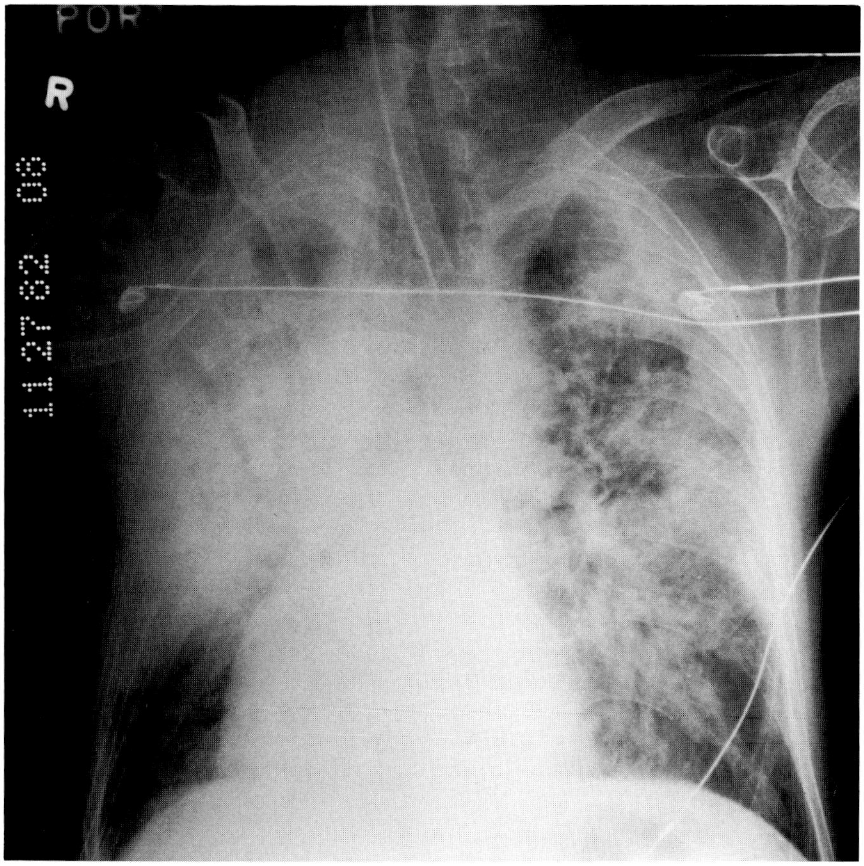

Endotracheal Tube Malplacement

Clinical Information

This 59-year-old blind male deaf-mute with a continuing fever, dehydration, hypotension, and pneumonia was transferred from a nursing home with an endotracheal tube (ETT) in place. A large amount of rust-colored "sputum" was aspirated from the ETT. Although the ETT was removed, the patient rapidly went downhill and died. Autopsy showed extensive bilateral pneumonia and esophageal ulcerations at the location of the malplaced ETT.

Roentgen Findings

A portable anteroposterior film of the chest obtained shortly after admission shows an ETT located lateral to the right side of the laryngeal margin. It evidently is not within the trachea and apparently terminates in the esophagus. No inflated cuff is seen. The esophagus is not distended. Extensive bilateral pneumonic infiltrates are clearly visible.

Comments

The distal end of a properly placed ETT should be located near the level of T3 when the patient's neck is in a neutral position. Flexion and extension of the neck can displace the tip of the ETT for a distance of about 3 cm. A neutral attitude of the neck will project the mandible near the level of C6. It will project over T1 or lower with neck flexion and above C3 with neck extension (2). The ETT in an adult should lie about 5 cm above the carina in the middle third of the trachea. The carina is situated at approximately the T6 level. The vocal cords are located at the C5–C6 level.

Overinflation of the cuff of the ETT, which is situated 1–2 cm proximal to its tip, will damage the tracheal wall. An overinflated tube is evident from radiolucent lateral bulges and an overall diameter that exceeds that of the tracheal lumen. Pathologic studies indicate that bruising of the pharynx during intubation is rather frequent, although pharyngeal perforation is relatively uncommon and usually occurs in one of its lateral sinuses or the posterior wall (3). The short distance (less than 6 cm) between the carina and the larynx in the average neonate causes ETT malposition to occur quite often in this age group. The ETT most commonly is inserted too far inferiorly. An esophageal location of the tip of an ETT is a fairly frequent malposition that usually is recognized promptly. An obturator esophageal airway has been developed for use by relatively untrained individuals (4). It is designed to be placed within the esophagus. Its proper use involves inflation of a distal cuff to prevent gastric dilatation and aspiration of gastric contents while permitting simultaneous aeration of the lungs through more proximal orifices in the tube. Malplacement of an obturator esophageal airway within the trachea obviously prevents any aeration to occur if the cuff is inflated. The esophagus can be perforated by either a standard ETT or an obturator airway. This complication is usually initially manifested radiologically by cervical and/or mediastinal emphysema.

The most frequent abnormal location of an ETT tube, said to occur in about 10% of intubated individuals, is termination of its distal tip within the right mainstem bronchus. This can lead to left-sided atelectasis and overexpansion of the right lung. The bevelled distal end of an ETT can abut against the lateral tracheal wall of an infant (1). This is especially likely to occur when the tube orifice faces in a direction opposite to that of the infant's head. Such an occurrence is exaggerated by neck flexion and a high position of the tube. It leads to relative obstruction of the airway with a consequent reduction in air flow. A radiologist obviously must determine whether the location of an ETT is appropriate and be aware of the appearance and possible consequences of frequently encountered malpositions.

Source Materials

1. Brasch RC, Held GP, Hecht ST. Endotracheal tube orifice abutting the tracheal wall: A cause of infant airway obstruction. Radiology 141:387, 1981.
2. Goodman LR, Conrardy PA, Laing F, Singer MM. Radiographic evaluation of endotracheal tube position. AJR 127:433, 1976.
3. Hirsch M, Abramowitz HB, Shapira S, Barki Y. Hypopharyngeal injury as a result of attempted endotracheal intubation. Radiology 128:37, 1978.
4. Smith JP, Bodai BI, Seifkin A, et al. The esophageal obturator airway. A review. JAMA 250:1081, 1983.

Case 40

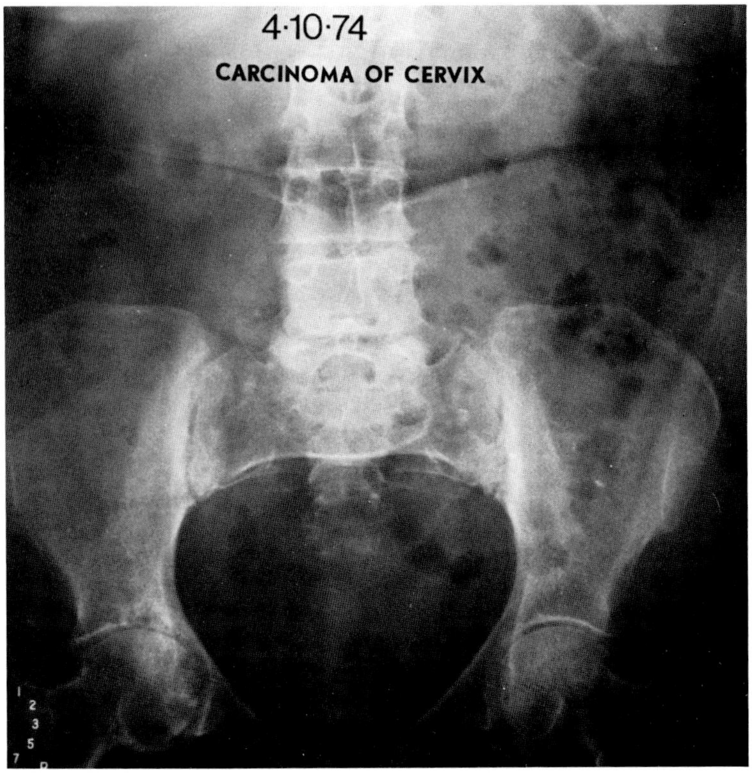

A

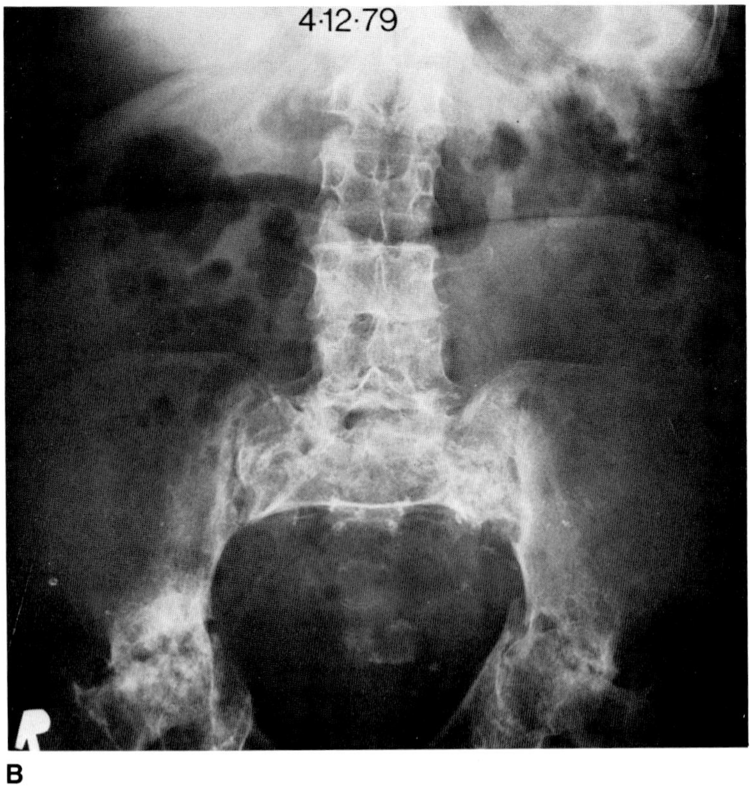

B

Radiation Osteonecrosis

Clinical Information

This 67-year-old white female received cobalt-60 irradiation and cesium implants in 1974 for treatment of a carcinoma of the cervix. A total dose of 8500 rads was delivered. Although the cancer was cured, she subsequently developed severe radiation osteonecrosis.

Roentgen Findings

An abdominal film (A) obtained in 1974 at the time of her radiation therapy shows no significant abnormality other than mild degenerative changes in her right hip joint. Extensive radiation osteonecrosis is evident by 1979 (B). There are pathologic fractures in the medial aspects of both acetabulae. The changes of aseptic necrosis are seen in the right proximal femur, which demonstrates considerable bony resorption of both the head and the femoral neck. The iliac bones and sacrum display splotchy, patchy densities, which are limited to the area of irradiation. Serial films during the 5 years between 1974 and 1979 showed inexorable progression of these abnormalities.

Comments

Radiation osteitis and radiation atrophy of bone have been used as synonyms for radiation osteonecrosis (2,3). This condition apparently results from endothelial damage to small blood vessels as well as suppression of normal osteoblastic activity. No bony damage is expected with a dose below 3000 rads, although osseous death usually occurs if the dose exceeds 5000 rads. The latent period for these changes to appear is at least 3 years. The process will stabilize by 7 years.

The major complications that can befall irradiated bone are infections, fractures, and radiation-induced sarcomas. Fractures are relatively common. They usually are asymptomatic unless the affected bone bears weight. As a matter of fact, the absence of pain is a distinguishing feature. These fractures may heal but nonunion and pseudoarthrosis are common. Bone biopsy can be a risky procedure, because it may be followed by the development of a fracture or infection (1). Infection causes pain, lysis of bone, and possibly soft tissue calcifications. Rapid bone dissolution without evidence of infection is highly suspicious of malignancy, particularly if there is an associated soft tissue mass. Pain usually attends the development of radiation-induced, metastatic, or recurrent malignancy. About half of all radiation-induced malignancies are osteosarcomas (4). Most of the remainder are fibrosarcomas and chondrosarcomas. Radiation-induced malignancy does not develop until at least 11 years have elapsed from the time of the initial therapy.

The radiologic findings of radiation osteonecrosis can vary in different portions of the body. Lysis of the lateral third of the clavicle may follow irradiation to the upper chest or shoulder girdle. Radiation osteonecrosis of the pelvis leads to a coarse, mottled trabecular pattern than has been described as "pagetoid." Aseptic necrosis of the femoral head and multiple fractures are common. There may be sizable lytic areas scattered throughout the involved area. The x-ray changes of radiation osteonecrosis are characterized by limitation to the treatment port. This is an important observation.

Source Materials

1. Edeiken B, deSantos LA. Percutaneous needle biopsy of the irradiated skeleton. Radiology 146:653, 1983.
2. Howland WJ, Loeffler RK, Starchman DE, Johnson RG. Postirradiation atrophic changes of bone and related complications. Radiology 117:677, 1975.
3. Paling MR, Herdt JR. Radiation osteitis: A problem of recognition. Radiology 137:339, 1980.
4. Smith J. Radiation-induced sarcoma of bone: Clinical and radiographic findings in 43 patients irradiated for soft tissue neoplasms. Clin Radiol 33:205, 1982.

Case 41

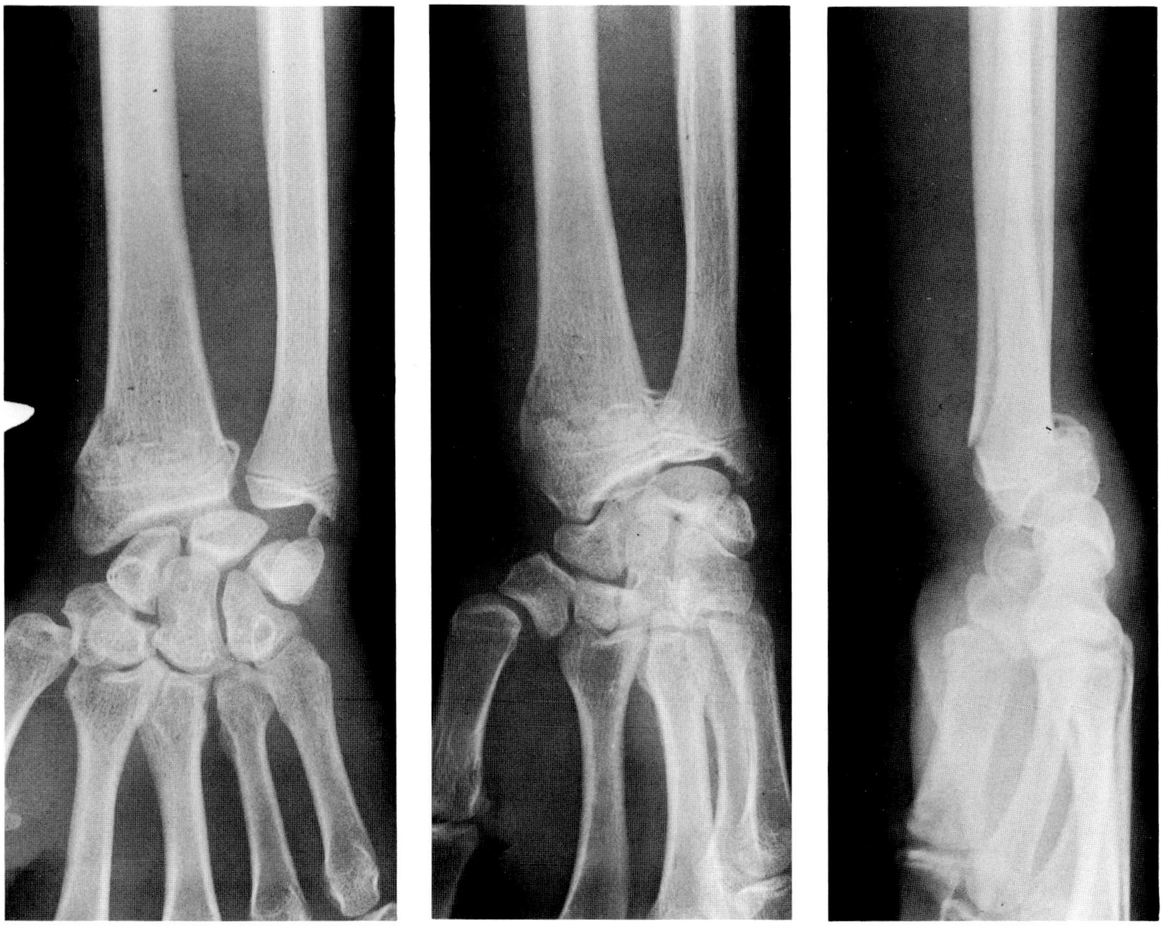

A B C

Colles' Fracture

Clinical Information

This 20-year-old white male fell and landed on his outstretched right hand. The injury resulted in pain, limitation of motion, and deformity of the right wrist.

Roentgen Findings

Films of the right wrist (A–C) show a Colles' fracture through the distal end of the radius. The fracture is impacted on its dorsal aspect. The articular surface of the radius is tilted posteriorly. There is little, if any, radial shortening. No significant radial shift is seen. The ulnar styloid has been avulsed.

Comments

A Colles' fracture characteristically leads to dorsal tilting of the distal radius. There often is shortening of the radius with radial and/or dorsal displacement of the distal fragment. An associated avulsion of the ulnar styloid is present in 60% of these injuries. The fracture line may enter either the radioulnar or the radiocarpal joint, or both. It is sharply outlined or mildly distracted on the volar radial surface with impaction and often comminution on the dorsal side. This injury occurs most frequently in older women, a finding probably related to osteoporosis.

There are several variations of distal radial fractures. Volar tilting of the fractured fragment has been called a Smith's fracture or even a reversed Colles'. Fracture of the articular radial rim with dislocation of the carpus is known as a Barton's fracture, whereas an isolated fracture of the radial styloid has been called a Hutchinson's or chauffeur's fracture. The latter injury often occurred while cranking an automobile.

Avulsion of the radial styloid as a component of a Colles' fracture is frequently associated with carpal instability (3). Treatment is designed to overcome radial displacement and to return its length to near normal. The dorsal tilt usually can be corrected. Overcoming radial displacement is more difficult. Therapeutic results depend more upon the correction than the severity of the injury or the type of immobilization (4). Fractures that enter the radiocarpal or radioulnar joints have a higher incidence of post-traumatic arthritis. Shortening of the radius can cause ulnar dislocation, which can lead to median nerve palsy. On rare occasions there is delayed rupture of the extensor pollicis longus tendon or a shoulder-hand type of reflex sympathetic dystrophy. Although nonunion is infrequent, a Colles' fracture must be followed carefully with radiographs, since settling at the fracture site or even collapse is not rare.

A Colles' fracture can be evaluated adequately with properly positioned anteroposterior and lateral films of the wrist. There may be displacement of the pronator quadratus fat pad (1). The distal ends of the dorsal and lateral aspects of the articular surface of the radius normally extend slightly beyond their volar and medial counterparts, respectively, and create an angle of 5–15° between lines perpendicular to the long axis of the radius and the radial articular surface on both the anteroposterior film (radial angle) and the lateral film (dorsal angle). The dorsal angle is often reversed. This injury not only tilts the radius dorsally but often leads to radial shortening as well as radial displacement. Dorsal and radial displacement at the fracture site vary independently of each other, but all of the other deformities relatively parallel one of these changes. Consequently, a Colles' fracture can be adequately evaluated from the dorsal angle and the radial shift (4).

Source Materials

1. MacEwan DW. Changes due to trauma in the fat plane overlying the pronator quadratus muscle. A radiologic sign. Radiology 82:879, 1964.
2. Rogers LF. Radiology of Skeletal Trauma, Vol 2. Churchill Livingstone, New York, 1982, pp 505–509.
3. Rosenthal DI, Schwartz M, Phillips WC, Jupiter J. Fracture of the radius with instability of the wrist. AJR 141:113, 1983.
4. van der Linden W, Ericson R. Colles' fracture. How should its displacement be measured and how should it be immobilized? J Bone Joint Surg 63A:1285, 1981.

Case 42

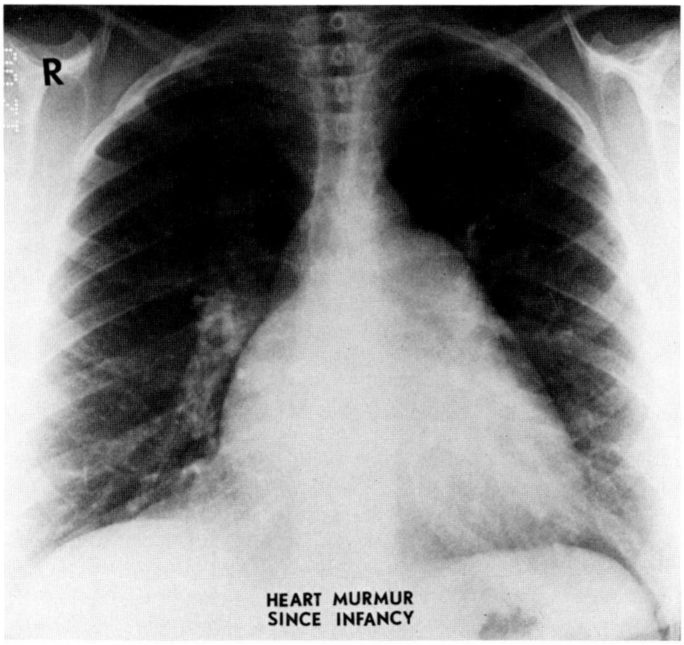

A

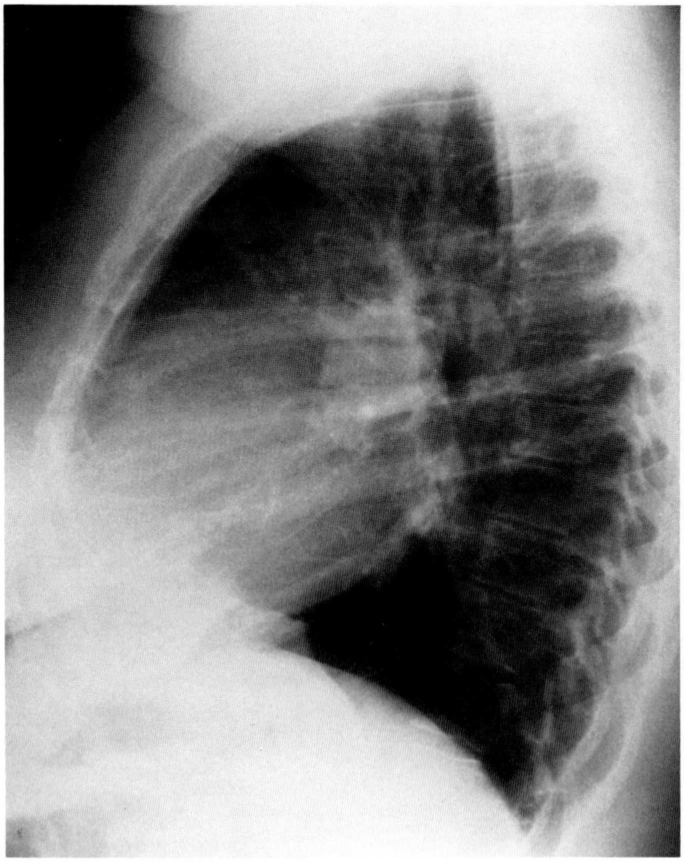

B

Atrial Septal Defect

Clinical Information

This 22-year-old acyanotic female had been known to have a heart murmur since infancy. She had experienced the onset of mild dyspnea on exertion at the age of 18. A recent cardiac catheterization established the presence of an atrial septal defect (ASD) with a 3:1 left-to-right shunt. The ASD was surgically closed and her symptoms disappeared.

Roentgen Findings

The heart is moderately enlarged and displays a globular configuration (A). There is prominence of the upper anterior portion of the cardiac contour on the lateral film (B). This appearance suggests right ventricular hypertrophy. The main pulmonary artery is strikingly enlarged, but the aortic knob is hardly visible. Large vascular shadows indicating a large left-to-right shunt extend from the hila into the lateral thirds of both lung fields. These findings are characteristic of an ASD.

Comments

A defect in the septum secundum, the most frequently encountered type of ASD, is a common congenital anomaly. Blood shunts from the left atrium into the right atrium through the defect. This abnormality is much more common in females than in males. The condition may not be diagnosed until adulthood, because most individuals with a secundum ASD have few, if any, symptoms early in life and the associated murmurs may not be striking. Some of these defects close spontaneously. Partial anomalous pulmonary venous return to the right atrium causes the same disturbance in physiology as does an ASD. An ASD is a frequent component of the Holt-Oram syndrome and the Ellis-van Creveld syndrome. Surgery is indicated for a persistent ASD that causes a significant left-to-right shunt.

Patients with an ASD do not develop increased pulmonary arteriolar resistance so early in life as do individuals with either a patent ductus arteriosus or a ventricular septal defect. It is held that the low-pressure shunt of an ASD creates much less kinetic disturbance and consequent mechanical damage than does the high-pressure shunt of a patent ductus or a ventricular septal defect. The shunts of both of these lesions are directed into or very near the pulmonary artery. Nevertheless, a patient with an ASD who survives beyond 40 years is very likely to develop an elevated pulmonary arteriolar resistance, reverse the direction of the shunt, and become cyanotic (2). The heart will usually remain enlarged with striking radiologic prominence of the main pulmonary artery.

The posteroanterior chest film is usually normal if the left-to-right shunt is small. A sizable shunt in which pulmonic blood flow is at least twice the systemic flow is commonly associated with an enlarged globular heart and shunt vascularity. The cardiac enlargement is right-sided, since the shunted blood completely bypasses the left ventricle and the aorta. Marked enlargement of the right ventricle can cause posterior displacement of the left ventricle and the left atrium (4). The pulmonary artery is very prominent, and the aortic knob appears diminutive, although angiographic studies have shown the aorta to be relatively normal in size. An ASD can be strongly suspected from radiographic findings evident on chest films. Echocardiography can provide valuable additional information (3). Cardiac catheterization and angiocardiography may be required for a definitive diagnosis.

Source Materials

1. Daves ML. Cardiac Roentgenology. Shadows of the Heart. Year Book, Chicago, 1981, pp 267–281.
2. Forfang K, Simonsen S, Andersen A, Efskind L. Atrial septal defect of secundum type in the middle-aged. Am Heart J 94:44, 1977.
3. Lieppe W, Scallion R, Behar VS, Kisslo JA. Two-dimensional echocardiographic findings in atrial septal defect. Circulation 56:447, 1977.
4. Ringertz H, Youker J, Carlsson E. Displacement of left ventricle in atrial septal defect. Acta Radiol 19:281, 1978.

Case 43

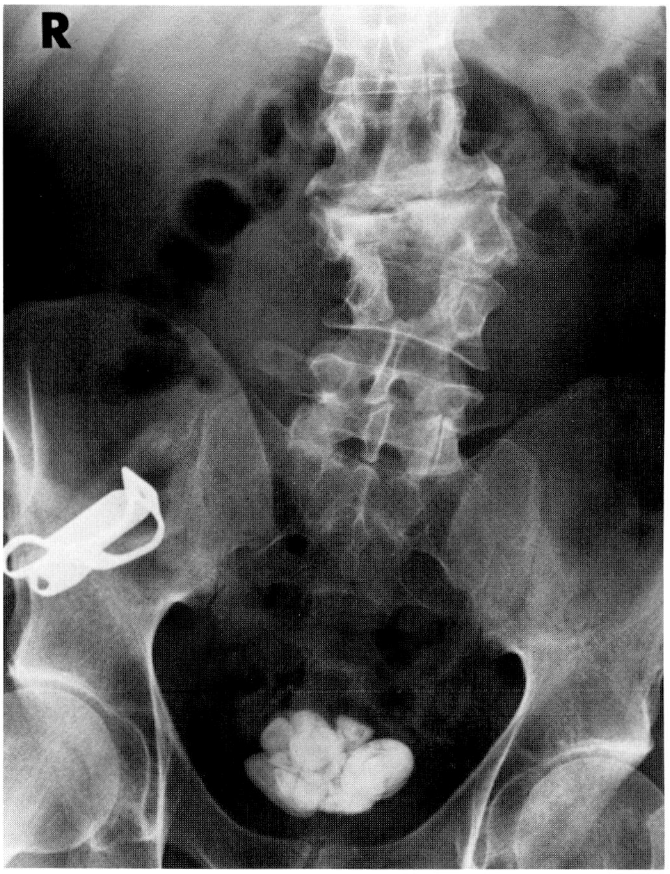

A

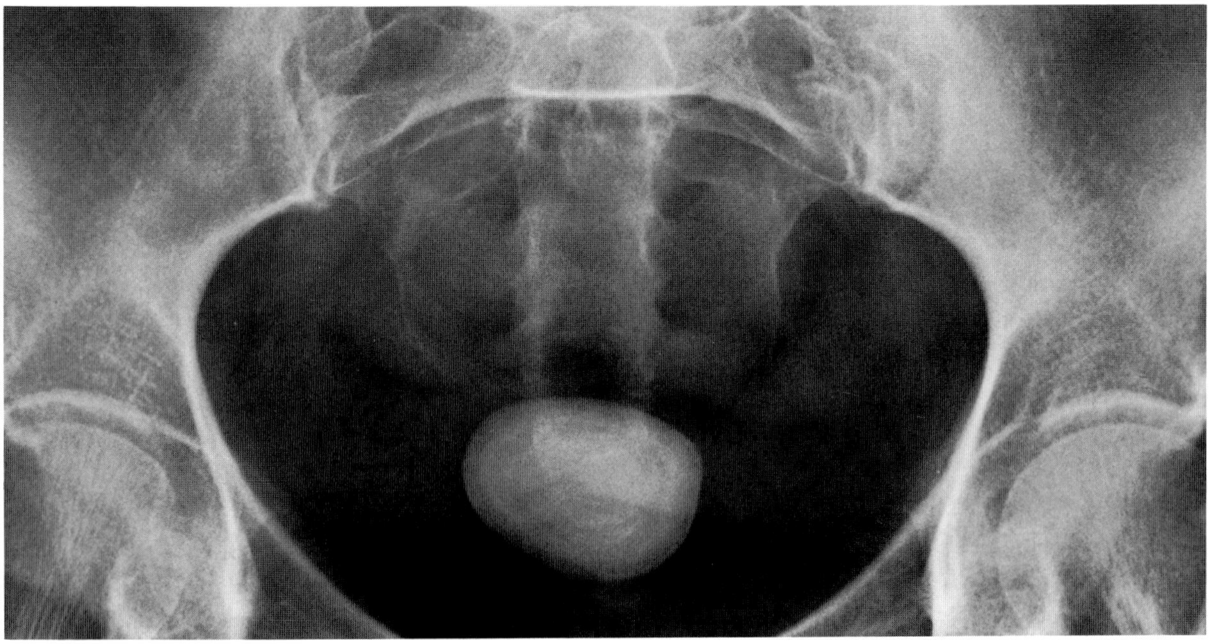

B (another patient)

Urinary Bladder Calculus

Clinical Information

This 37-year-old male had been paraplegic from the L3 level following a fall years ago. He had suffered repeated urinary tract infections.

Roentgen Findings

An abdominal film (A) shows a healed fracture of the third lumbar vertebral body. Multiple urinary bladder stones are seen within the bony pelvis.

Comments

Bladder stones are much more frequent in men than in women. Ninety-eight percent of bladder stones seen in males in the United States are associated with infection, obstruction, or both (3). The obstructive lesions include bladder neck obstruction, neurogenic bladder, vesical diverticula, and, in women, cystoceles. Foreign bodies in the bladder such as a broken-off Foley catheter or objects introduced through the urethra can form secondary calculi due to encrustations on their surface. Stones can reach the urinary bladder from the upper urinary tract. These are called migrant calculi.

Primary endemic bladder stone disease is characterized by absence of a known predisposing factor. These stones do not recur after removal. This condition was common in Europe and other Western countries during World War I but has now largely disappeared from these areas. Endemic stones are now commonly seen in Middle and Far Eastern countries. These stones are especially common in children, often before the age of 5 years. They affect rural and village children seven times more often than urban children. Diet may be an etiologic factor, since these stones are more common in socioeconomically deprived children. Primary stones can be very large (1). Bladder stones can cause pain and hematuria. These symptoms are worse when the bladder is near empty. Removal of the stones is the only effective therapy. This usually requires surgery but sometimes the calculi can be crushed or dissolved.

Bladder stones may be small, large, multiple, or single. They may have various shapes and can change their location with different positions of the patient. The latter fact can be an important differential diagnostic consideration on x-ray studies. A laminated calcific density in the midline of the body pelvis is diagnostic of a bladder calculus (see film B, from another patient). The appearance of the so-called burr or jackstone variety of urinary vesical calculus, which is composed almost entirely of calcium oxalate, is equally pathognomonic. The name of the latter results from its many projecting prongs. Stones in the urinary bladder are missed more frequently than elsewhere in the urinary tract. Lack of appropriate scrutiny is a major consideration in these errors. Another is the relative radiolucency of cystine and uric acid stones. Shadows of the bony sacrum and feces in the colon can obscure stones. Calcification in other viscera, such as prostatic calculi at the base of the bladder, can simulate vesical stones. Rectal suppositories can lead to diagnostic errors (2). Bladder stones must be differentiated from calcific encrustations upon cystitis, bladder tumors, or postirradiation changes. Stones lying partially within bladder diverticula can be dumbbelled in shape.

Source Materials

1. Brodman HR, Brodman LEB. Giant vesical calculus. (Letter to editor). JAMA 240:1338, 1978.
2. Lesher DR, Scott RL. Pitfalls to avoid: Radiopaque suppositories mimicking bladder calculi. J Assoc Can Radiol 30:54, 1979.
3. Witten DM, Myers GH Jr, Utz DC. Emmett's Clinical Urography, Vol II. W.B. Saunders, Philadelphia, 1977, pp 1338–1349.

Case 44

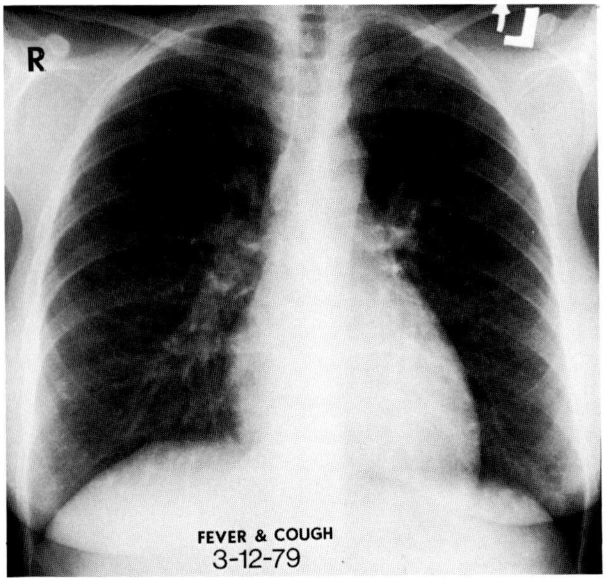

A

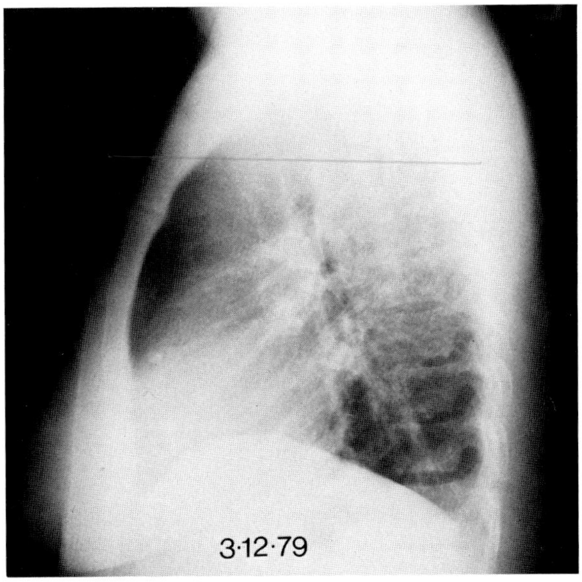

B

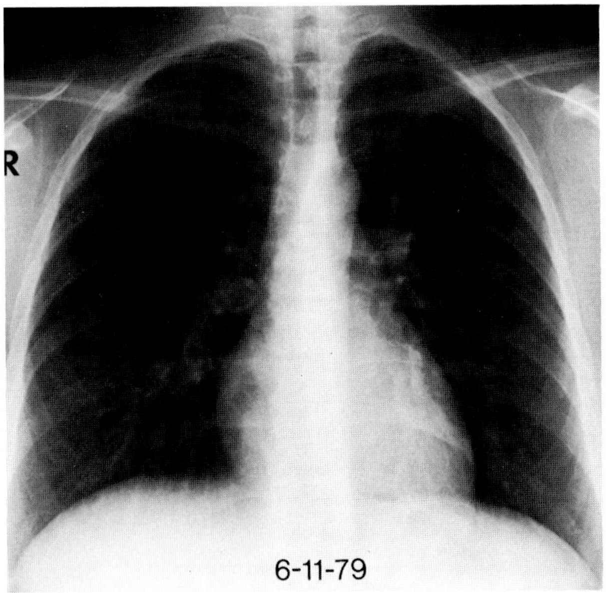

C

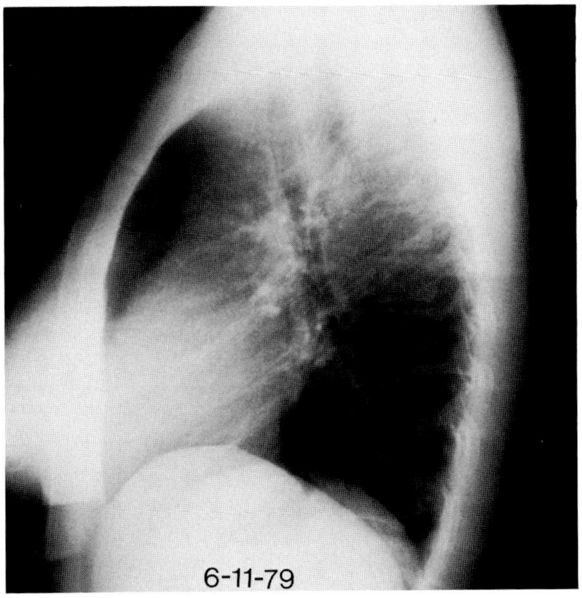

D

Silhouette Sign

Clinical Information

This 20-year-old college student had complained of fever, cough, and left-sided chest pain lasting 48 hours. The complaints disappeared after 5 days of therapy.

Roentgen Findings

The posteroanterior chest film (A) shows no indubitable abnormality, although the left diaphragmatic leaf behind the heart is not sharply defined. The lateral film (B) clearly depicts the right diaphragm. The anterior portion of the left diaphragmatic leaf is faintly visible on the original radiograph, but no remnant of the posterior left diaphragm is seen. There is questionable density in the posterior costophrenic sulcus. Radiographs obtained 3 months later (C,D) show no abnormality. Both diaphragmatic leaves are clearly evident on the lateral film.

Comments

Although the silhouette sign had been mentioned since the early 1930s, it was reported in 1950 by Felson and Felson (1) and subsequently has been associated with this name. The radiologic sign refers to the disappearence of a soft tissue margin that normally is visible. The terminology of the silhouette sign is a bit irregular in that the finding, in fact, refers to a loss of a normal silhouette. Soft tissue margins are visible on chest films because of differences in the densities of two contiguous structures. For example, the heart border is evident because its shadow is of soft tissue density and abuts more radiolucent air-containing lung tissue. If by chance the air in the medial segment of the right middle lobe, which is adjacent to the right heart border, is replaced by a pneumonic infiltrate, its density will approximate that of the heart and the margin between the two is lost. A silhouette sign can localize abnormalities on a posteroanterior chest film without recourse to a lateral radiograph. It can be applied to many structures within the chest and elsewhere (2). The sign is not invariably dependable. Felson has stated that approximately 3% of normal posteroanterior radiographs show obliteration of a portion of the heart border. Pectus excavatum frequently leads to loss of the right border of the heart, which is displaced toward the left and no longer abuts pulmonary tissue.

Although Felson maintains that contact between tissues is necessary to produce the silhouette sign, this has been refuted by Tuddenham, who demonstrated similar roentgen results produced experimentally without direct contact (4). Longuet et al. also believe contact is not necessary (3). They hold that visibility of a border depends upon the effective atomic numbers, densities, and thickness of the radiographed tissues. Although the niceties of physics may not require absolute physical contact, it is virtually impossible for biologic tissues to display perfect contour conformity without contact. Practically speaking, contact nearly always exists in the presence of a positive silhouette sign.

Source Materials

1. Felson B, Felson H. Localization of endothoracic lesions by means of the posteroanterior roentgenogram: The silhouette sign. Radiology 55:63, 1950.
2. Foote GA, Meredith HC. The silhouette sign and the inferior vena cava. Radiology 133:583, 1979.
3. Longuet R, Phelan J, Tanous H, Bushong S. Criteria of the silhouette sign. Radiology 122:581, 1977.
4. Tuddenham WJ. Problems of perception in chest roentgenology: Facts and fallacies. Radiol Clin North Am 1:277, 1963.

Case 45

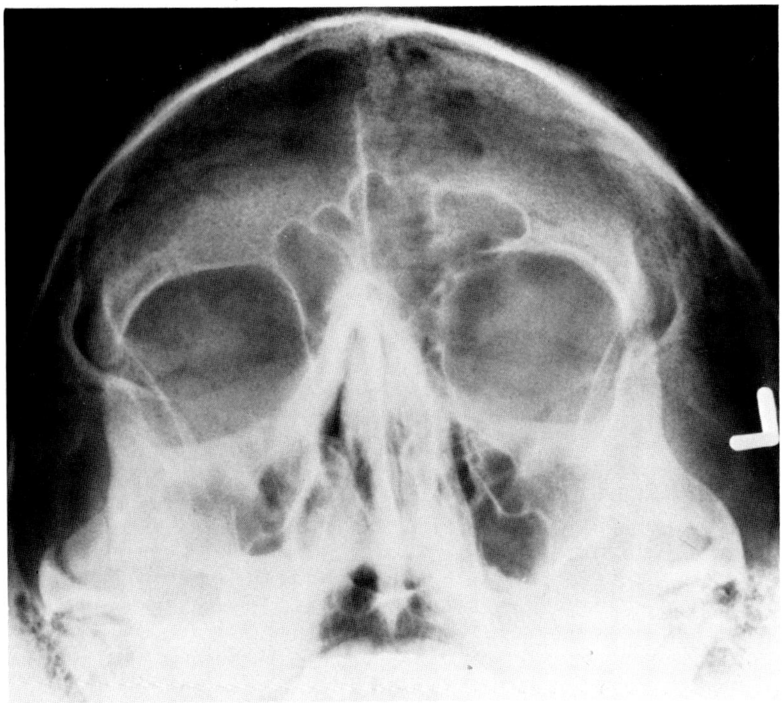

A

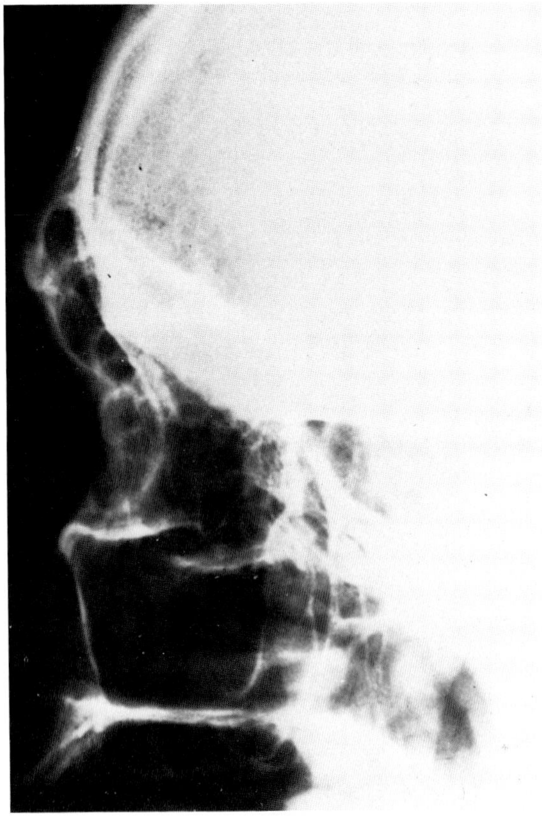

B

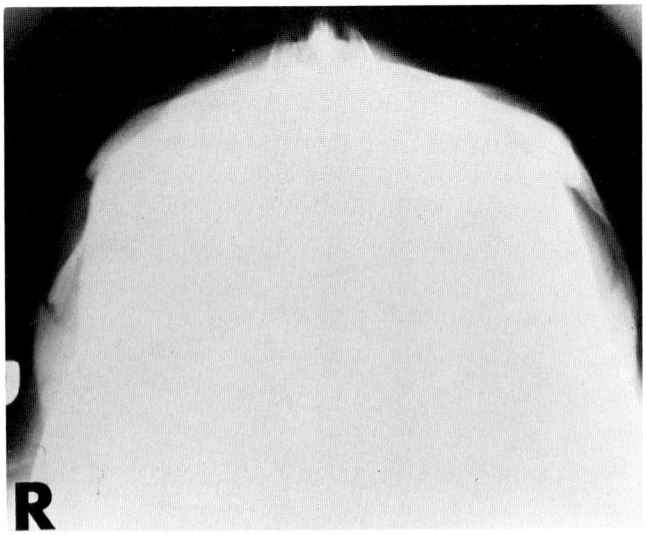

C

Tripod Fracture

Clinical Information

This 30-year-old male was struck in the right side of the face during a fist fight. At the time of hospital admission 12 hours later he had blood in the right nostril and complained of double vision and headaches, as well as difficult, painful right-sided jaw motion. The right side of his face was swollen and anesthetic and the right zygomatic arch depressed. He recovered without sequelae following open reduction and internal fixation.

Roentgen Findings

Selected facial bone films (A–C) show separation of the right zygomaticofrontal suture with mild medial displacement of the temporal process of the zygoma. The zygomatic arch is fractured in two places and depressed. Fractures involving the right orbital floor and lateral wall of the right maxillary antrum are less evident. The right antrum contains a fluid level and the body of the zygoma is mildly depressed. These changes are typical of a tripod fracture.

Comments

A tripod fracture is characterized by separation of the zygomaticofrontal and zygomaticotemporal sutures with a fracture near the zygomaticomaxillary suture. The body of the zygomatic bone is rarely fractured because its processes are less sturdy and break more easily. This injury has been also known as a trimalar fracture, malar eminence fracture, or zygomaticomaxillary complex fracture. It is the most common fracture of the midface and usually results from a direct blow to the malar bone.

Swelling, paresthesia of the affected side of the face, epistaxis, difficulty in opening and closing the mouth, and double vision are common symptoms. The affected side of the face may be flattened from depression of the zygomatic bone. Limitation of jaw movement is due to depression of the temporal process of the zygomatic arch. Anesthesia or paresthesia of the affected portions of the face results from involvement of the infraorbital nerve as it passes through the infraorbital foramen. The pupils may not be at the same level secondary to displacement of the frontal process of the malar bone. Diplopia can result from trapping of the extraocular muscles between the fracture edges. These symptoms can be corrected with proper reduction and fixation (3). Antibiotics and decongestants are indicated initially.

An appropriate radiologic examination for facial injury should include Waters, Caldwell, lateral, and basal views (1). An exaggerated Towne view is sometimes helpful to study the zygomatic arches. Separation of the zygomaticofrontal suture is best seen on the Caldwell projection. Fractures or separations near the zygomaticotemporal suture are best seen on the basal view (4). The other component of the tripod complex is a fracture located along the lower orbital border and/or the lateral maxillary wall. There usually is abnormal antral density due to bleeding. Rotation of the principal fragment of the zygomatic bone is manifested by medial or lateral displacement of the frontal process of the zygomatic bone at the zygomaticofrontal suture with depression of the lateral portion of the infraorbital rim. This may obscure the infraorbital foramen on the affected side. Posterior displacement, if present, may only be seen on a basal view. Details of the bony derangements can be shown in exquisite detail with computed tomography (2). Grooves for the anterior superior and posterior superior alveolar nerves, which run along the upper and lateral maxillary antral wall, respectively, must not be mistaken for fractures. These lines have sometimes been called maxillary pseudofracture lines.

Source Materials

1. Daffner RH, Apple JS, Gehweiler JA. Lateral view of facial fractures: New observations. AJR 141:587, 1983.
2. Gentry LR, Manor WF, Turkski PA, Strother CM. High-resolution CT analysis of facial struts in trauma: 2. Osseous and soft-tissue complications. AJR 140:533, 1983.
3. Gerlock AJ, Sinn DP. Anatomic, clinical, surgical, and radiographic correlation of the zygomatic complex fracture. AJR 128:235, 1977
4. Rogers LF. Radiology of Skeletal Trauma, Vol 1. Churchill Livingstone, New York, 1982, pp 229–242.

Case 46

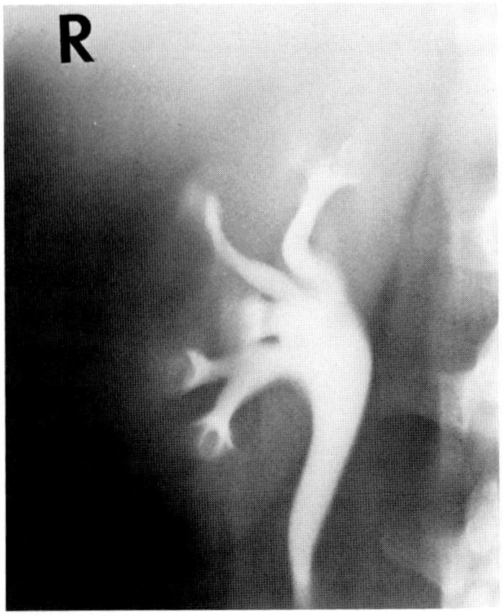

A

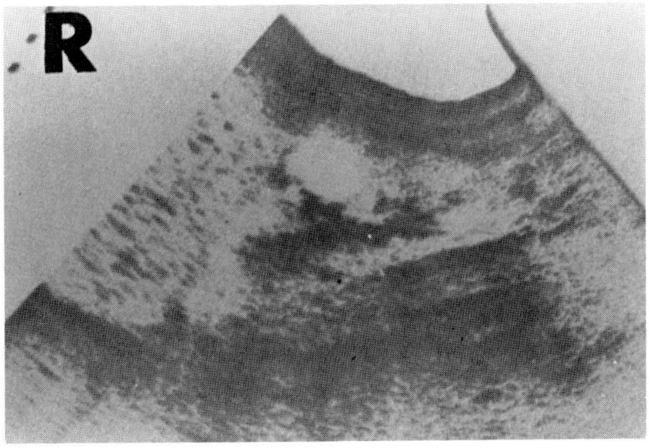

B

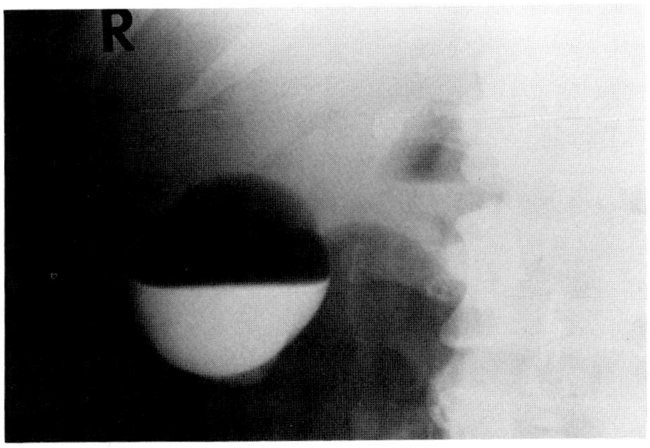

C

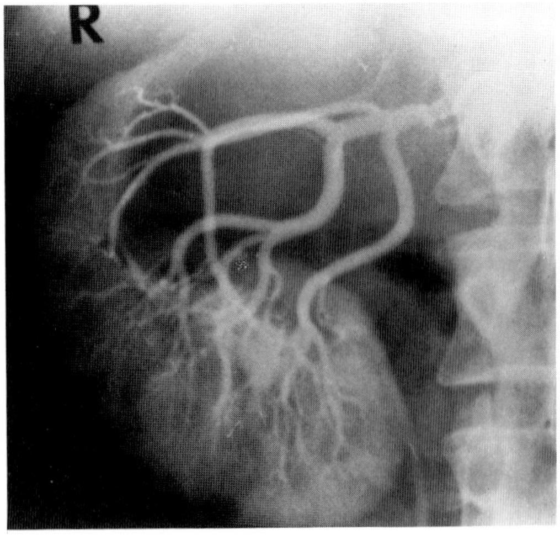

D (another patient)

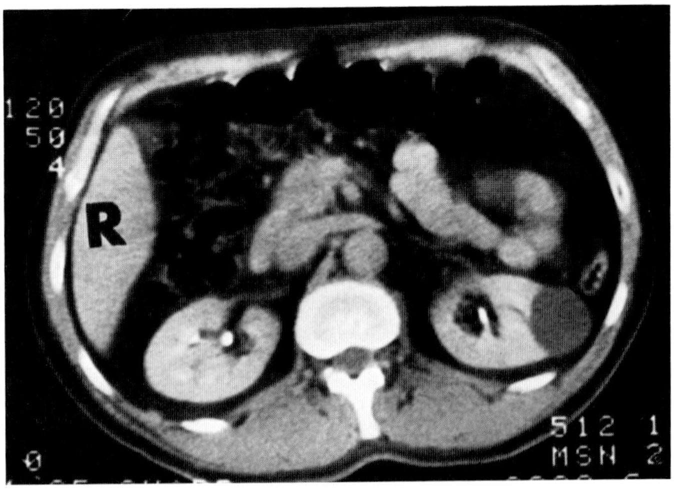

E (a third patient)

Simple Renal Cyst

Clinical Information

This 42-year-old female had no symptoms relative to her renal cyst.

Roentgen Findings

An intravenous urographic nephrotomogram (A) shows a small radiolucent lesion along the anterolateral aspect of the midportion of the right kidney. The middle calyces are displaced medially. An ultrasonic study (B) demonstrates a well circumscribed exophytic cystic mass inseparable from the right kidney. Films following cyst aspiration and opaque medium instillation (C) show a thin, smooth wall without a localized irregularity.

Comments

Simple renal cysts are rare before the age of 40 but increase in both number and size with increasing age. About 50% of individuals beyond 50 have these lesions, indicating a degenerative etiology (1). Age and chronic hemodialysis are the only factors associated with an increased incidence of renal cysts (4). The cysts may be multiple or multiocular and contain amber or straw-colored transudate. The cyst wall is formed by fibrous tissue. Its lining is composed of discontinuous flattened epithelium. Hemorrhage or infection complicates about 10% of simple renal cysts. There may be calcification in the cyst wall, although calcification within a renal mass not localized to the wall is more suggestive of malignancy. Most cysts are asymptomatic. Fifteen percent may cause a palpable mass or hematuria. Hypertension and polycythemia are rare. Specific treatment is usually not indicated. Simple renal cysts must be distinguished from parapelvic cysts that distort the central collecting system.

Intravenous urography and nephrotomography show simple renal cysts as smoothly outlined radiolucent lesions, usually peripheral in location, with sharply demarcated margins. The renal parenchyma appears to grasp the cyst. This is the well known "claw" sign. Angiography in another patient (D) shows an avascular renal cyst which had a negative epinephrine response. Unfortunately, 15% of renal cell carcinomas as well as many abscesses are also avascular. Cyst puncture can establish the diagnosis with about 97% accuracy. Cystography following aspiration reveals a uniform smooth wall in all projections. The aspirated fluid is clear, straw-colored or amber, has a negative cytology, contains little if any fat, and has a lactate dehydrogenase (LDH) level below that measured in the blood. Tumor or abscess fluid is murky or bloody. Tumor fluid often demonstrates a positive cytology. There is measurable fat and a low LDH if the lesion is malignant. The LDH level is elevated with an abscess. Findings of enhanced through transmission, absence of internal echoes, a clearly demarcated posterior wall, a spherical or ovoid shape, and a smooth outline are highly dependable sonographic signs of a renal cyst if all are present (2). Computed tomographic criteria of a homogeneous lesion of water density, a smooth interface with the adjoining renal parenchyma, and absence of contrast enhancement or measurable wall thickness as seen on the left (E) in still another patient approach an accuracy of 100%, but this procedure is hardly indicated when other modalities can be employed (3). An x-ray diagnosis is highly dependable if the radiologic findings are characteristic. Unfortunately, up to 20% of simple cysts lead to findings that in some ways mimic a renal malignancy. These patients require extensive diagnostic procedures, possibly including surgery.

Source Materials

1. Laucks SP, McLachlan MSF. Aging and simple cysts of the kidney. Br J Radiol 54:12, 1981.
2. Pollack HM, Banner MP, Arger PH, et al. The accuracy of gray-scale renal ultrasonography in differentiating cystic neoplasms from benign cysts. Radiology 143:741, 1982.
3. McClennan BL, Stanley RJ, Nelson GL, et al. CT of the renal cyst: Is cyst aspiration necessary? AJR 133:671, 1979.
4. Scanlon MH, Karasick SR. Acquired renal cystic disease and neoplasia: Complications of chronic hemodialysis. Radiology 147:837, 1983.

Case 47

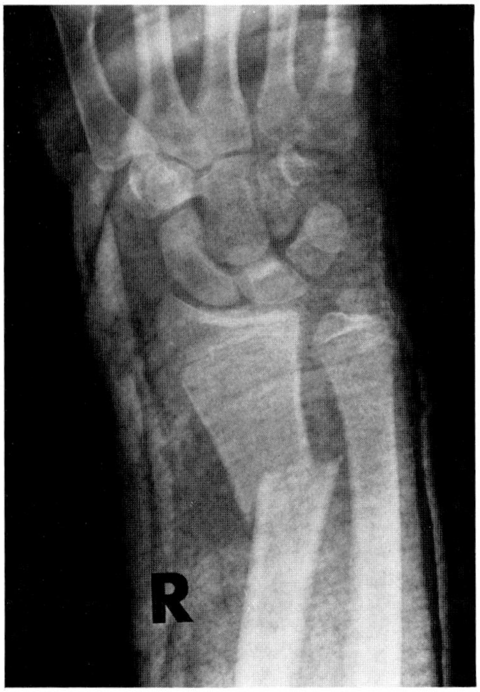

A

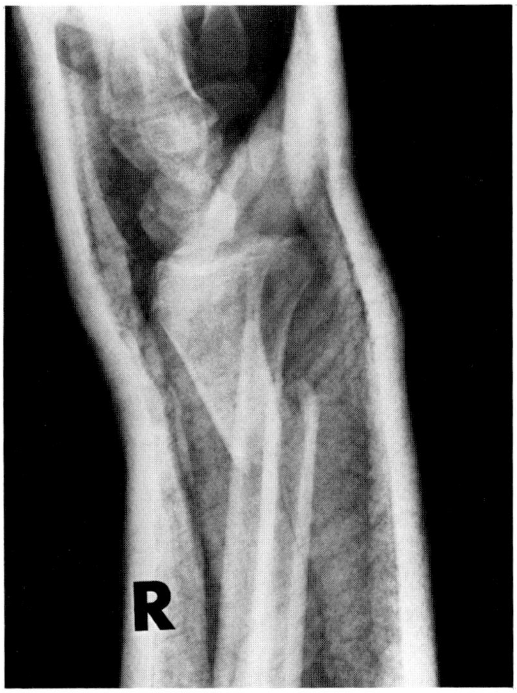

B

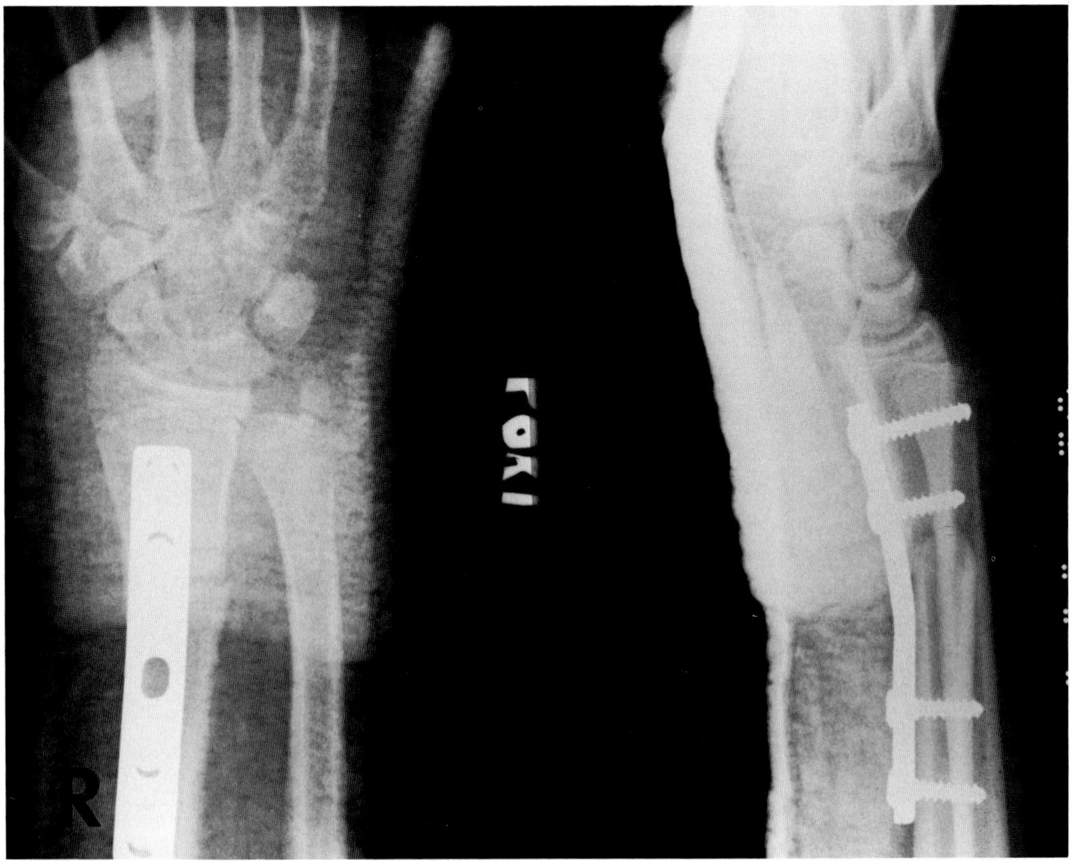

C

Galeazzi's Fracture-Dislocation

Clinical Information

This 12-year-old boy was transferred from another hospital after having injured his right wrist and forearm. A plaster cast had been applied. Treatment involved open reduction and internal fixation (see film C).

Roentgen Findings

Films of the right wrist (A,B), still in a plaster cast, show a fracture of the distal radius with sharp volar angulation. There is dislocation of the radioulnar joint with the ulnar head displaced in a volar direction. The ulnar styloid is also fractured. Films after open reduction and internal fixation show the radial fracture in good alignment and the ulnar dislocation to have been reduced (C).

Comments

A Galeazzi's fracture-dislocation is an uncommon injury seen with approximately the same frequency as a Monteggia's fracture (see Case 19). The two have similarities in their pathogenesis since the radial and ulnar shafts are held together by a tight interosseous membrane (2). Therefore, a fracture with angulation of either bone will force the other to either fracture, bend, or dislocate. A Monteggia's fracture is characterized by a proximally angulated ulnar fracture with dislocation of the radial head and elbow. The Galeazzi corollary is a fracture of the distal radius with angulation and dislocation or subluxation of the ulnar head at the radioulnar joint. These similarities are further emphasized by the fact that a Galeazzi's fracture-dislocation sometimes has been called a reverse Monteggia's fracture, as well as a Piedmont fracture or a Darrach-Hughston-Milch fracture. It is apparent that an adequate evaluation of an angulated fracture of either forearm bone must include films of the elbow and wrist. A Galeazzi's fracture-dislocation usually results from falling on an outstretched, extremely pronated hand. This injury leads to pain, swelling, and wrist deformity with restricted pronation and supination. Open reduction and internal fixation are the usual treatment. The ulnar reduction is frequently unstable even after apparently appropriate management.

Normal relationships at the distal end of the forearm on a posteroanterior projection show the head of the ulna to be situated 1–2 cm proximal to the distal radial surface, from which it is separated by 1–2 mm. A radiologic examination is difficult to interpret if the wrist is not placed in a true lateral position (4). The radius normally overlaps the ulna, and the posterior surface of the head of the ulna on a properly positioned lateral film parallels the posterior plane of the triquetrum. A determination that a true lateral position has been achieved can be ascertained by comparing a similar view of the other forearm.

The radial fracture usually occurs near the junction of its middle and distal thirds. The ulna can be subluxed or completely dislocated either anteriorly or posteriorly. This abnormality at the distal radioulnar joint is often missed. Subluxation or dislocation always occurs in the same direction as the apex of the radial fracture's angulation. The triangular cartilage at the distal end of the ulna is always disrupted when a patient suffers a Galeazzi's fracture-dislocation. This ligament is the primary stabilizing factor of the distal radioulnar joint (3). Injection of contrast medium into the radiocarpal joint will show it to extend abnormally into the radioulnar joint (1). The triangular cartilage is also ruptured when the ulnar styloid is avulsed.

Source Materials

1. Demos TC. Bone Radiology Case Studies. Slack, Inc., Thorofare, NJ, 1982, pp 293–296.
2. Mikić Z. Galeazzi fracture-dislocations. J Bone Joint Surg 57A:1071, 1975.
3. Ogden JA, Beall JK, Conlogue GJ, Light TR. Radiology of postnatal skeletal development. IV. Distal radius and ulna. Skeletal Radiol 6:255, 1981.
4. Rogers LF. Radiology of Skeletal Trauma, Vol 2. Churchill Livingstone, New York, 1982, pp 493–497, 513–517.

Case 48

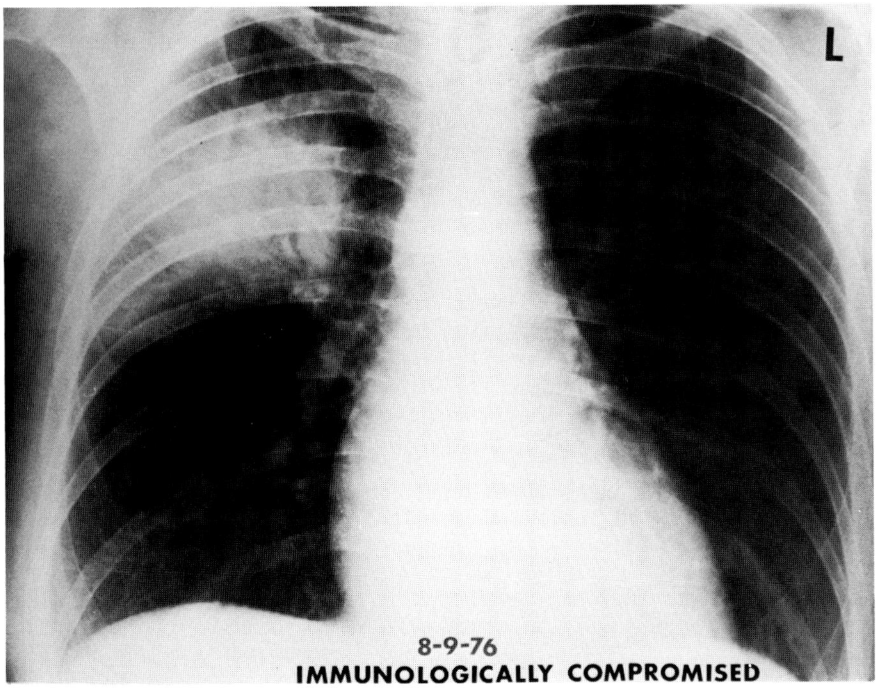

A

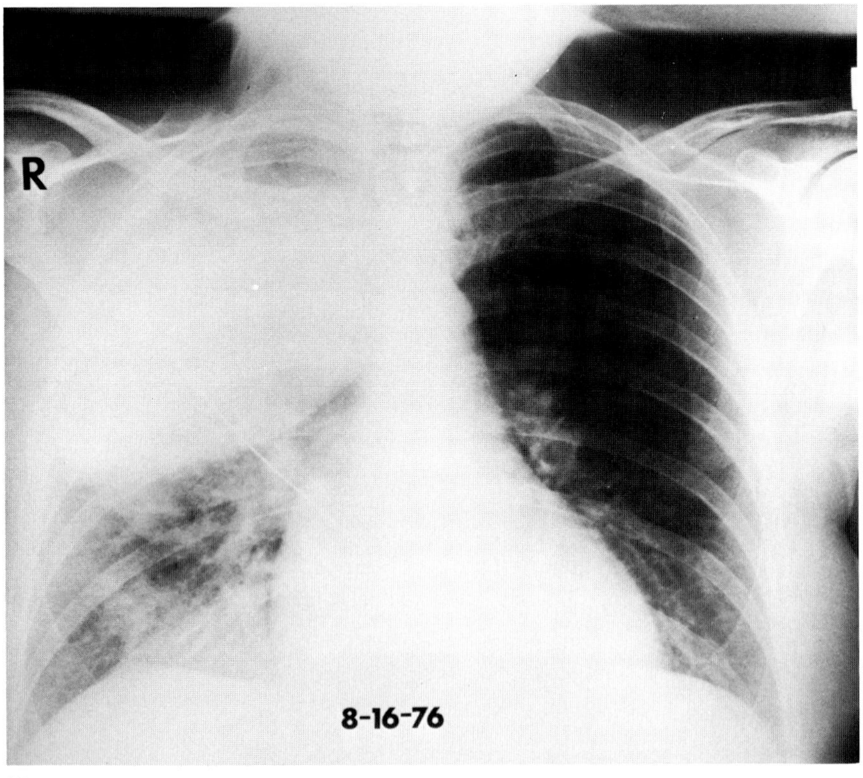

B

Friedlander's (Klebsiella) Pneumonia

Clinical Information

This 53-year-old female had received long-term steroid therapy for systemic lupus erythematosis. She was hospitalized for treatment of a fever, cough, and right-sided chest pain. There was massive growth of *Klebsiella pneumoniae* from her sputum. Antibiotic and supportive therapy led to a slow resolution of the pneumonia with some residual loss of volume and mild fibrosis in the right upper lobe.

Roentgen Findings

A posteroanterior chest film (A) shows an area of pneumonic density in the right upper lobe. Air bronchograms are evident within the density. Film B shows opacity of almost all of the right upper lobe with bulging of the minor fissure between the right upper and right middle lobes. Some pneumonic infiltrate is also present in the right cardiophrenic angle.

Comments

Klebsiella pneumoniae is a nonmotile, Gram-negative, encapsulated rod. The pneumonia caused by this organism was originally described by Friedlander, accounting for the name often used to designate this condition. The clinical substrate upon which an acute klebsiella pneumonia develops, along with typical radiologic findings, often permits an etiologic diagnosis. This acute infection most frequently occurs in an elderly, diabetic, alcoholic, or immunologically compromised patient (1). It is seen more commonly in black than in white individuals. Klebsiella pneumonia is rare in infants and children. It is a relatively common nosocomial infection that can be spread by contaminated hospital equipment. The acute process produces symptoms that are very similar to those of pneumococcal pneumonia. The patient usually complains of chills, fever, pleural pain, and a productive cough. Bacteremia is common. About a third of these individuals produce a very distinctive currant jelly, gelatinous sputum. The process may develop rapidly. In fact, death can ensue within 48 hours. The mortality of klebsiella pneumonia approximates 50%, although some newer antibiotics have improved the prognosis. Complicating pleural effusion and empyema are frequently encountered. The acute inflammatory process may be necrotizing and lead to cavitation. In fact, massive gangrene of an entire lobe can occur. Healing is nearly always associated with some volume loss and scar formation.

The chronic form of klebsiella pneumonia is usually engrafted upon chronic bronchopulmonary disease, often tuberculosis or obstructive airway disease. The symptoms of a chronic infection are much milder than those of acute klebsiella pneumonia. Positive sputum cultures can be expected to persist in the chronic form of the disease.

The radiologic findings in klebsiella pneumonia may be much like those of acute pneumococcal pneumonia. The consolidation is usually located in one of the upper lobes, particularly the right. No satisfactory explanation has been offered for this preferential location, which is especially noteworthy since most other Gram-negative pneumonias tend to involve the lower lobes (4). The inflammatory process can create enough inflammatory exudate to increase the volume of the affected lobe. This results in bulging of the related interlobar fissures. Although a bulging fissure is a long-revered hallmark of klebsiella pneumonia, this finding is often absent and can be caused by other disease processes. Nevertheless, a bulging fissure, particularly if small abscesses indicative of a necrotizing pneumonia are also seen, is highly suggestive of klebsiella pneumonia (2). The diagnosis is particularly likely if there is an associated pleural effusion or empyema.

Source Materials

1. Blank N, Castellino RA, Shah V. Radiographic aspects of pulmonary infection in patients with altered immunity. Radiol Clin North Am 11:175, 1973.
2. Felson B, Rosenberg LS, Hamburger M Jr. Roentgen findings in acute Friedlander's pneumonia. Radiology 53:559, 1949.
3. Genereux GP, Stilwell GA. The acute bacterial pneumonias. Semin Roentgenol 15:9, 1980.
4. Unger JD, Rose HD, Unger GF. Gram-negative pneumonia. Radiology 107:283, 1973.

Case 49

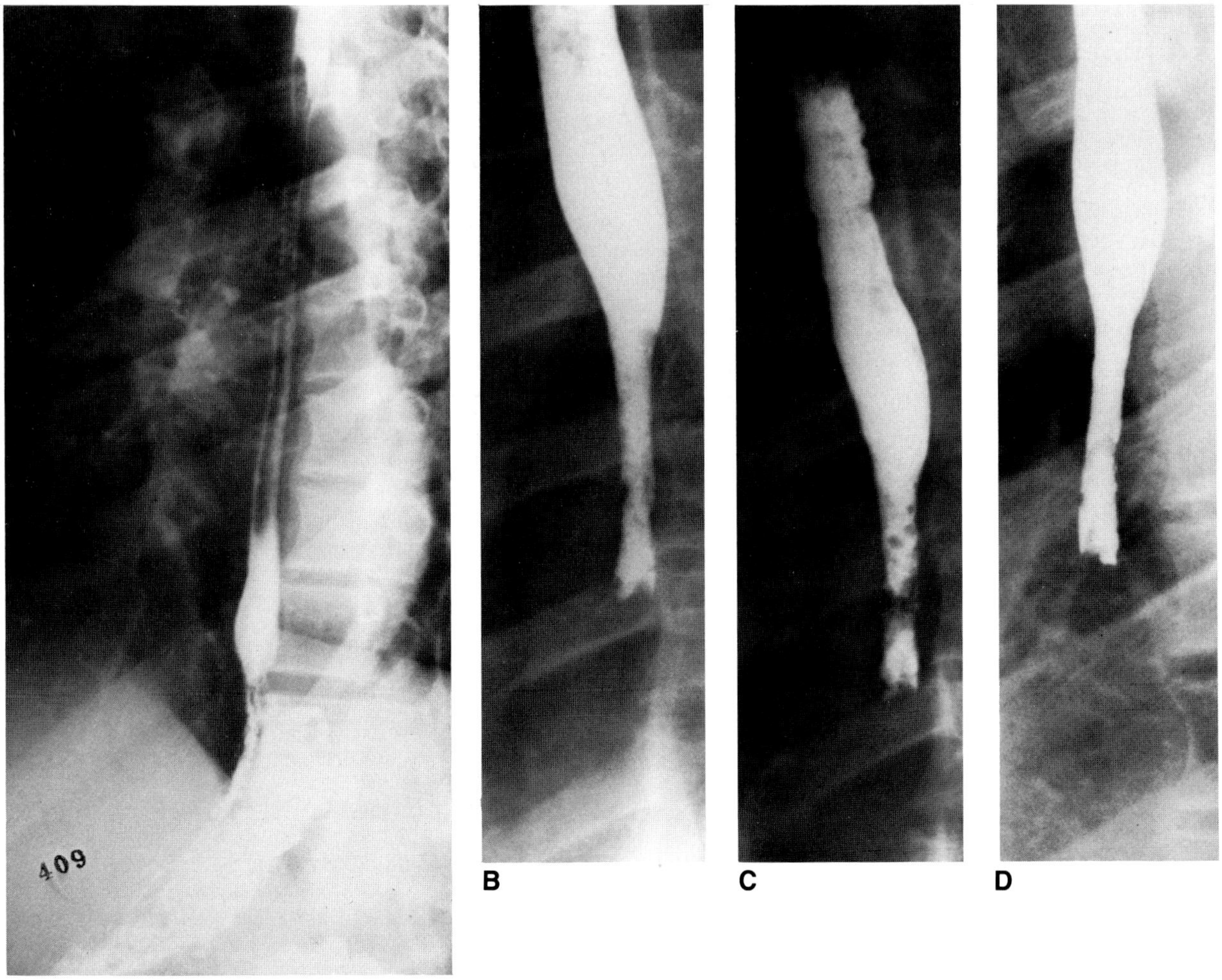

A B C D

Esophageal Lye Stricture

Clinical Information

This 21-year-old male had undergone repeated esophageal dilatations for dysphagia since ingesting a lye solution at 2 years of age.

Roentgen Findings

Barium swallows (A–D) show the opaque material to pass readily into the stomach. A small hiatus hernia is evident. There is a long segment in the middle and distal portions of the esophagus that is rather severely but smoothly constricted.

Comments

Ingestion of caustic lye occurs as an accidental event in a child or as a suicidal attempt in an adult, who often is deranged. Cleaning solutions in common use, such as Liquid-Plumr, contain a high concentration of sodium hydroxide. Some resemble milk; others are clear. It has been estimated that 5000 children accidentally ingest caustic lye each year in the United States (1). The degree of damage depends upon the amount and concentration of the lye solution ingested and the duration of its tissue contact. The mouth, pharynx, esophagus, and stomach may be affected, but the predominant effects usually are evident in the esophagus. The points of damage do not correlate to areas of normal esophageal narrowing. Immediate treatment with weak acids is not very effective, although rinsing and dilution are recommended. Antibiotics are indicated, and the early administration of steroids is said to diminish the severity of eventual strictures. Dilatations with bougienage may be effective in patients with esophageal narrowing from scar formation, but esophageal rupture can occur, particularly in children (3). Some patients require esophageal replacement.

Three stages of caustic esophageal damage are recognized. The first is acute necrosis during the first 4 days. Ulceration and granulation follow between the third and the fifth day. This is the period when the esophagus is most likely to rupture. Stricture formation, which occurs in up to 30% of these individuals, begins in the third or fourth week.

Plain films soon after lye ingestion may be negative. They can show pneumomediastinum or evidence of mediastinal widening or inflammation. An adequate contrast study of the esophagus may be impossible, or even contraindicated, at this time. Blurring of the esophageal margins is an early x-ray finding. There may be streaks and collections of contrast material held up for long periods within the ulcerated esophagus and its surrounding soft tissues. Persistent dilatation results from esophageal atony and may herald impending perforation. Radiologic examinations after stricture formation reveal the narrowed area, which varies in length from about 1 cm up to the entire length of the esophagus. The involved segment is usually long, may be multiple, and is often located in the middle of the esophagus. No definite mucosal folds are seen at the most narrowed points, which no longer exhibit peristaltic activity. Narrowed areas are usually concentric and smoothly tapering, although they may have overhanging edges. A diverticulum is occasionally seen in the area of narrowing. A rather large percentage of affected children subsequently develop a hiatus hernia as the stricture forms and the esophagus shortens (2). Lack of a hiatus hernia in association with any esophageal stricture suggests the narrowing may be due to malignancy (4). Nodularity in the strictured area raises the possibility of carcinoma. Malignancy has been seen with some frequency following ingestion of lye, especially by children. It takes up to 40 years after the initial insult to develop a carcinoma, which has a very poor prognosis. Radiologic changes similar to those caused by caustics can follow the ingestion of corrosive acids.

Source Materials

1. Benirschke K. Time bomb of lye ingestion? Am J Dis Child 135:17, 1981.
2. Franken EA Jr. Caustic damage of the gastrointestinal tract: Roentgen features. AJR 118:77, 1973.
3. Glick ME. Clinical course of esophageal stricture managed by bougienage. Dig Dis Sci 27:884, 1982.
4. Ho C-S, Rodrigues PRD. Lower esophageal strictures, benign or malignant? J Can Assoc Radiol 31:110, 1980.

Case 50

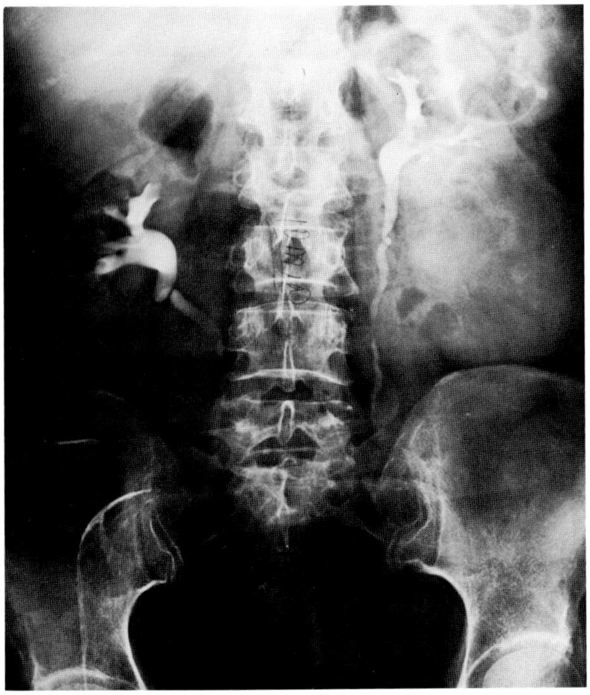

A

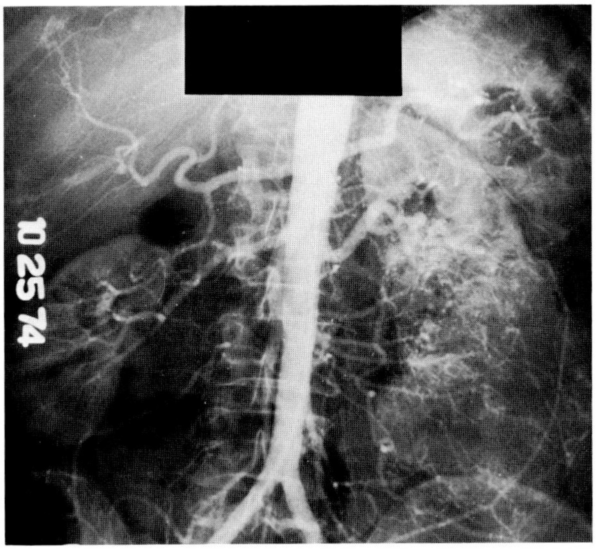

B

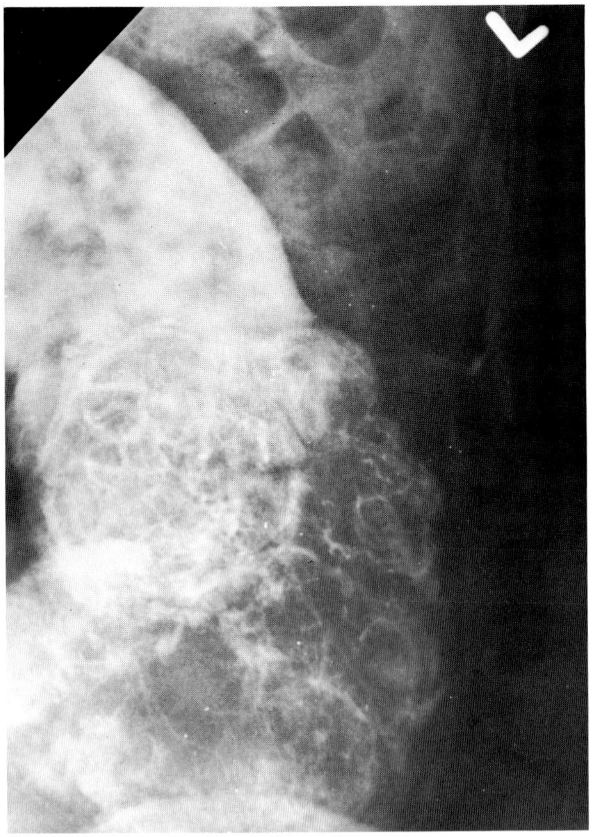

C

Renal Cell Carcinoma

Clinical Information

This 68-year-old white female had lost 20 pounds over the preceding year. The surgically removed left kidney contained a very large, partially necrotic, hemorrhagic renal cell carcinoma (clear cell type) in its lower pole.

Roentgen Findings

The 10-minute film of an intravenous urogram (A) shows a 10 $\times$ 12 cm mass at the lower pole of the left kidney. It compresses and distorts the lower calyces. An aortogram reveals a hypervascular mass with areas of necrosis, vascular pooling (B), and tumor vessels (C), which did not respond to epinephrine.

Comments

A renal cell carcinoma is the most frequently encountered malignant kidney tumor. Affected patients are usually beyond the age of 50 years. There is a 3:1 male predominance. A triad of flank pain, hematuria, and an abdominal mass is seen in 15% of these patients. The initial symptom often relates to a metastasis. Tumor growth can be slow or rapid. The lungs are the most common and earliest site of metastases, although the tumor can spread via the bloodstream to any organ. Bone metastases are usually lytic. Renal cell carcinomas may be clear cell or granular cell in type and often become necrotic. They may cause several systemic responses, including a leukemoid reaction, polycythemia, eczema, hypertension, hypercalcinuria, peripheral neuropathy, myopathy, plasmocytosis, amyloidosis, and an otherwise unaccountable fever. Survival varies between 10–60% and depends upon the stage of the tumor at the time of diagnosis. Radical nephrectomy is the only treatment that offers a significant hope of cure.

Most renal cell carcinomas are initially discovered as an abnormal mass during intravenous urography. Plain radiographs may show an increase in renal size and a distorted kidney outline. About 10% will reveal calcification, which usually is central and stippled, amorphous, or mottled but can be peripheral and somewhat curvilinear (2). An intravenous urogram usually demonstrates an indistinctly outlined mass that distorts or amputates adjacent calyces. The collecting system can be compressed or invaded. Severely affected kidneys may not function. A dependable diagnosis often requires additional studies. In most institutions the next procedure is a sonogram to determine whether the mass is cystic or solid. Indisputable sonographic evidence of a benign renal cyst may obviate the need for additional studies, although further differentiation is possible with cyst aspiration and possibly radiographs after instillation of an opaque medium. Ultrasonic studies reveal a renal cell carcinoma as a mass with irregular contours. There may be various types of internal echoes, poor sound transmission, and no clearly defined distal wall (1). Detailed information can be obtained in solid masses with computed tomography (CT) and/or angiography (3). Most of these tumors display increased vascularity at angiography, although 15% are hypovascular or avascular. Normal renal vessels can be curved, stretched, encased, or amputated. There may be multiple small, tortuous tumor vessels that do not respond to epinephrine; pooling of the contrast material; and arteriovenous shunting with rapid filling of the renal veins. Collateral circulation to surrounding structures via capsular vessels may be evident. Sometimes tumor can be seen within the renal vein. CT reveals a renal cell carcinoma as a mass with irregular margins and a density greater than that of a renal cyst. There may be obliteration of the perinephric fat. Large metastatic or hyperplastic lymph nodes are sometimes seen. CT occasionally can identify tumor within the renal vein or the inferior vena cava. CT is especially helpful in staging. These procedures when used in concert can provide an accurate diagnosis in virtually all patients with a renal mass.

Source Materials

1. Coleman BG, Arger PH, Mulhern CB Jr, et al. Gray-scale sonographic spectrum of hypernephromas. Radiology 137:757, 1980.
2. Daniel WD Jr, Hartman GW, Witten DM, et al. Calcified renal masses. A review of ten years experience at the Mayo Clinic. Radiology 103:503, 1972.
3. Weyman PJ, McClennan BL, Stanley RJ, et al. Comparison of computed tomography and angiography in the evaluation of renal cell carcinoma. Radiology 137:417, 1980.

Case 51

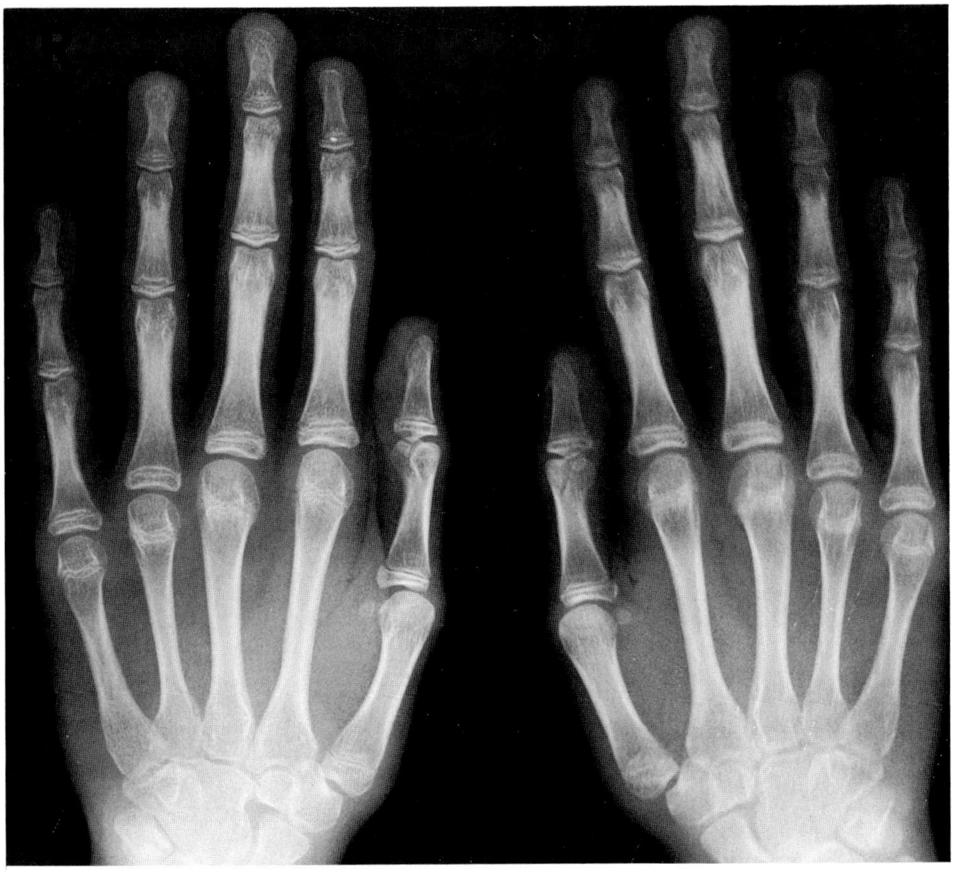

Arachnodactyly

Clinical Information

This 14-year-old white male was admitted for syncopal episodes. He had pectus excavatum and normal intelligence. It was felt he had an incomplete form of Marfan's syndrome.

Roentgen Findings

All of the fingers are long, relatively thin, and gracile. The soft tissues surrounding the bones are sparse. The metacarpal index is 9.4.

Comments

Arachnodactyly (spider fingers) is characterized by elongated metacarpals and phalanges. These bones have a thin cortex and a delicate trabecular pattern. The increase in bone length is not accompanied by a commensurate increase in width. Consequently, the bones are slender. The metacarpal index, which is the ratio of the sum of the lengths of metacarpals 2–5 to the sum of the widths of their midshaft diameters, normally ranges between 5.4 to 7.9 (3). In arachnodactyly this number varies from 8.4 to 10.4. The toes and metatarsals are also long.

The term arachnodactyly is sometimes used synonymously with Marfan's syndrome. This is not appropriate, since arachnodactyly can occur with other conditions and even in the absence of any additional underlying abnormality. Patients with arachnodactyly are often "double-jointed." The thin, long, tapered fingers are hypermobile. It is possible for these patients to fold a thumb across the palm, grasp it with the fingers, and have the end of the thumb protrude from the ulnar side of the hand (4).

Marfan's syndrome is a hereditary connective tissue disorder characterized by arachnodactyly, a high arched palate, dislocated lens, pectus excavatum, scoliosis, and varied cardiovascular disorders such as aneurysmal dilatation of the aorta, a dissecting aneurysm, or mitral valve prolapse. Arachnodactyly is also seen with homocystinuria, which is another hereditary (autosomal recessive) disease, which features dislocation of the lens, mental retardation, a tendency toward vascular thrombosis, and osteoporosis (see Case 2). In this condition a deficiency of cystathionine synthetase causes a metabolic block that leads to the accumulation of homocystine in the blood, which subsequently is excreted in the urine. Disturbed ratio of growth of the carpal bones causes enlargement of the capitate and hamate bones with hypoplasia of the lunate.

In another disease, congenital contractural arachnodactyly, the lengthened digits are associated with scoliosis, contractures, and characteristic abnormalities in the earlobes (2). These patients do not have ocular or cardiovascular defects. The entity is an autosomal dominant trait and has been confused with Marfan's syndrome. In addition, arachnodactyly is occasionally seen with multiple endocrine adenomatosis (MEA) type IIB (1). This is the same condition as multiple endocrine neoplasia (MEN). It must be distinguished from Sipple's syndrome, which is MEA type IIA. Features of MEA type IIB include arachnodactyly with marfanoid body habitus, multiple mucosal neuromas, medullary thyroid carcinoma, and pheochromocytomas. It obviously is necessary to be aware of the different clinical syndromes that can be associated with arachnodactyly so appropriate investigations can be initiated in patients who present this finding. As mentioned above, some patients may have arachnodactyly in the absence of any significant additional abnormality.

Source Materials

1. Block MB, Roberts JP, Kadair RG, et al. Multiple endocrine adenomatosis type IIB. Diagnosis and treatment. JAMA 234:710, 1975.
2. Nai-Kiong H, Teng-Kew K. Congenital contractural arachnodactyly. Am J Dis Child 133:639, 1979.
3. Parish JG. Radiographic measurements of the skeletal structure of the normal hand. Br J Radiol 39:52, 1966.
4. Steinberg I. A simple screening test for the Marfan syndrome. AJR 97:118, 1966.

Case 52

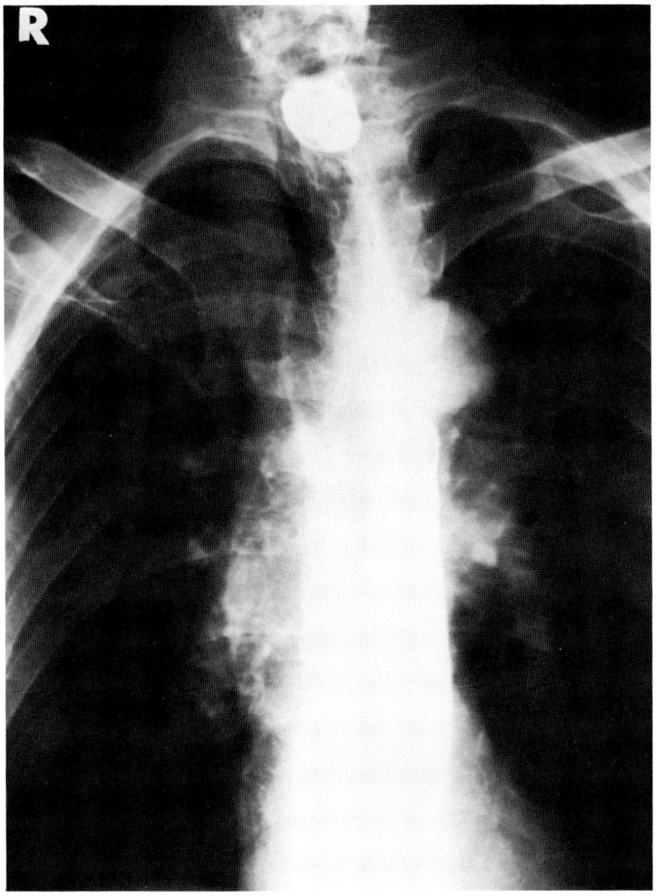

A

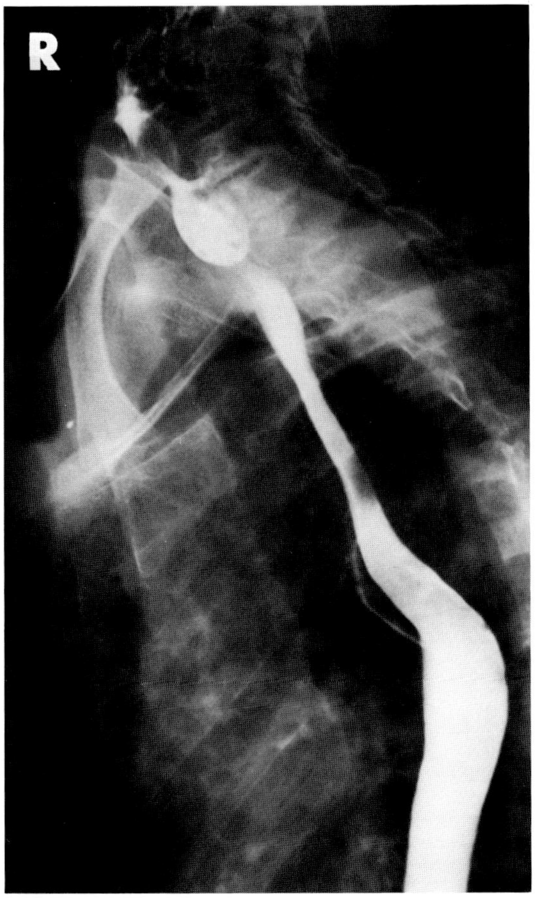

B

Zenker's Diverticulum

Clinical Information

This 55-year-old white female had suffered for 1 month with increasing dysphagia, which had progressed to the point that she was vomiting most of her food. Surgical excision of a Zenker's diverticulum cured her symptoms.

Roentgen Findings

Barium swallows reveal a smooth diverticulum extending almost directly posteriorly from the pharyngoesophageal junction at the level of C7 (A,B). The diverticulum contains retained food and measures about 3 cm in greatest diameter. It inclines inferiorly and compresses and displaces the esophagus. It was noted fluoroscopically to fill immediately with the first swallow of barium, which subsequently overflows into the esophageal lumen.

Comments

A Zenker's diverticulum has variously been described as a posterior hypopharyngeal pouch, a pharyngoesophageal diverticulum, or a proximal esophageal diverticulum. All of these diverticula are pulsion in type, arise directly in the midline, and extend posteriorly, usually toward the left. They invariably arise immediately below the inferior pharyngeal constrictors near the transverse fibers of the cricopharyngeus through a triangular weak space located at the junction of the pharynx and the esophagus. Incoordination of the peristaltic muscular activity that propels a bolus of food into the proximal esophagus with relaxation of the cricopharyngeus muscle is thought to underlie the development of a Zenker's diverticulum (2–4), although some do not feel this is the basic abnormality (1). It is commonly held that the cricopharyngeus muscle, being a true sphincter, is normally contracted and guards the proximal opening of the esophagus (2). If swallowing is properly coordinated, the cricopharyngeus relaxes as the bolus of food arrives. If this does not occur quite soon enough or if the muscle contracts too soon, excessive pressure is exerted against the weak space just proximal to the cricopharyngeus. Eventually the mucosa and submucosa will dissect between the muscle fibers and form a pulsion diverticulum. The diverticulum then extends downward between the spine and the esophagus.

A Zenker's diverticulum is not seen in children or young adults. It is most commonly encountered beyond 60 years of age and is seen most frequently in males (1). About 5% of asymptomatic individuals more than 40 years of age have some incoordination in the swallowing mechanism. Such changes can be seen cineradiographically in about 90% of elderly individuals. These abnormal findings are not necessarily associated with symptoms. A Zenker's diverticulum can be evident radiologically in the absence of complaints, but it causes dysphagia in about 2% of people with this symptom (3). It is the only diverticulum affecting the esophagus that often causes symptoms. These symptoms vary in severity from very mild difficulty to complete obstruction due to compression by the diverticulum when it is filled with food. These patients may complain of regurgitation and aspiration of the contents of the diverticulum, particularly at night. Myotomy of the cricopharyngeus muscle may be effective in overcoming the incoordination of swallowing and conceivably could prevent the eventual development of a Zenker's diverticulum. Once a symptomatic Zenker's diverticulum is formed, relief can come only from a diverticulectomy.

Radiologic findings of this condition are diagnostic. Plain films may show a fluid level or a soft tissue density in the posterior upper mediastinum if the diverticulum is large enough. These diverticula vary a great deal in size and tend to extend downward and toward the left. Barium swallows fill the diverticulum immediately and eventually overflow into the esophagus. The diverticulum is smooth-lined but may contain filling defects due to retained food. If the diverticulum is large enough it will compress and obstruct the esophagus.

Source Materials

1. Knuff TE, Benjamin SB, Castell DO. Pharyngoesophageal (Zenker's) diverticulum: A reappraisal. Gastroenterology 82:734. 1982.
2. Seaman WB. Cineroentgenographic observations of the cricopharyngeus AJR 96:922, 1966.
3. Seaman WB. Pharyngeal and upper esophageal dysphagia. JAMA 235:2643. 1976.
4. White IL. Severe complication of a Zenker's diverticulum with endoscopic diverticulotomy rescue. Laryngoscope 91:708, 1981.

Case 53

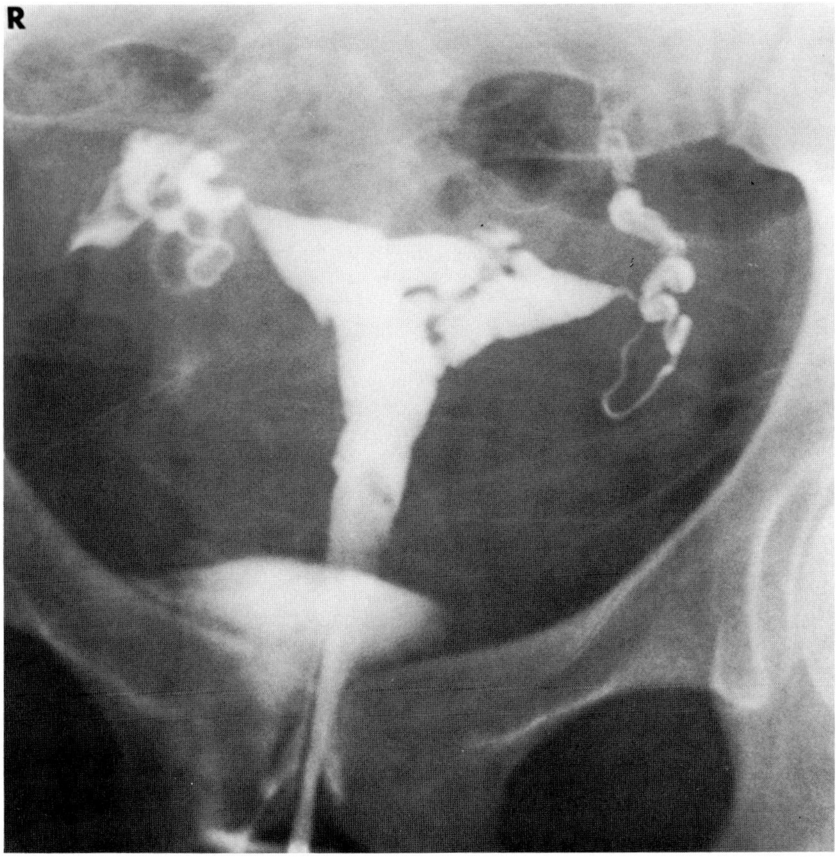

A

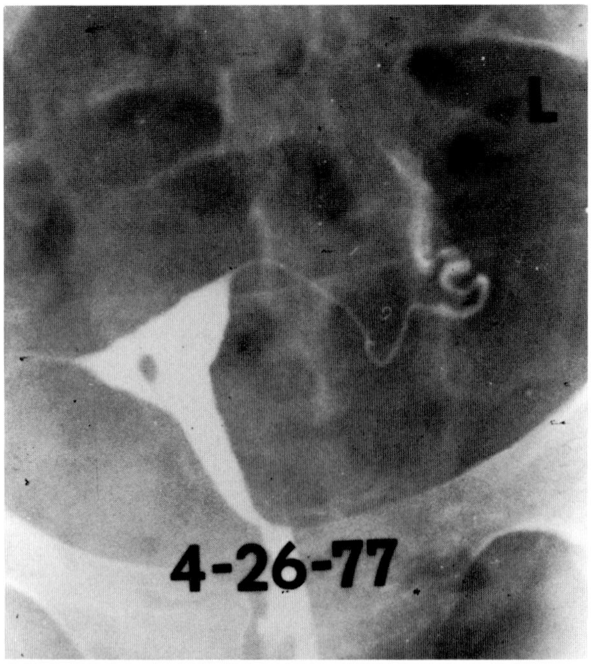

B (another patient)

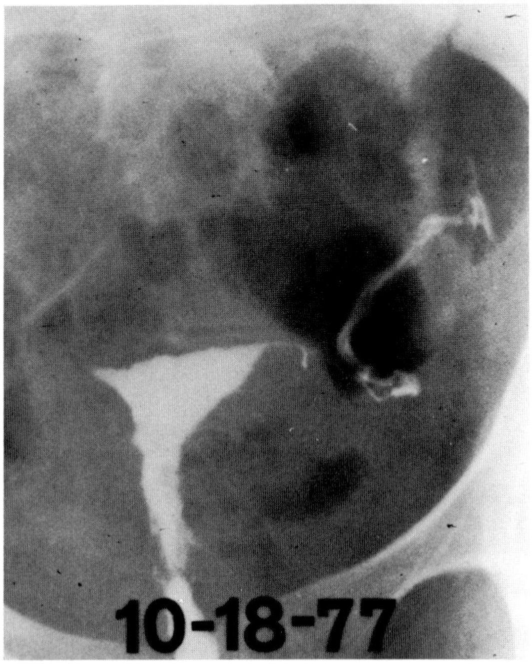

C (same patient as in B)

Asherman's Syndrome

Clinical Information

This 23-year-old black female had two normal pregnancies that were followed by four consecutive spontaneous abortions, each of which was completed by dilatation and curettage.

Roentgen Findings

A hysterosalpingogram shows good filling of the uterus and both Fallopian tubes. The opaque material outlines a sharply marginated, rather narrow, but irregular filling defect in the left half of the uterus. The defect in general is oriented in a vertical direction and runs from near the cervical os to the left side of the dome of the uterus. A few lateral extensions are visible along its course. This x-ray appearance is characteristic of Asherman's syndrome or intrauterine synechiae.

Comments

Asherman's syndrome is characterized by intrauterine adhesions, abnormal menstrual flow, and infertility or habitual abortion. The adhesions are usually caused by iatrogenic manipulations, usually curettage, frequently in a postpartum uterus. Some cases are thought to follow radiation therapy or endometrial infection. The number of the adhesions varies from a single synechia to, at times, total obliteration of the entire uterine cavity. Many cases of Asherman's syndrome have been reported. It has been said these patients have no difficulty in becoming pregnant, although it is more commonly held that this condition distinctly decreases the likelihood of pregnancy (3). All agree that patients with Asherman's syndrome, if they become pregnant, are likely to abort. Pregnancies are also often beset with abnormal implantation, abnormal fetal presentation, or premature delivery (3).

Appropriate treatment is lysis of the adhesions, usually by curettage, and introduction of an intrauterine contraceptive device until the endometrium has regenerated. This is variably successful. Although the patients after treatment may subsequently become pregnant, only about half carry the pregnancy to term. It has been shown that recurrent uterine adhesions develop frequently, sometimes in different locations (2). This raises the possibility that intrauterine adhesions are in fact only a local manifestation of a more generalized endometrial fibrosis (2).

The x-ray appearance of Asherman's syndrome is quite characteristic and marked by sharply demarcated, often linear, filling defects that do not change their size or shape with increasing quantities of opaque medium or the pressure exerted during its injection. This condition can be differentiated from a congenital septum because the latter is situated near the middle of the uterus. The appearance of Asherman's syndrome may be simulated by mucosal hyperplasia, but increasing the pressure of injection will overcome these filling defects. Tuberculosis is much more likely to cause strictures and to deform the uterus. At times an adhesion can look much like a polyp (B). Hysterosalpingographic evidence in such cases is not conclusive. The patient shown in B was treated by surgical lysis with disappearance of this filling defect as shown in C. Unfortunately, she continued to abort spontaneously.

Source Materials

1. Bergman P, Wehlin L. Post-traumatic intra-uterine synechiae. Acta Radiol 49:453, 1958.
2. Polishuk WZ, Sadovsky E. Syndrome of recurrent intrauterine adhesions. Am J Obstet Gynecol 123:151, 1975.
3. Topkins PT. Traumatic intrauterine synechiae. The Asherman syndrome. Am J Obstet Gynecol 83:1599, 1962.

Case 54

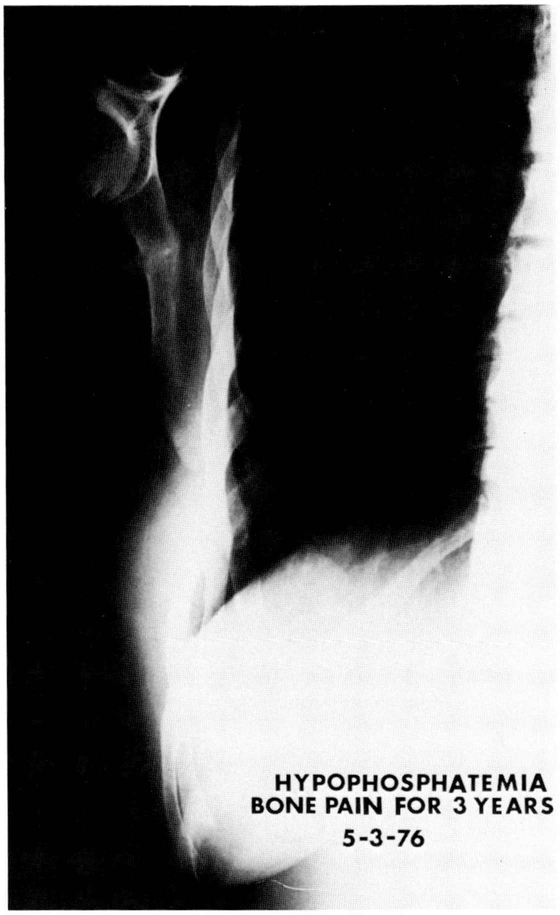

A

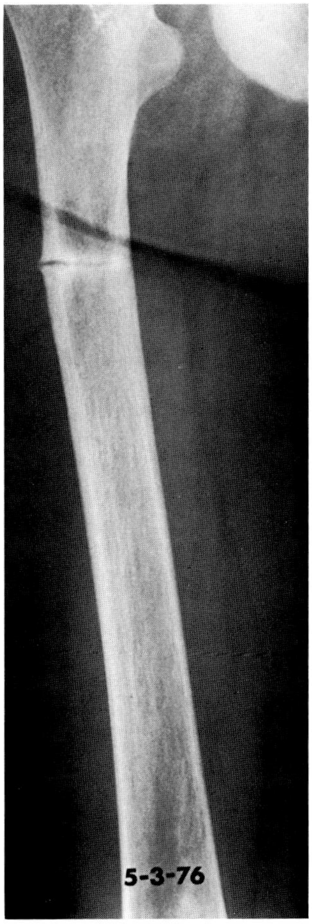

B

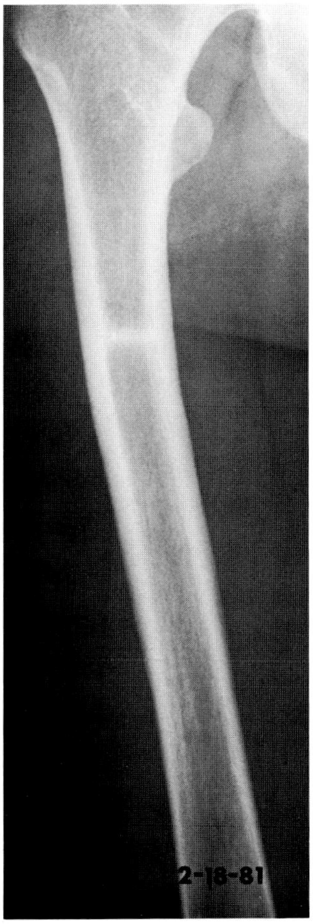

C

Adult Onset Nonfamilial Hypophosphatemic Vitamin D-Resistant Osteomalacia

Clinical Information

This 27-year-old white female had complained of bone pain for 3 years. Her bones were not bowed or otherwise deformed. No one in her family had a similar disease. She responded well to therapy for hypophosphatemic osteomalacia.

Roentgen Findings

Anteroposterior films of the right ribs (A) and right femur (B) show multiple pseudofractures. The femoral fracture runs transversely across the upper third of the femoral shaft. Several lower ribs are fractured in the anterior axillary line, although they are not well shown on the print. The lateral scapular margin also shows a pseudofracture. Similar pseudofractures were present on the opposite side. The cortices of the visualized bones are thin and poorly defined, and the medullary trabecular pattern is mildly striated. A film of the right femur (C) obtained almost 5 years later, after therapy, shows the pseudofracture to have healed and the cortex to have returned to normal thickness and appearance.

Comments

Adult onset nonfamilial hypophosphatemic vitamin D-resistant osteomalacia (AONHO) is an unusual form of osteomalacia (1,3) characterized by hypophosphatemia and symptoms that include muscle weakness and bone pain. It probably represents a defect that develops in the renal tubules and permits loss of phosphate in the urine with secondary hypophosphatemia. It is not hereditary. The condition does not manifest itself until adulthood. This late onset prevents the bone deformities that attend osteomalacia that is active during the period of growth. Loss of height may occur due to collapse of several vertebral bodies.

Vitamin D-resistant osteomalacia can lead to spinal stenosis in adulthood (2). The serum alkaline phosphatase is elevated. Calcium levels in the blood are normal but the phosphate is low. Urine phosphate is markedly elevated. There also may be glycosuria, which accounts for the fact that this condition is sometimes called phosphate diabetes. AONHO was formerly treated with large quantities of vitamin D, which often caused vitamin D intoxication with abundant soft tissue calcifications. Current treatment involves oral phosphates with the addition of calcium and less vitamin D. Tumors, usually benign soft tissue and vascular tumors, have been associated with AONHO (3). Removal of these tumors has led to disappearance of the hypophosphatemia and osteomalacia. The pathogenic connection between the tumor and the osteomalacia is unknown. There are also reports of spontaneous cure of this type of osteomalacia.

The radiographic findings are typical and characterized by pseudofractures (Looser's zones), widespread osteomalacia, thin and poorly defined cortical bone, and a coarse trabecular pattern of the cancellous bone. The extremity bones are neither shortened nor bowed. This is an important point in the radiologic differentiation of AONHO from familial hypophosphatemic vitamin D-resistant osteomalacia. The vertebral bodies may show "codfish" collapse. AONHO must be distinguished from the major causes of osteomalacia, which include deficiency states, absorptive defects, and osteomalacia secondary to renal disease (4). These conditions usually do not show hypophosphatemia. AONHO can be differentiated from Fanconi's syndrome because the latter leads to dwarfing and anemia. AONHO has the same biochemical findings as familial hypophosphatemic vitamin D-resistant osteomalacia, although in the latter condition there is early onset, short stature, excellent muscular development, overgrowth of bone at tendinous and ligamentous insertions, x-linked inheritance, and small ossicles in the carpus. The familial type less frequently shows pseudofractures.

Source Materials

1. Dent CE, Stamp TCB. Hypophosphatemic osteomalacia presenting in adults. Q J Med 158:303, 1971.
2. Masel JP, Cartwright DW, Latham SC. Hypophosphataemic vitamin D-resistant rickets—a cause of spinal stenosis in adults. Australas Radiol 25:264, 1981.
3. Robertson A. Case of the winter season. Semin Roentgenol 18:5, 1983.
4. Turner ML, Dalinka MK. Osteomalacia: Uncommon causes. AJR 133:539, 1979.

Case 55

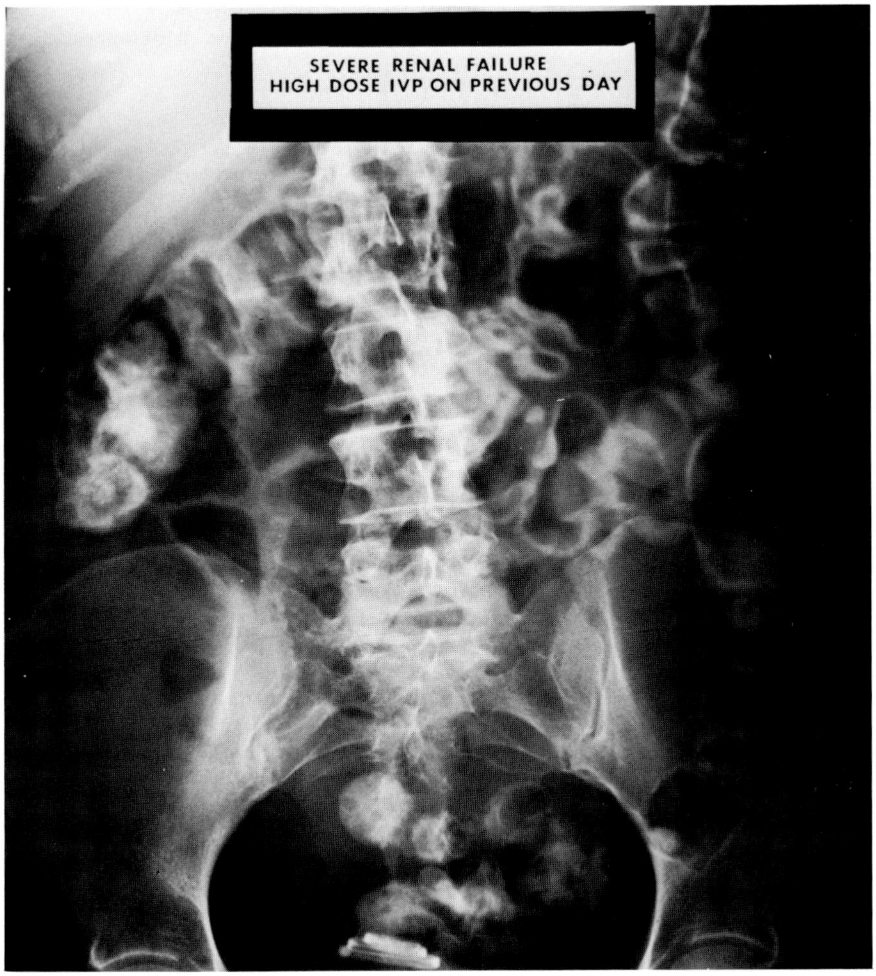

Vicarious Excretion of a Urographic Contrast Agent

Clinical Information

This 30-year-old white female with severe renal failure had a high-dose intravenous urogram on the day before this film of the abdomen was exposed. No renal excretion of the opaque was visualized. The patient suffered no ill effects from this examination.

Roentgen Findings

A film of the abdomen shows much of the colon to be opacified by an evenly dispersed radiopaque contrast agent. No opaque medium is seen within the urinary tract. An incidental intrauterine contraceptive device is seen.

Comments

An occasional patient with severe renal failure will excrete sufficient urographic contrast agent through the gastrointestinal tract during high-dose intravenous urography to afford radiologic visibility of the gallbladder or colon. The gastrointestinal tract can serve as a substitute pathway of excretion when the kidneys cannot perform this function. Under such circumstances much of the contrast agent is excreted by the liver. A smaller amount is excreted by the small intestines. Even less excretion of the opaque agent occurs in the saliva, sweat, tears, and gastric juices. Although such vicarious excretion is often evident on x-ray studies by visualization of the colon, the large bowel does not excrete the material. The colon becomes opacified because it absorbs water from the intestinal contents, increasing the colonic concentration of the opaque agent.

The site of excretion of iodine-containing contrast agents largely depends upon their ability to bind plasma proteins. Those compounds that avidly bind plasma proteins are preferentially excreted by the liver; those that do not are excreted by the kidneys. The availability of an unsubstituted position 5 on the benzene ring encourages plasma protein binding and consequent hepatic excretion. Approximately half of the patients who had intravenous urography with some of the older contrast agents showed a degree of gallbladder opacification. Such an event is much less common with current urographic contrast agents. In fact, alternate pathways of excretion are rarely seen in the absence of renal failure or urinary tract obstruction.

Diatrizoate compounds in current use are excreted almost entirely by the glomeruli if the patient has normal renal function. Alternate routes come into use if renal function is impaired. There is, however, no clear relationship between the severity of the renal failure and the amount of excretion that occurs vicariously. In fact, a few cases have been recorded in which renal function has been normal yet the gallbladder became opacified. There have been several cases with unilateral renal damage or unilateral ureteric obstruction who demonstrated gallbladder visualization. There is no satisfactory explanation for this route of excretion under such circumstances. Although the excretion of the urographic contrast agent is markedly prolonged in the presence of renal failure, the likelihood of toxic reactions is not strikingly increased. The addition of severe liver damage to renal failure does not seem to increase the possibility of an adverse effect. Nevertheless, there are those who feel urography is contraindicated in the face of combined hepatic and renal failure. It is generally agreed that the development of a reaction in a patient with poor kidney and liver function calls for ridding the body of the contrast medium as quickly as possible by hemodialysis.

Source Materials

1. Kohler R, Edgren J. Gallbladder filling by urographic sodium metrizoate. Acta Radiol 12:184, 1972.
2. Lautin EM, Friedman AC. Vicarious excretion of contrast media. JAMA 247:1608, 1982.
3. Shea TE, Pfister RC. Opacification of the gallbladder by urographic contrast media. Reflection of an alternate excretory pathway. AJR 107:763, 1969.
4. Talner LB. Urographic contrast media in uremia. Physiology and pharmacology. Radiol Clin North Am 10:421, 1972.

Case 56

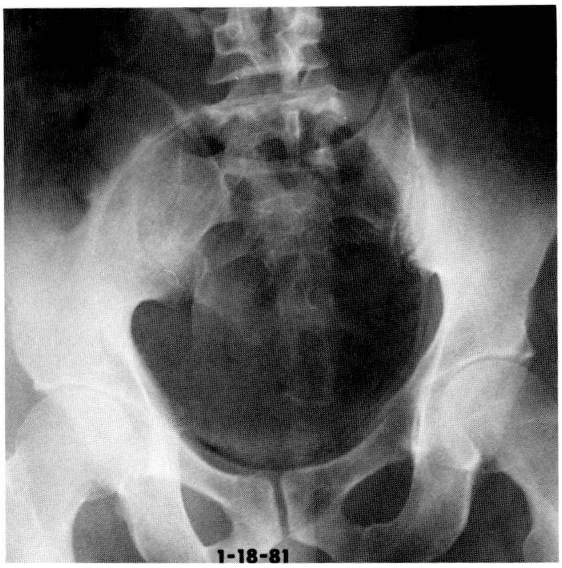

A

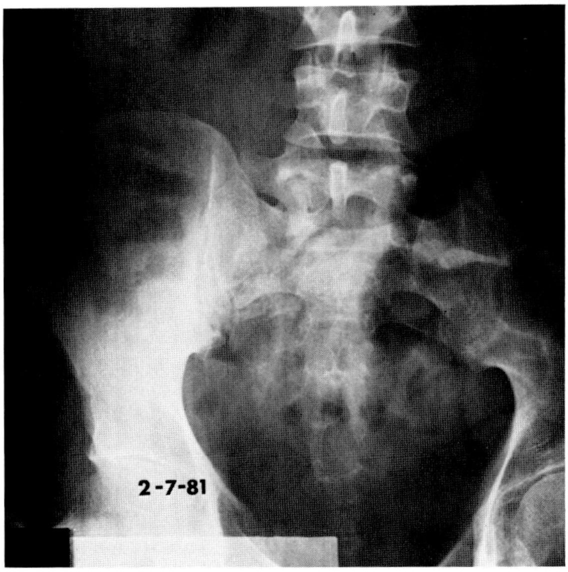

B

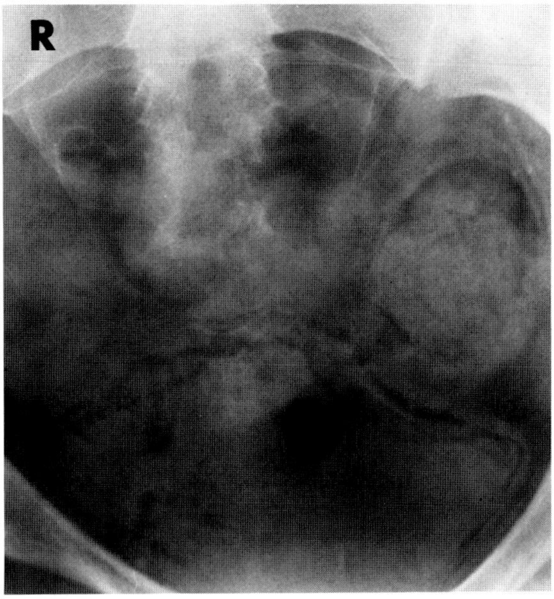

C (another patient)

Emphysematous Cystitis

Clinical Information

This 34-year-old white male nondiabetic had undergone two operations during the previous 2 weeks. These procedures had been required following an automobile accident. He developed gross hematuria and pneumaturia 1 day before film A was obtained. A Foley cathether had been in place throughout his hospitalization. It had been clamped for an unknown period of time before this radiograph was obtained. His symptoms and radiologic abnormalities disappeared with antibiotic therapy (film B).

Roentgen Findings

A supine film of the lower abdomen (A) shows mild intestinal ileus. A thin line of radiolucency is seen in the pelvis. It inscribes a circle that measures about 14 cm in diameter and encloses an area that is slightly more lucent than the surrounding soft tissues. This line of radiolucency represents air in the wall of a dilated urinary bladder. Air within the bladder lumen accounts for its slightly decreased density. The intraluminal gas was confirmed by cystography (not shown) and accounts for the pneumaturia. These x-ray findings are diagnostic of emphysematous cystitis. Film B shows all of the gas to have disappeared.

Comments

Emphysematous cystitis results from infection in the urinary bladder wall by gas-producing bacteria, most commonly *E. coli* or *Aerobacter aerogenes,* although many different organisms, including clostridia, have been cultured from patients with this condition (4). These organisms produce carbon dioxide and hydrogen as well as lactic and butyric acids through the fermentation of glucose. Some bacteria can produce gas from urine albumin in the absence of glycosuria. Although patients with emphysematous cystitis may have pneumaturia in addition to gas in the bladder wall, it is the latter that must be seen to establish the radiologic diagnosis. Intramural gas is necessary for the diagnosis, because many other conditions such as instrumentation, trauma, and fistulae can lead to gas within the lumen of the urinary bladder. The bladder wall gas is located in submucosal vesicles. These vesicles vary in size up to 1 cm in diameter. They are surrounded by hemorrhagic areas in a thickened bladder wall.

Patients with emphysematous cystitis complain of dysuria and frequent urination. They occasionally have gross or microscopic hematuria. Pneumaturia is not common. The disease is more common in women. Most of the patients are beyond middle age, and about half have longtime diabetes with glycosuria. The average duration of the diabetes is about 14 years. Many patients have associated urinary retention due to prostatic hypertrophy, bladder diverticula, or a neurogenic bladder. Treatment involves antibiotics for the infection and control of the diabetes. The prognosis is relatively good. The gas usually will disappear from both the urine and the bladder wall within a few days.

As mentioned above, the decisive x-ray finding is gas within the wall of the urinary bladder. The gas appears as a narrow radiolucent stripe, which usually entirely encircles the bladder. This is a diagnostic x-ray finding. There are no differential diagnostic possibilities. There may be gas within the lumen of the bladder in addition to the intramural stripe of radiolucency. With contrast studies it is possible to show that the bladder wall is thickened and has a cobblestone appearance. Another example of this condition is shown (C) in a different patient.

Source Materials

1. Bailey H. Cystitis emphysematosa. 19 cases with intraluminal and interstitial collections of gas. AJR 86:850, 1961.
2. Fainfold JE, Hansen CO, Rigler LG. Cystitis emphysematosa. Review of the literature and report of four cases diagnosed by roentgen examination. Radiology 61:346, 1953.
3. Holesh S. Gas in the bladder. Cystitis emphysematosa. Clin Radiol 20:234, 1969.
4. West TE, Holley HP Jr, Lauer AD. Emphysematous cystitis due to *Clostridium perfringens.* JAMA 246:363, 1981.

Case 57

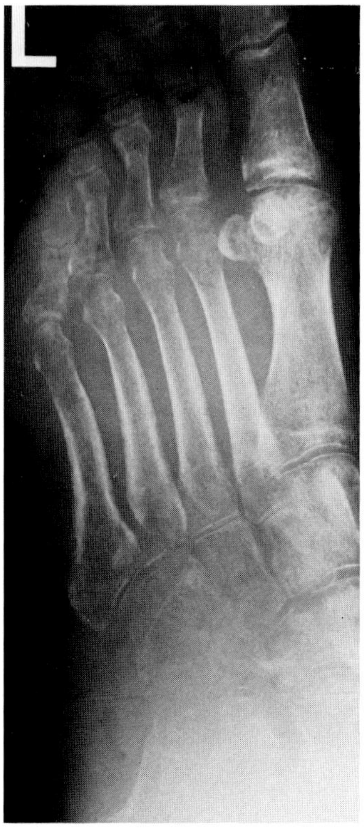

A

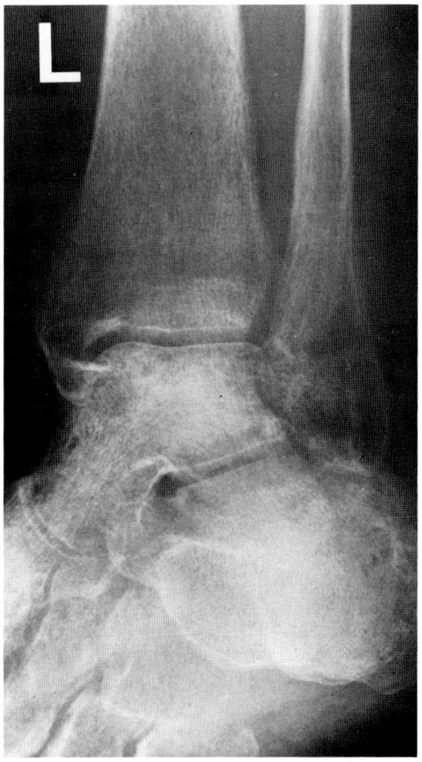

B

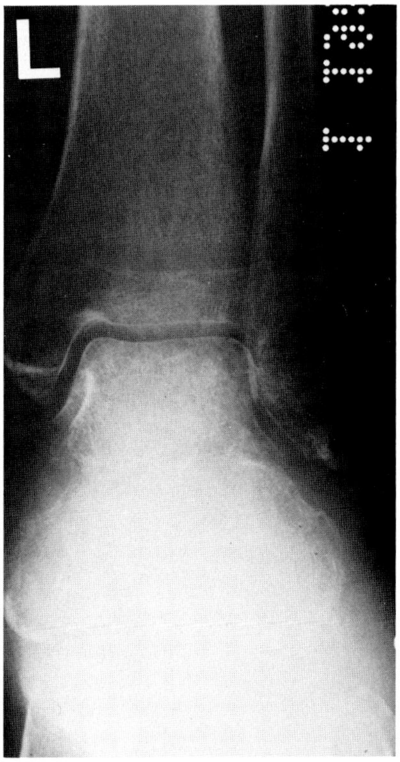

C

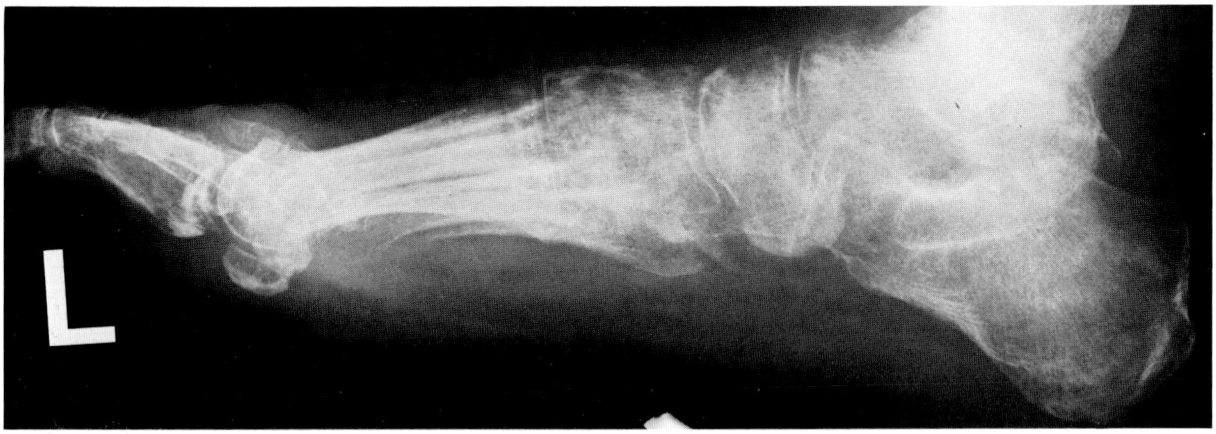

D

Reflex Sympathetic Dystrophy Syndrome (Sudeck's Atrophy)

Clinical Information

This 48-year-old male noted pain, swelling, and increased temperature in his left foot and ankle about 1 week after he fell and twisted his left ankle. These symptoms slowly cleared with symptomatic therapy over the next 6 months.

Roentgen Findings

Films of the left foot and ankle (A–D) show some soft tissue swelling and striking splotchy osteopenia. The latter is most marked in the tarsal bones and periarticular regions. The osteopenic radiolucency is particularly noticeable where it parallels the cortex and the closed epiphysis at the distal end of the tibia. The third, fourth, and fifth metatarsals show some cortical striations or tunneling and mild endosteal scalloping.

Comments

The reflex sympathetic dystrophy syndrome (RSDS), also called causalgia, Sudeck's atrophy, shoulder-hand syndrome, and post-traumatic osteoporosis, was first recognized as an entity in 1864. Sudeck described the radiographic features in 1900 (4). This condition most commonly results from trauma, which is usually mild, but it can follow other conditions such as osteoarthritis, which may affect the peripheral nerves. About 25% of patients with RSDS have no known antecedent incident. Some sort of stimulus to an afferent nerve is required to initiate an abnormal reflex. Symptoms apparently result from an abnormal sympathetic innervation and secondary vascular changes. Usually an entire extremity distal to the point of injury is affected, although at times only a portion is involved (3). The lower extremity is more frequently affected than the upper. Clinical features include pain, restricted motion, vasomotor instability, and secondary skin changes. The pain is usually of a severe, aching character and is aggravated by immobilization. The shoulder-hand syndrome seen after cardiac surgery or a myocardial infarction has features very similar to RSDS.

X-ray findings always include soft tissue swelling and bony changes caused by acute osteopenia. The changes of RSDS are particularly striking in the carpus and tarsus. This aggressive loss of bone density is characterized by accelerated remodeling. Patchy, irregular radiolucencies, especially in the highly vascularized periarticular regions and near the epiphyseal-metaphyseal junctions, are invariably present, although all of the affected bones may reveal reduced mineral content. Accelerated osteopenia is further manifested by thinning of the cortex with endosteal scalloping. Intracortical tunneling is a characteristic finding (2). The accelerated osteoclasis in cortical bone may lead to a striated appearance that simulates periosteal new bone formation—so-called pseudoperiostitis (1). Subchondral cortical erosions in the periarticular region are occasionally seen. There may even be minimal subperiosteal bony resorption.

Identical x-ray findings may be seen in other entities such as acute disuse osteoporosis, hyperparathyroidism, or even at times osteomalacia, Cushing's syndrome, multiple myeloma, metastatic cancer, or thyrotoxicosis. All are due to acutely developing osteopenia. Differentiations between the several causes of this x-ray appearance, as well as its variations, are largely a matter of the rate of osteoclastic activity and the associated clinical signs and symptoms. The clinical features of RSDS are highly characteristic.

Source Materials

1. Forrester DM, Kirkpatrick J. Periostitis and pseudoperiostitis. Radiology 118:597, 1976.
2. Genant HK, Kozin F, Bekerman C, McCarty DJ, Sims J. The reflex sympathetic dystrophy syndrome. A comprehensive analysis using fine detail radiography, photon absorptiometry, and bone and joint scintigraphy. Radiology 117:21, 1975.
3. Helms CA, O'Brien ET, Katzberg RW. Segmental reflex sympathetic dystrophy syndrome. Radiology 135:67, 1980.
4. Sudeck P. Ueber die acute entzündliche Knochenatrophie. Arch Klin Chir 62:147, 1900.

Case 58

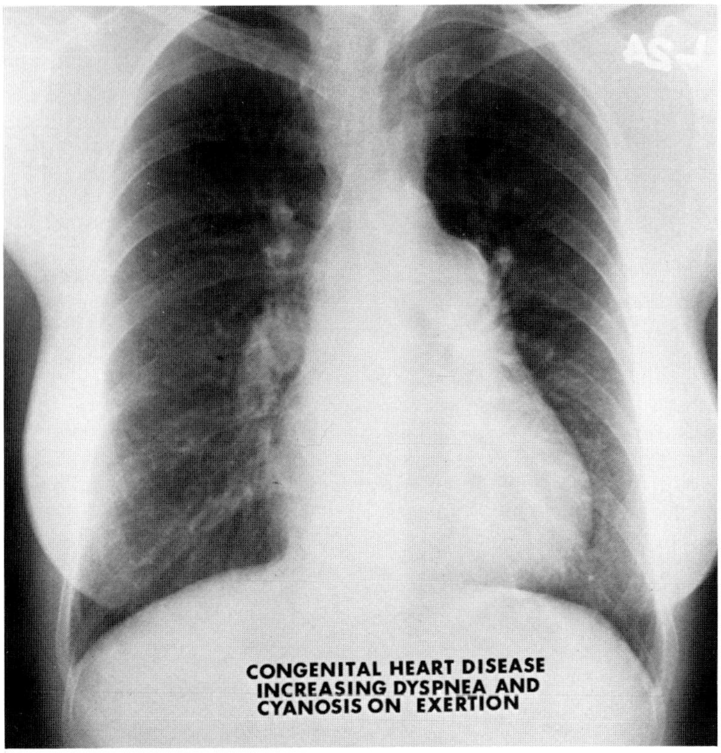
AS-L
CONGENITAL HEART DISEASE
INCREASING DYSPNEA AND
CYANOSIS ON EXERTION

A

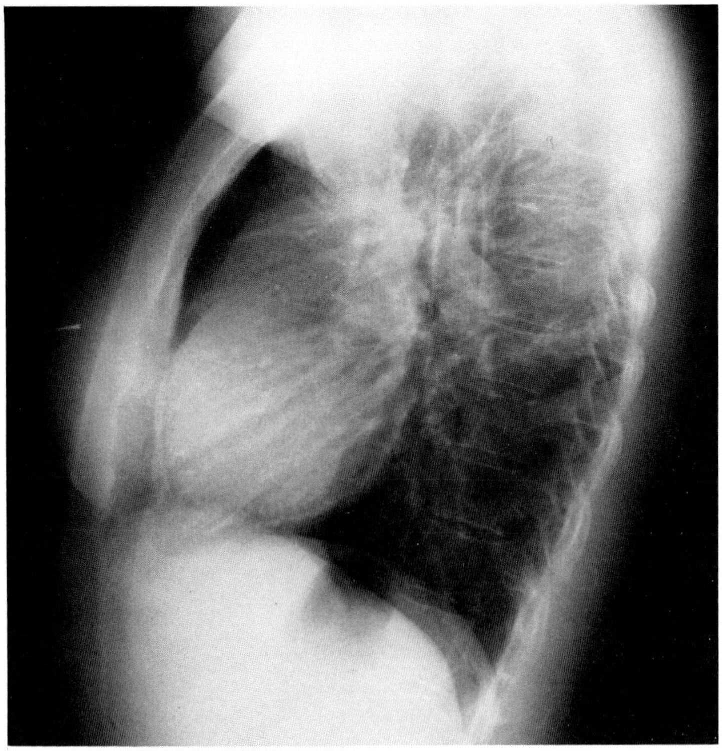

B

Eisenmenger Syndrome

Clinical Information

This 30-year-old female with known congenital heart disease noted increasing dyspnea and recurrent hemoptyses. Subsequent study revealed a ventricular septal defect, bidirectional shunting, and equal pressures in the pulmonary and systemic arteries.

Roentgen Findings

Chest films (A,B) show mild cardiomegaly. The central pulmonary arteries are enlarged, taper rapidly, and are calcified. The lung fields are clear.

Comments

In 1897 Eisenmenger described a congenital anomaly comprised of a ventricular septal defect and aortic overriding. This anomaly has become known as Eisenmenger's complex. It was subsequently noted that patients with a long-standing left-to-right shunt can reverse its direction following the development of increased pulmonary arteriolar resistance, a situation that has been called Eisenmenger syndrome or physiology (4). This series of events is seen in all left-to-right shunts but is especially common and appears earliest with a ventricular septal defect or patent ductus arteriosus. The increased kinetic disturbance in the pulmonary arteries occasioned by the high pressure of the shunted blood in these anomalies apparently accounts for the difference.

A newborn has rather thick, somewhat cuboidal pulmonary arterial endothelium to discourage pulmonary blood flow during fetal life. Shortly after birth the endothelium normally becomes flattened, decreasing pulmonary resistance. Failure of the pulmonary endothelium to flatten may cause high pulmonary resistance from birth. Patients with a long-standing left-to-right shunt may eventually develop permanent changes in their pulmonary arterioles that lead to increased vascular resistance, which can reach systemic levels and cause the left-to-right shunt to reverse its direction. In actual fact, the ratio of pulmonary to systemic flow usually approaches unity. Patients with Eisenmenger syndrome are characteristically cyanotic, dyspneic, and clubbed. There may be recurrent hemoptyses, which is the cause of death in almost a third of these patients. They usually die within the third to fifth decades of life. Surgical mortality is extremely high.

The typical x-ray changes of Eisenmenger syndrome are prominent central pulmonary arteries with rapid peripheral diminution in their size (pruned tree appearance). Some of the smaller vessels may be somewhat tortuous. Calcium may be present in the central pulmonary artery (1,2). The calcification, primarily seen with a patent ductus or a ventricular septal defect, indicates a long-standing left-to-right shunt has led to pulmonary hypertension. Not all patients who develop Eisenmenger physiology show the typical x-ray changes enumerated. At times the heart and lung fields appear normal. It is sometimes possible to suggest the location of the original left-to-right shunt that led to the Eisenmenger syndrome. With a ventricular septal defect the size of the heart may become virtually normal as the shunt is balanced or reversed. An atrial septal defect, on the other hand, usually maintains considerable cardiomegaly and a large pulmonary artery, especially in comparison with the size of the aorta. The heart may become somewhat smaller but does not so nearly approach normality as can occur with a ventricular septal defect.

Source Materials

1. Gutierrez FR, Moran CJ, Ludbrook PA, et al. Pulmonary arterial calcification with reversible pulmonary hypertension. AJR 135:177, 1980.
2. Mallamo JT, Baum RS, Simon AL. Diffuse pulmonary artery calcifications in a case of Eisenmenger's syndrome. Radiology 99:549, 1971.
3. Rees RSO, Jefferson KE. The Eisenmenger syndrome. Clin Radiol 18:366, 1967.
4. Wood P. The Eisenmenger syndrome or pulmonary hypertension with reversed central shunt. Br Med J 2:701, 1958.

Case 59

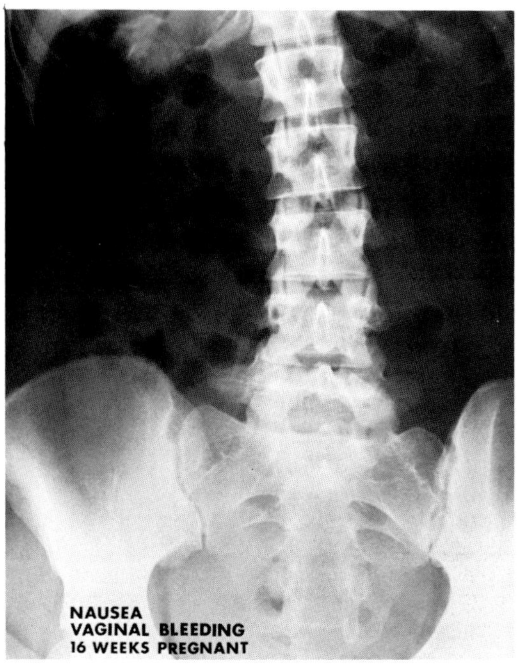

A

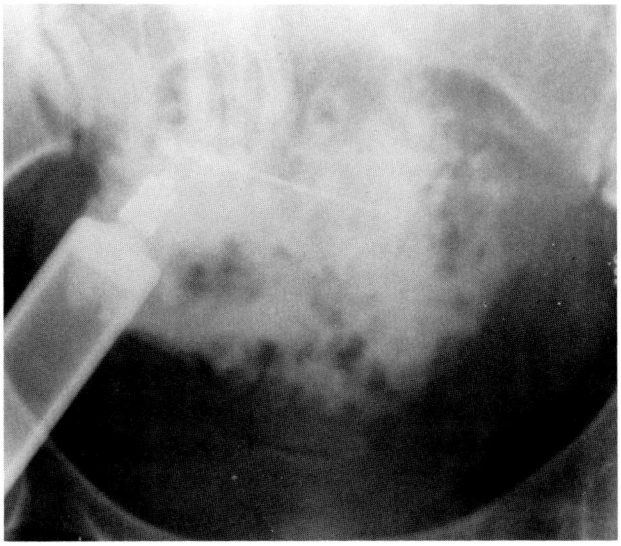

B

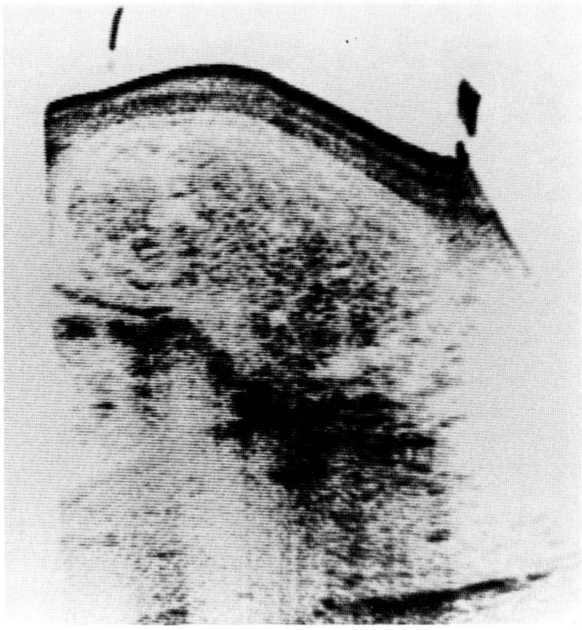

C (another patient)

Hydatidiform Mole

Clinical Information

This 22-year-old female was 16 weeks pregnant by date of last menstruation, but her uterine size corresponded to 20–22 weeks. Her human chorionic gonadotropin titer was very high. A hydatidiform mole was successfully removed.

Roentgen Findings

A film of the abdomen (A) shows no bony fetal parts. A pelvic soft tissue mass, evidently the uterus, extends to the top of the fifth lumbar vertebra. It is much larger than would be expected with a 16-week pregnancy. An amniogram (B) shows numerous smooth filling defects.

Comments

A hydatidiform mole appears to be a true neoplasm. The exact series of events that occasion a molar pregnancy is unknown. Present theories indicate that a spontaneous or missed abortion leaves residual trophoblastic tissue within the uterus, which forms the mole. In the Western world a hydatidiform mole is seen once in 2000 pregnancies, but in some parts of Asia the incidence is 1 in 200. This difference is unexplained. The characteristic clinical manifestations of hydatidiform mole include a uterus that is larger than expected from the date of the last menstruation, bleeding, and exaggerated symptoms of pregnancy, particularly nausea. Occasionally bits of grapeskin-like tissue are passed. This situation usually becomes evident between the fourth and fifth months.

Hydatidiform mole is the least malignant of three related conditions, the others being choriocarcinoma destruens (invasive mole) and choriocarcinoma. All have similar clinical histories and x-ray findings. All are characterized by a marked elevation of human chorionic gonadotropin in the blood. An occasional mole (up to 5%) is reported in a live pregnancy (2). It is generally presumed these cases represent a twin pregnancy in which one degenerated into a hydatidiform mole and the other survived. Twenty to thirty percent of hydatidiform moles are associated with a thecal lutein cyst or cysts, apparently due to the stimulation of the human chorionic gonadotropin. Appropriate treatment consists of curettage and, if the woman desires no further pregnancies, a total hysterectomy. Some patients develop pulmonary edema during the evacuation of the molar pregnancy. This may be due at times to trophoblastic embolization (1). The success of treatment is evident by a decrease in the human chorionic gonadotropin levels to normal. If this does not occur within 8 weeks, it is presumed the patient has a malignant process, either choriocarcinoma destruens or choriocarcinoma, and is treated with methotrexate and actinomycin D. A cure can be expected.

X-ray studies show no fetal parts and a larger uterus than expected from the date of the last menstruation. The diagnosis is confirmed by ultrasonography and an elevated human chorionic gonadotropin titer (3). Ultrasound (see film C from another patient) shows very evenly dispersed echoes throughout the enlarged uterus. This is referred to as a "snowstorm" pattern. There are occasionally lucent structures, which represent hydropic vesicles. This appearance is different from a degenerating placenta, which has a more coarse and uneven pattern and shows an amniotic cavity and varying amounts of calcification, which are not seen with a mole.

Source Materials

1. Huberman RP, Fon GT, Bein ME. Benign molar pregnancies: Pulmonary complications. AJR 138:71, 1982.
2. Naumoff P, Szulman AE, Weinstein B, et al. Ultrasonography of partial hydatidiform mole. Radiology 140:467, 1981.
3. Requard CK, Mettler FA Jr. The use of ultrasound in the evaluation of trophoblastic disease and its response to therapy. Radiology 135:419, 1980.

Case 60

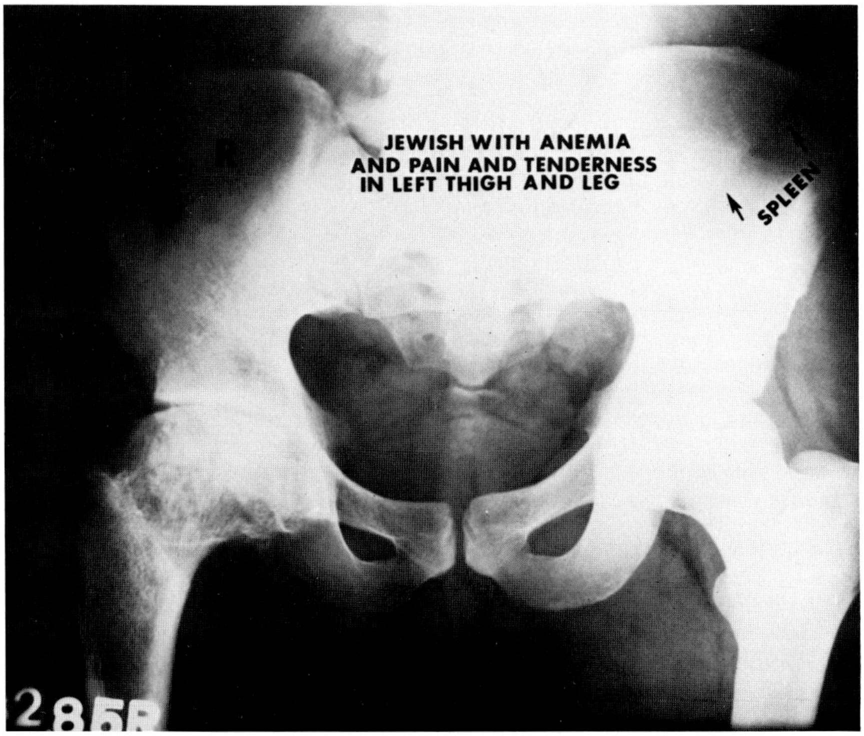
JEWISH WITH ANEMIA
AND PAIN AND TENDERNESS
IN LEFT THIGH AND LEG
SPLEEN
285R

A

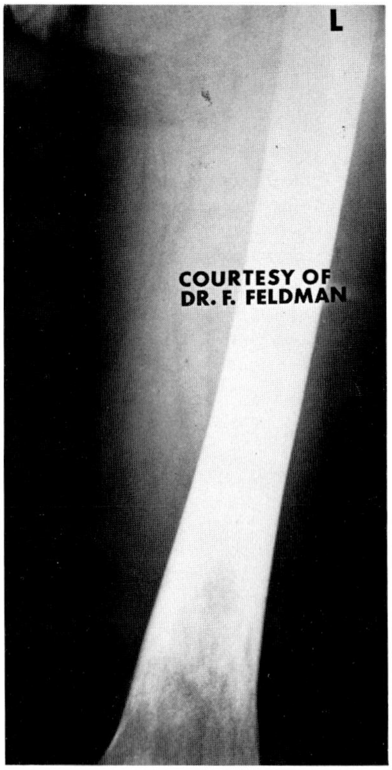
L
COURTESY OF
DR. F. FELDMAN

B

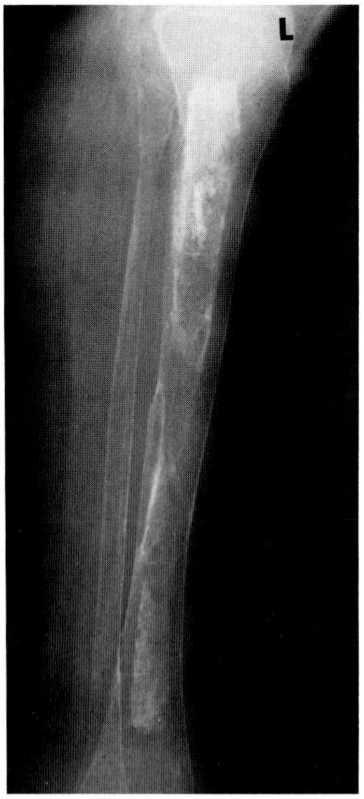
L

C

Gaucher's Disease

Clinical Information

This 22-year-old Jewish woman was anemic and had suffered from pain in her left leg for 2 years. Bone marrow studies showed abundant Gaucher cells.

Roentgen Findings

A film of the pelvis and lower abdomen (A) shows the spleen to be markedly enlarged. There is aseptic necrosis of the right femoral head. A film of the left lower extremity (B) reveals the diaphysis of the distal left femur to be somewhat expanded and osteopenic. The left tibia (C) shows striking calcification of a "bone within a bone," representing an old bone infarct. Calcified infarcts were also visible in the left calcaneus and talus.

Comments

Gaucher's disease is a hereditary metabolic disorder characterized by the accumulation of abnormal lipids, primarily kerasin, within enlarged reticuloendothelial cells located in the bone marrow, lymph nodes, liver, spleen, and other organs. The diagnosis is usually proved by the discovery of these cells in the bone marrow, although they are occasionally seen in the peripheral blood. Most patients with Gaucher's disease are Jews, although cases have been reported in all races (3).

The disease may be acute but usually is chronic. The acute type affects infants, who usually die within the first year of life from deposits of Gaucher cells within the central nervous system. Unlike in the chronic form, the bones are spared in acute Gaucher's disease. Chronic Gaucher's disease becomes clinically manifested in adolescence. The usual symptoms include vague systemic complaints, abdominal fullness due to enlargement of the spleen and liver, weight loss, and a characteristic yellowish pigmentation in the conjunctiva and the skin, especially on the lower extremities. A bleeding tendency is common. There may be episodes of bone pain due to infarction, which can lead to tenderness and increased temperature, suggesting osteomyelitis (2). An elevated serum acid phosphatase is quite common. These patients also have an increased incidence of gallstones. Patients with Gaucher's disease usually die by the age of 50, although survival to old age is not uncommon. Death often results from bleeding or infection, to which these patients are liable due to crowding of the bone marrow and spleen by Gaucher cells. Splenectomy may accelerate the bony changes (4).

The radiologic manifestations of this condition include hepatosplenomegaly. The spleen tends to be relatively larger than the liver. The bone changes result from crowding of the marrow spaces with Gaucher cells (1). Osteoporosis is seen in bones that contain red marrow because the bony trabeculae and endosteal cortex are resorbed by the Gaucher cells. There may be circumscribed radiolucent defects, which suggest metastatic carcinoma or multiple myeloma. Sclerotic areas can be seen. They apparently represent areas of osseous metaplasia. The abundance of Gaucher cells can enlarge the ends of the bones and lead to a Florentine or Erlenmeyer flask appearance, which, in association with aseptic necrosis of a related femoral head, is quite diagnostic. These abnormal bones break fairly easily but for some reason seem to heal more rapidly than normal. Collapse of a vertebral body may occur when the disease is severe. Gaucher's disease often leads to bone infarction from compression or actual infiltration of blood vessels. Occasionally a bone infarction can lead to a "bone within a bone" appearance. At times the necrotic bone calcifies. Periosteal reaction may overlie areas of acute bone infarction. The lungs may show mottled interstitial densities in the absence of mediastinal lymphadenopathy, atelectasis, pneumothorax, or pleural effusion. The diagnosis of Gaucher's disease is easily made if the condition is considered.

Source Materials

1. Greenfield GB. Bone changes in chronic adult Gaucher's disease. AJR 110:800, 1980.
2. Miller JH, Ortega JA, Heisel MA. Juvenile Gaucher disease simulating osteomyelitis. Case report. AJR 137:880, 1981.
3. Novy SB, Natelson E, Stuart L, Whitlock L. Gaucher's disease in a black adult. AJR 133:947, 1979.
4. Rose JS, Grabowski GA, Barnett SH, Desnick RJ. Accelerated skeletal deterioration after splenectomy in Gaucher type I disease. Case report. AJR 139:1202, 1982.

Case 61

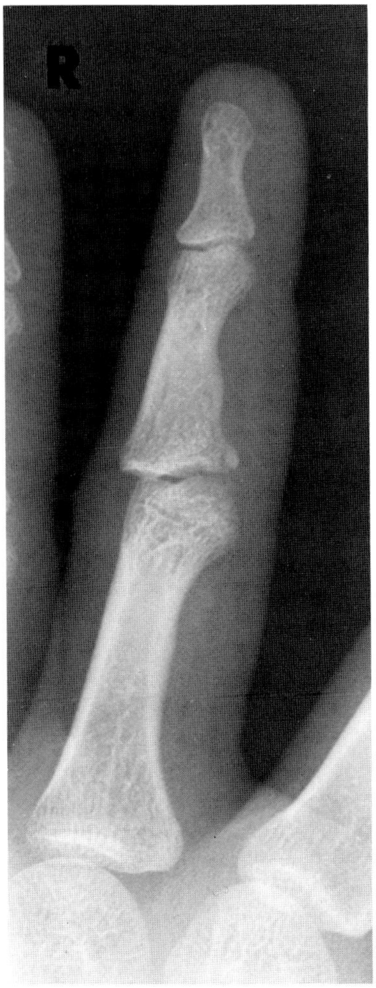

A

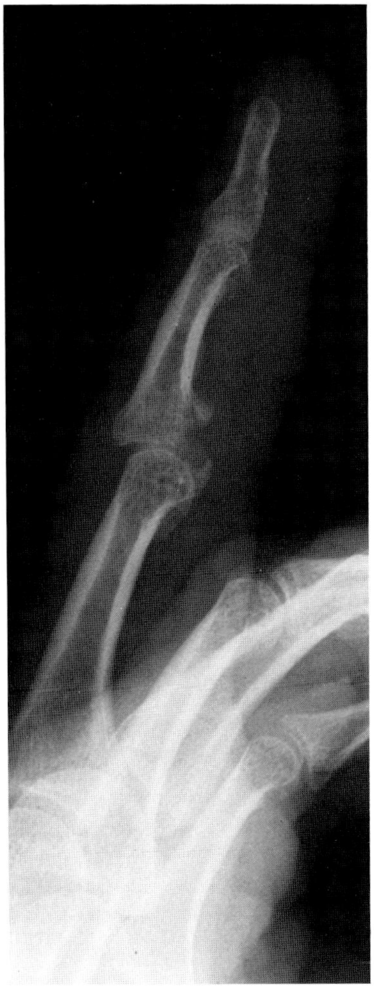

B

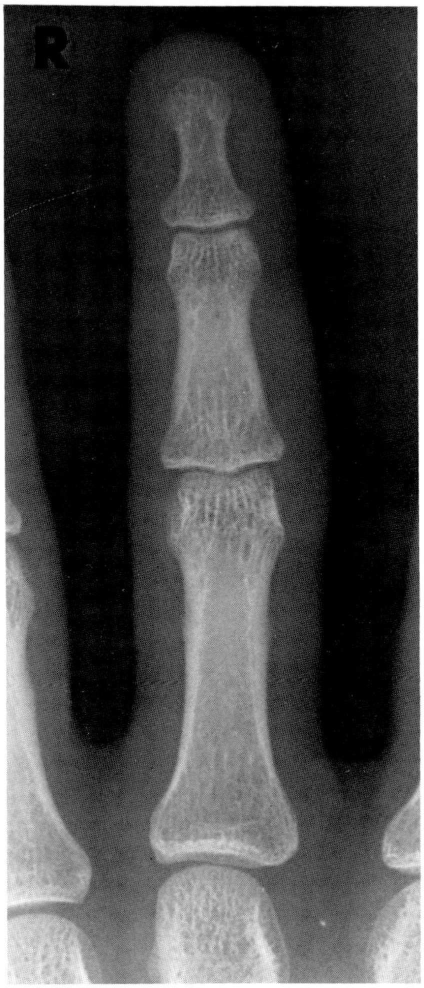

C

Volar Plate Fracture

Clinical Information

This 22-year-old male college student suffered a hyperextension injury of the ring finger of the right hand while playing basketball. The resulting subluxation was reduced and the finger was splinted in flexion. Recovery was uneventful.

Roentgen Findings

Films of the ring finger of the right hand (A–C) show soft tissue swelling around the proximal interphalangeal joint, where there is dorsal subluxation of the middle phalanx. A small chip fracture involves the proximal palmar edge of the middle phalanx.

Comments

The volar plate comprises the major portion of the palmar aspect of the fibrous capsule of the proximal interphalangeal joint (1). Since the volar plate is not bony, the term volar plate bony fracture is somewhat of a misnomer, although this injury is often associated with an avulsion. The volar plate is attached along a continuous broad edge, the volar lip, to the proximal edge of the middle phalanx. This fibrous structure divides proximally into two lateral bands called the checkrein ligaments, which attach to each side of the palmar aspect of the distal portion of the proximal phalanx. The function of the volar plate is to prevent hyperextension. This fibrous structure is quite strong. It has been said that 19 kg of force is required to rupture an isolated volar plate. A volar plate also exists on the palmar surface of the distal interphalangeal joints but is most often injured at the proximal interphalangeal articulations.

Fracture of a volar plate is relatively frequent. The majority of such injuries result from hyperextension, most frequently incurred during athletic activities such as basketball, baseball, or football (4). The fibrous volar plate may be ruptured, although frequently there is an associated bony avulsion, usually from the proximal palmar edge of the middle phalanx (3). Occasionally there is an avulsion from the palmar aspect of the proximal phalanx or from the dorsal surface of either the proximal or the middle phalanx. An associated subluxation or dislocation of the proximal interphalangeal joint is often present. The size of the avulsed fragment can vary from a tiny fleck of bone up to half of the surface of the middle phalangeal portion of the proximal interphalangeal articulation. The phalanges on the ulnar side of the hand are involved somewhat more often than are those on the radial side. Simple fixation is usually adequate treatment. This is best accomplished by a splint that limits extension but permits flexion (2). Open reduction is indicated if more than 30% of the joint is affected. Late complications of improper treatment are instability and lack of pinch power. Traumatic arthritis, flexion contracture, or a swan-neck deformity can occur.

A volar plate injury can often be diagnosed clinically from a history of hyperextension injury associated with tenderness on the palmar surface of the proximal interphalangeal joint and pain caused by passive hyperextension of this articulation. There nearly always is swelling around the proximal interphalangeal joint. X-ray examination often shows an avulsion fracture, frequently with dorsal subluxation. The bony fragment usually is best seen on the lateral projection, although occasionally the injury is more accurately delineated with an oblique view. Careful scrutiny and good films may be needed to see a tiny bony avulsion. Failure to discover this type of injury can lead to considerable disability.

Source Materials

1. Gad P. The anatomy of the volar part of the capsules of the finger joints. J Bone Joint Surg 49B:362, 1967.
2. McElfresh EC, Dobyns JH, O'Brien ET. Management of fracture-dislocation of the proximal interphalangeal joints by extension-block splinting. J Bone Joint Surg 54A:1705, 1972.
3. Nance EP Jr, Kaye JJ, Milek MA. Volar plate fractures. Radiology 133:61, 1979.
4. Roemer FJ. Hyperextension injuries to the finger joints. Am J Surg 80:295, 1950.

Case 62

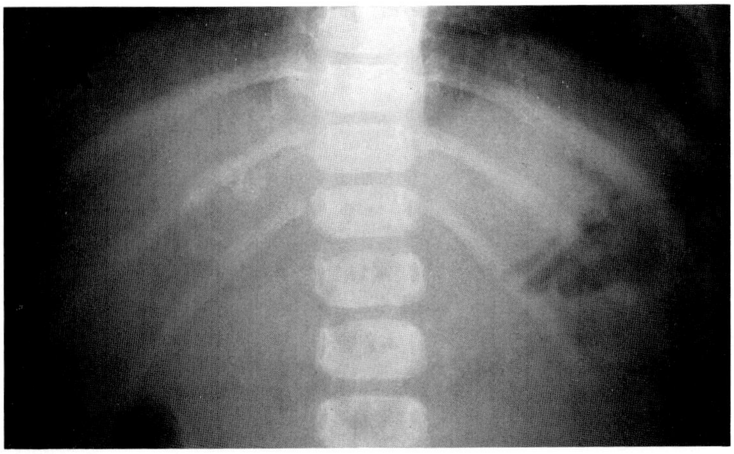

A

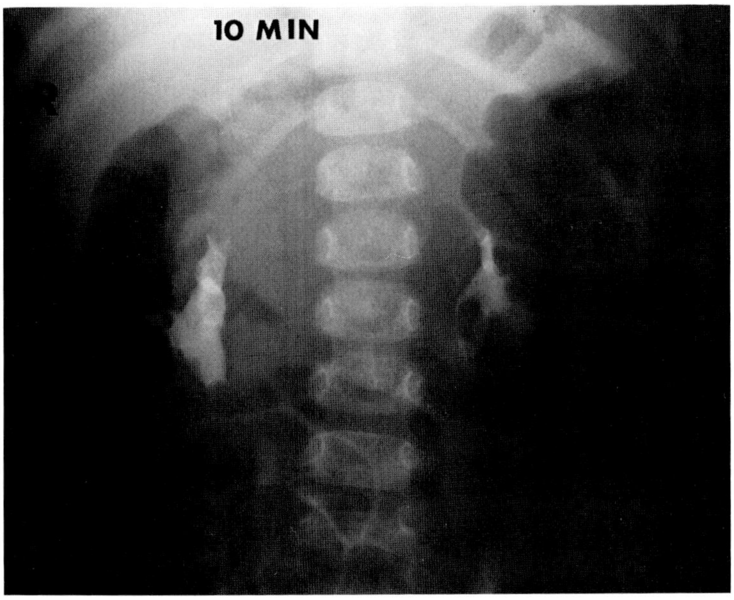

B

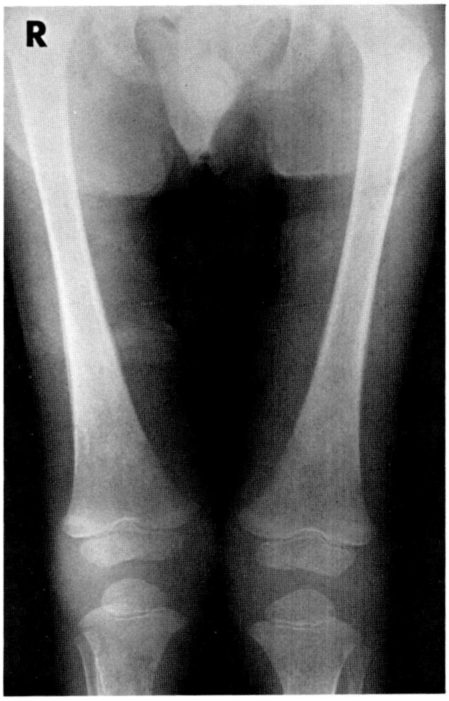

C

Neuroblastoma

Clinical Information

The mother of this 27-month-old white male discovered a right-sided upper abdominal mass. The radiologic diagnosis of a neuroblastoma was confirmed at surgery.

Roentgen Findings

Flocculent calcification in the upper quadrant lies above a nondisplaced normal right kidney (A, B). An anteroposterior film of both thighs and knees (C) shows periosteal reaction overlying bilaterally similar and symmetrical mottled bony destruction in the distal thirds of both femora. Similar destruction is evident in the upper tibiae.

Comments

Neuroblastoma is the most common malignant neoplasm of infants and children, especially newborns. Along with Wilms' tumor it forms the great bulk of childhood retroperitoneal malignancies. More than 50% of retroperitoneal neuroblastomas in newborns originate in the adrenals, though an adrenal origin is somewhat less frequent in older children. About 25% of all neuroblastomas do not originate in the adrenals, and a similar percentage are diagnosed during the first year of life. Most are discovered before the age of 5.

Three-quarters of all patients with this tumor have metastases at the time of diagnosis. These tumors occasionally produce catecholamines. Their metabolites may be found in the urine, and there can be associated symptoms of sweating, diarrhea, and tachycardia. In fact, the mother of an infant born with a neuroblastoma may complain of these symptoms, which resemble eclampsia, from catecholamines that cross the placenta. Tumor spread is by both hematogenous and lymphatic routes. The bones, lymph nodes, and liver are frequent sites of metastases. Pulmonary metastases are uncommon, a differential point between neuroblastoma and Wilms' tumor. Osseous metastases occur in only 2% of neonates but are present in two-thirds of children over 2 years of age. Subcutaneous metastases, noted almost exclusively in infants, are associated with a relatively good prognosis. Retroorbital metastases lead to exophthalmos and periorbital ecchymosis. Intracranial spread frequently localizes along the sutural lines and causes separation, which is not the result of increased intracranial pressure. Neuroblastoma in situ is an incidental autopsy finding in about 1.5% of children who die of other causes. Treatment includes surgery, radiation, and chemotherapy. A few neuroblastomas apparently maturate into benign ganglioneuromas. The overall survival is about 35%. Prognosis is better the younger the patient is at the time of diagnosis. Liver metastases have a better prognosis than bony or pulmonary metastases.

Half of adrenal neuroblastomas show calcification. An adrenal neuroblastoma commonly displaces the kidneys downward and laterally. Wilms' tumor usually distorts the collecting system and frequently displaces the renal pelvis medially and anteriorly. The renal pelvis may be both compressed and displaced by an adrenal neuroblastoma. The displacement is important, since other retroperitoneal tumors tend to rotate the kidney and compress but not displace the renal pelvis (3). A left adrenal neuroblastoma may mimic a pancreatic tumor. Bony metastases appear as mottled destruction, which can resemble Ewing's tumor, and are often bilaterally symmetrical (2). There frequently is associated periosteal proliferation. Computed tomography and ultrasound can be valuable and may be the only method by which a diagnosis is reached (2, 4). Technetium-99m methylene diphosphonate shows uptake in the soft tissues of a neuroblastoma. This finding is said to be pathognomonic of a neural crest neoplasm (1). Radiologic examinations occasionally are positive for metastases when scans are normal.

Source Materials

1. Podrasky AE, Stark DD, Hattner RS, et al. Radionuclide bone scanning in neuroblastoma: Skeletal metastases and primary tumor localization of 99m Tc-MDP. AJR 141:469, 1983.
2. Stark DD, Brasch RC, Moss AA, et al. Recurrent neuroblastoma: The role of CT and alternative imaging tests. Radiology 148:107, 1983.
3. Stark DD, Moss AA, Brasch RC, et al. Neuroblastoma: Diagnostic imaging and staging. Radiology 148:101, 1983.
4. White SJ, Stuck KJ, Blane CE, Silver TM. Sonography of neuroblastoma. AJR 141:465, 1983.

Case 63

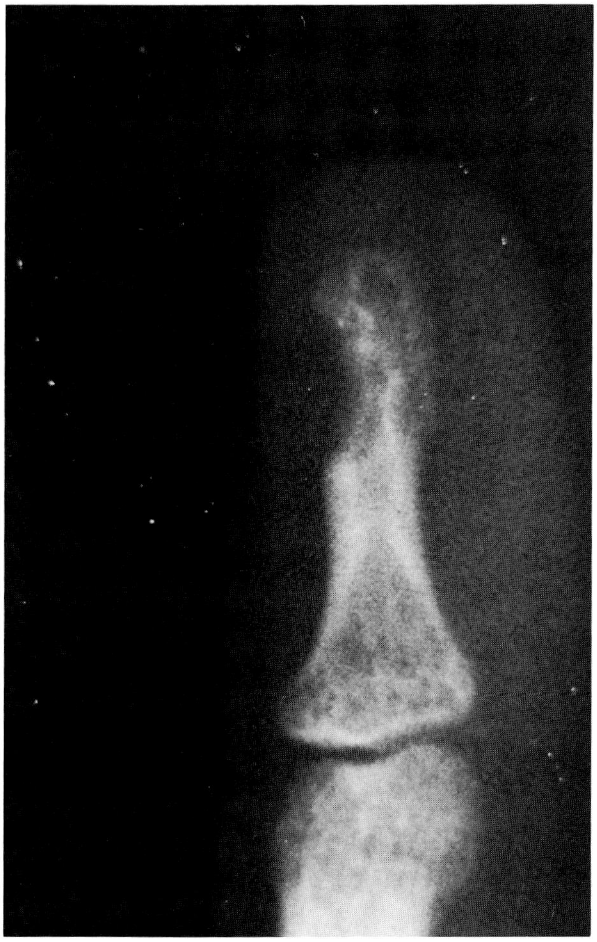

A

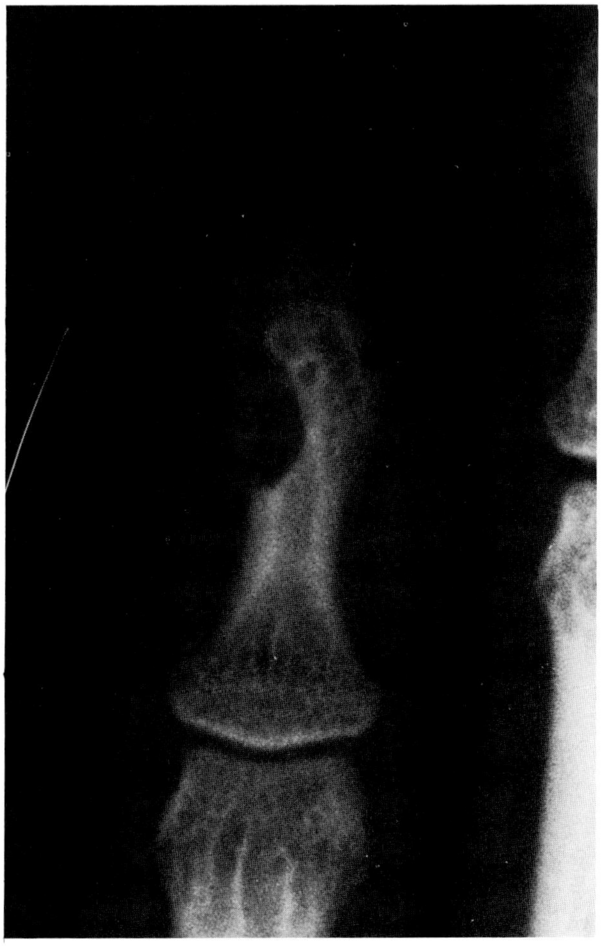

B

Glomus Tumor

Clinical Information

This 30-year-old white female came to medical attention because of an increasingly painful and sensitive terminal portion of the ring finger of her right hand. A tiny discolored area beneath the fingernail proved to be a glomus tumor. It was surgically removed with complete relief of the patient's symptoms.

Roentgen Findings

A small oval area of extrinsic bony destruction is seen in the ulnar and dorsal aspects of the tuft of the right ring finger (A, B).

Comments

Bone involvement by tumors of vascular origin, whether benign or malignant, is uncommon. Glomus (Latin for ball) tumors, or glomangiomas, represent fewer than 2% of all soft tissue tumors of the extremities. These tumors were mentioned in writings of Hippocrates and Galen. They are benign hamartomatous lesions characterized by hypertrophy of the specialized glomus apparatus, which is interposed in lieu of capillaries between the terminal arterioles and venules. The function of the glomus apparatus apparently involves the regulation of skin circulation and temperature control. Although widely distributed throughout the body in adults, glomus cells are not evident in infants less than 1 year of age and are seen in decreasing frequency after the age of 60. They are found in various parts of the upper and lower extremities, more commonly the upper (70%). In addition to glomus cells, glomangiomas contain smooth muscle, nonmyelinated nerve fibers, and connective tissue. The lesion is histologically encapsulated and never invasive. There is no associated inflammatory reaction.

A glomus tumor is a small, inconspicuous subcutaneous tumor, which develops slowly during adult life. Its diameter is 1 cm or less. The tumor is virtually always solitary and it is most common between the ages of 30 and 60. There is a slight male predominance, although a subungual location is particularly common in females. The lesion is located beneath a fingernail in 30% of cases. The skin is intact and the nail remains flat or only slightly raised. There may be a measure of discoloration, which ranges from red to blue, especially blue. The tumor may pulsate slightly and skin temperature can be elevated locally. These lesions are extremely tender. Excruciating burning or shooting pain, both local and referred up the extremity, occurs spontaneoulsy or is produced by pressure over the tumor. Heat, excessive cold, and even contact with clothing can become intolerable so that protection is required continuously day and night. Proper treatment involves surgical excision, which usually brings complete and immediate relief. There are reports of glomus tumors arising within bone, although this is rare (4). Difficulty may be encountered in determining whether these tumors actually arise within bone or are in fact soft tissue tumors that have subsequently eroded bone from pressure exerted by the extraosseous tumor.

Bony x-ray abnormalities are seen in about 20% of glomus tumors of the hands. These changes are characterized by erosion from extrinsic pressure, which nearly always is located in the tuft of a terminal phalanx. Consequently, the bony defect is smooth and concave without an overlying rim of bone. The margin of the lesion is smooth and marked by a narrowed zone of sclerosis. It most commonly is located on the dorsal aspect of the tuft. As is true in this case, the defect can be marginal. It also can appear as a through-and-through punched-out lesion that penetrates the full thickness of the bone. There may be some disuse osteoporosis. A glomus tumor must be differentiated from an epidermoid inclusion cyst, which can look quite similar, although the latter usually has a thin surrounding bony cortical surface and is not painful.

Source Materials

1. Carroll RE, Berman AT. Glomus tumors of the hand. J Bone Joint Surg 54A:691, 1972.
2. Mathis WH Jr, Schulz MD. Roentgen diagnosis of glomus tumors. Radiology 51:71, 1948.
3. Rypins EL. The roentgenologic aspects of the subungual glomus tumor. AJR 46:667, 1941.
4. Sugiura I. Intra-osseous glomus tumour. J Bone Joint Surg 58B:245, 1976.

Case 64

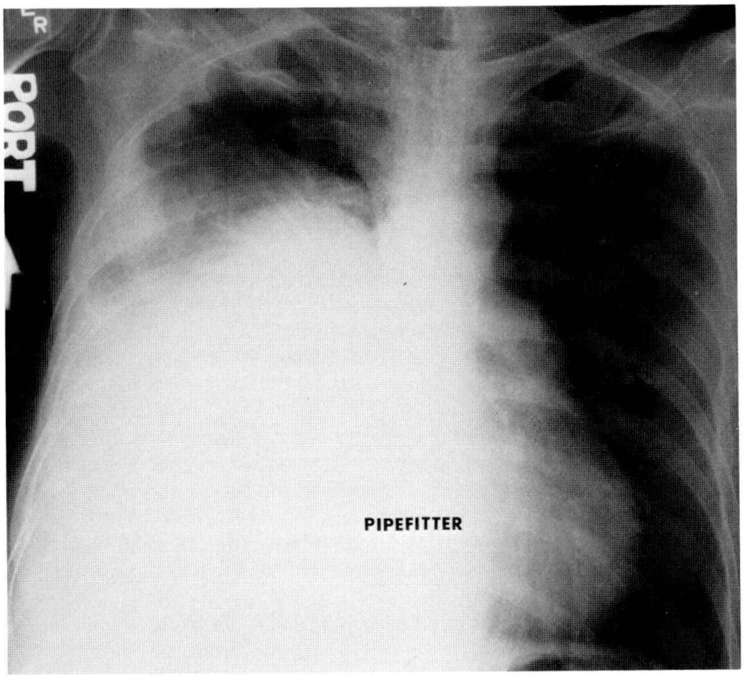

A

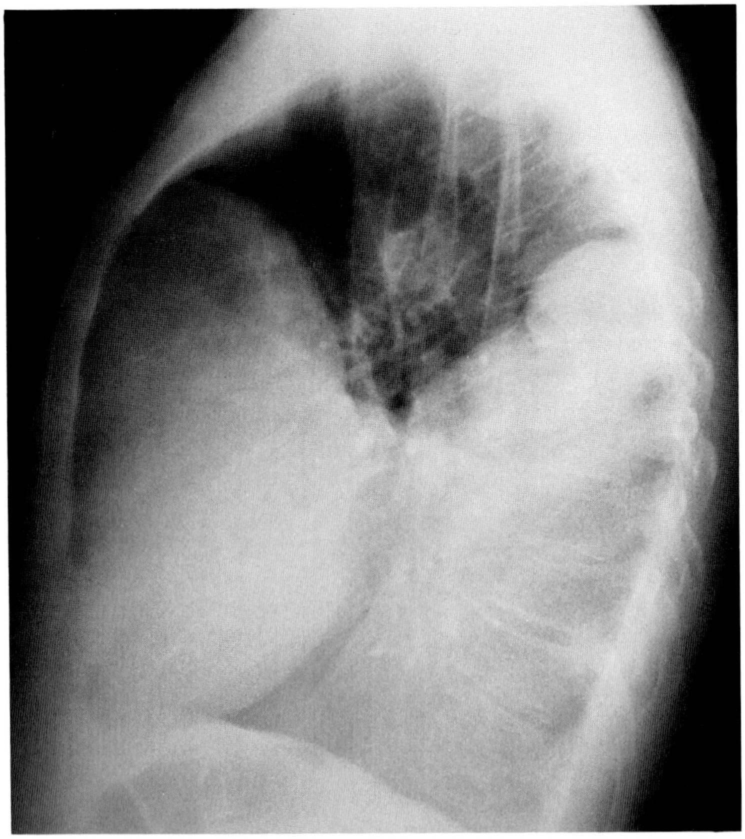

B

Mesothelioma

Clinical Information

This 60-year-old pipefitter was admitted for rapidly progressive shortness of breath and increasing cough. A pleural biopsy revealed a mesothelioma. His course was rapidly downhill with death occurring 5 weeks after these films were obtained.

Roentgen Findings

Anteroposterior (A) and lateral (B) chest films show the heart and left lung to be normal. The mediastinum is in the midline. There are multiple nodules of soft tissue density within the right hemothorax as well as evidence of pleural fluid. The latter was proved to be relatively small with a lateral decubitus film. Some of the soft tissue densities are quite large. Each approximates a pleural surface.

Comments

Mesotheliomas arise from the serous lining of a pleural, pericardial, or peritoneal cavity. Malignant mesotheliomas are increasing in frequency because of more extensive industrial use of asbestos. From 20% to 75% of patients with a malignant mesothelioma have an occupational or environmental exposure to asbestos (1). An association with smoking does not increase the incidence of mesothelioma as it does bronchogenic carcinoma. This suggests that irritation by the asbestos fibers may be etiologic in mesothelioma, whereas carcinogens are more likely of significance in bronchogenic carcinoma. Patients with malignant mesotheliomas usually do not have x-ray evidence of pneumoconiosis. The exposure needed to cause a mesothelioma apparently is less than that needed for asbestotic pneumoconiosis. Pleural calcification is uncommon. Malignant mesotheliomas can metastasize widely. Treatment is unsatisfactory.

A mesothelioma may be benign or malignant. Both usually develop between the ages of 30 and 60. A localized fibrous benign mesothelioma is less common and does not cause respiratory symptoms but can lead to pulmonary hypertrophic osteoarthropathy or hypoglycemia, both of which are said not to occur with malignant mesothelioma. There is no known association with asbestos exposure. Benign mesotheliomas can grow slowly to great size. They usually are not associated with a pleural effusion. These tumors are frequently pedunculated and can change position with respiration or alteration of the patient's posture (4). Such a change is virtually diagnostic. Complete resection cures a benign mesothelioma.

Malignant mesotheliomas usually form multiple nodules on a pleural surface. The involvement is usually unilateral. Cough, dyspnea, and chest pain are common. Most of these patients have a pleural effusion, which can be massive. Somewhat more than half of the effusions are sanguinous. The pleural effusion can displace the mediastinum (tension effusion), although prior fibrosis may have stabilized midline structures. The nodules along the chest wall or fissural surfaces are best seen after withdrawal of some pleural fluid followed by the introduction of air. It may be difficult to determine whether the nodular densities are tumor tissue or localized collections of pleural fluid. Pleural metastases may mimic a malignant mesothelioma, although unilaterality of the lesions strongly favors a primary pleural tumor. A hilar mass is occasionally evident and invasion of the chest wall is not uncommon. A malignant mesothelioma can extend medially to encircle and constrict the central hilar portions of the lung. Rib involvement is not rare (3). Computed tomography is of value in the diagnosis of these lesions (2).

Source Materials

1. Antman KH. Malignant mesothelioma. N Engl J Med 303:200, 1980.
2. Grant DC, Seltzer SE, Antman KH, et al. Computed tomography of malignant pleural mesothelioma. J Comput Assist Tomogr 7:626, 1983.
3. Steiner RM, Cooper MW, Brodovsky H. Rib destruction: A neglected finding in malignant mesothelioma. Clin Radiol 33:61, 1982.
4. Weisbrod GL, Yee AC. Computed tomographic diagnosis of a pedunculated fibrous mesothelioma. J Can Assoc Radiol 34:147, 1983.

Case 65

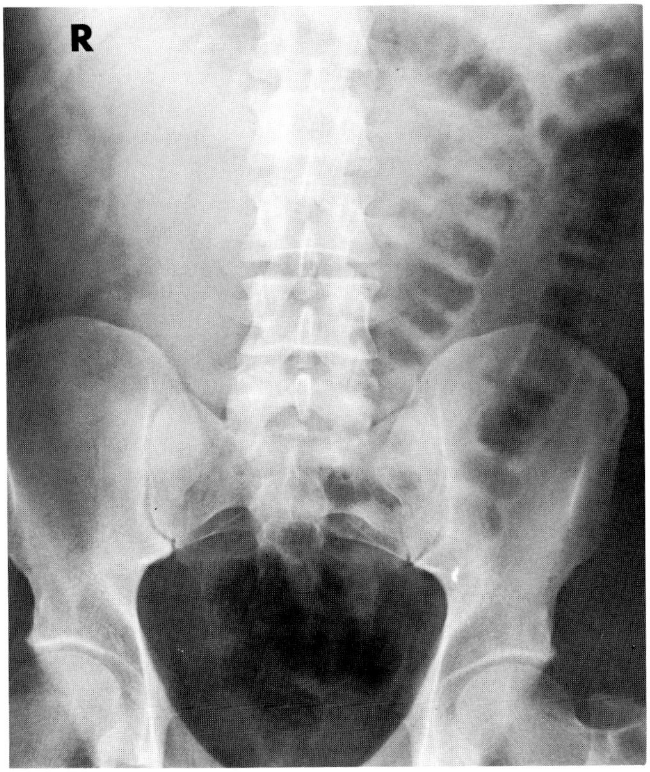

A

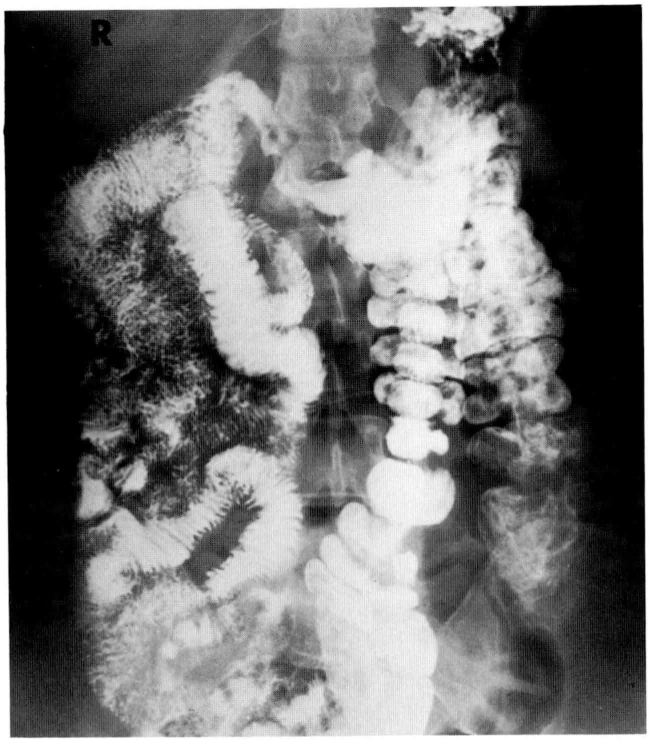

B

Intestinal Malrotation

Clinical Information

This 36-year-old male with hepatitis was admitted for abdominal pain.

Roentgen Findings

A flat film of the abdomen (A) shows ascending and descending colonic gas in the left side of the abdomen. A previous small bowel study (B) had revealed complete malrotation with the small bowel on the right and all of the colon on the left.

Comments

Colonic malrotation is a developmental abnormality that usually affects the small bowel as well as the colon. There are many variations of this condition. Each leads to a different anatomical location of the intestinal segments. These abnormalities usually represent incomplete intestinal rotation or complete lack of rotation. Normal attachment of the mesentery to the posterior abdominal wall does not occur. This leaves mobile portions of the gut, which are subject to volvulus. Symptoms, if any, can vary. Most acute episodes occur in neonates or children. Eighty percent of acute episodes occur within the first month of life, and nearly all present with persistent vomiting, which usually is bilious. These symptoms are almost always secondary to volvulus or Ladd's band. Malrotation in adults rarely causes symptoms. The complaint when present usually is intermittent abdominal cramping or pain, which results from transient volvulus. Such patients usually show no radiologic abnormality other than malrotation.

Normal intestinal rotation primarily involves two portions of the intestinal tract, the duodenojejunal segment and the cecocolic segment. Rotation of these two segments of the midgut, which includes all of the bowel from the middle of the duodenum to the distal transverse colon, occurs between the fifth and eighth weeks of fetal life (2). The duodenojejunal segment passes beneath the superior mesenteric artery to eventually find its normal location in the left upper quadrant after 270° of counterclockwise rotation. The cecocolic segment also undergoes 270° of rotation, which places the cecum in the right lower quadrant. The cecum is the last portion to reach a definitive location. All degrees of malrotation of each of these two segments and in all combinations can occur. Each may occur independently.

The x-ray findings of malrotation are diverse. Plain films may be normal but can show the colon in the left side of the abdomen and the small bowel in the right side. The exact location of each segment can be confirmed with barium studies. Ladd's bands usually affect the duodenum and are often found in symptomatic infants. Volvulus may lead to a mass and an abnormal corkscrew appearance of the small bowel as it twists around the superior mesenteric artery. Mucosal edema due to venous and lymphatic obstruction may be evident. Location of the duodenojejunal junction is important. It defines the rotation of the duodenojejunal segment. Rotation is complete if it is situated to the left of the spine without a z-shaped configuration (1). Partial malrotation is present when it overlies the spine. Location of the duodenojejunal junction to the right of the spine indicates no rotation of the proximal segment. Similarly, all of the colon to the left of the spine indicates total lack of rotation of the cecocolic segment. The angiographic findings of midgut volvulus in the adult are characterized by the "barber pole" sign and dilatation of the mesenteric veins. The "barber pole" sign results from twisting of the superior mesenteric artery (3). Midgut malrotation has been confused radiologically with intussusception, both from the x-ray appearance and from its symptoms (4). Evidence of malrotation elsewhere in the bowel should obviate this error.

Source Materials

1. Ablow RC, Hoffer FA, Seashore JH, Touloukian RJ. Z-Shaped duodenojejunal loop: Sign of mesenteric fixation anomaly and congenital bands. AJR 141:461, 1983.
2. Balthazar EJ. Intestinal malrotation in adults: Roentgenographic assessment with emphasis on isolated complete and partial nonrotations. AJR 126:358, 1976.
3. Griska LB, Popky GL. Angiography in mid-gut malrotation with volvulus. AJR 134:1055, 1980.
4. Schey WL. Malrotation simulating intussusception on barium enema. Pediatr Radiol 9:149, 1980.

Case 66

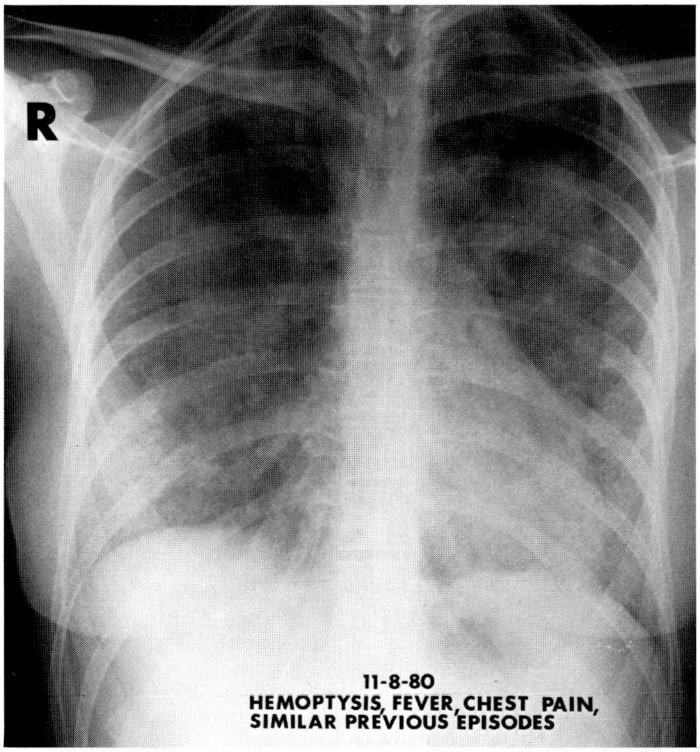
R
11-8-80
HEMOPTYSIS, FEVER, CHEST PAIN,
SIMILAR PREVIOUS EPISODES

A

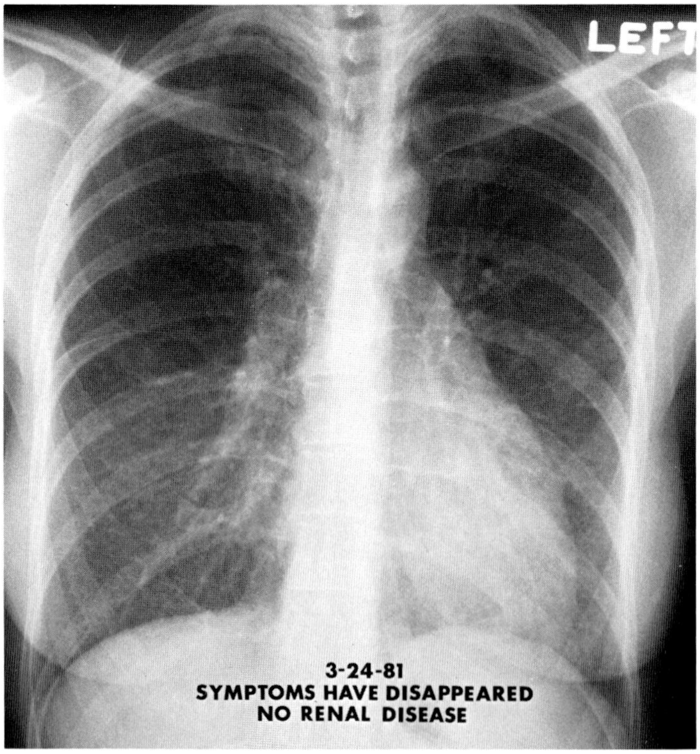
LEFT
3-24-81
SYMPTOMS HAVE DISAPPEARED
NO RENAL DISEASE

B

Idiopathic Pulmonary Hemosiderosis

Clinical Information

This 37-year-old white female had experienced several episodes of dyspnea, fever, cough, chest pain, and hemoptysis. She was experiencing a recurrence at the time the 11-8-80 film (A) was obtained. She had no renal disease or antiglomerular basement membrane antibodies. A lung biopsy was consistent with idiopathic pulmonary hemosiderosis (IPH).

Roentgen Findings

A posteroanterior chest film (A) shows fluffy alveolar densities occupying the lower two-thirds of both lungs. No pleural effusion is seen. The alveolar densities are not present on film B, taken when her symptoms had cleared. A faint, streaky granular density occupying the lower half of both lungs is poorly reproduced but clearly evident on the original film.

Comments

IPH is an uncommon disease characterized by hemoptysis, iron-deficiency anemia, and chest film abnormalities. Its cause is unknown, although many possibilities have been suggested. No consistent hereditary pattern exists for IPH, although two members of the same family have been affected (1). IPH was previously thought to particularly affect young individuals, especially females. It is now known that adults may have this condition, with adult males and females being affected in about equal frequency. Factors that precipitate the hemorrhage are unknown. Patients with this condition suffer recurrent episodes of shortness of breath, cyanosis, cough, hemoptysis, and chest or abdominal pain. Acute attacks last a few days and subside gradually. They can be fulminant and lead to death from pulmonary hemorrhage. Although IPH may cause few symptoms, pulmonary fibrosis, reduced pulmonary function, and even cor pulmonale can follow repeated hemorrhages. No consistently effective treatment exists. It has been said that death occurs on the average about 2½ years after the first symptoms (4). The pulmonary hemorrhage occurs distal to the cilia escalator. Consequently, hemorrhage can be present without hemoptysis, other symptoms, or an abnormal chest film. Carbon monoxide uptake is a simple procedure to detect fresh lung hemorrhage in such situations. Chromium tagging studies may show increased uptake over the lung fields when the disease is clinically inactive.

The diagnosis of IPH is primarily a matter of excluding other etiologies in a patient who has episodes of pulmonary hemorrhage and appropriate x-ray findings (2). There are numerous causes of pulmonary hemorrhage (3). These include mitral stenosis and congestive heart failure; various vasculitides such as periarteritis nodosa, Wegener's granulomatosis, or systemic lupus erythematosis, which can also cause renal disease; infection, particularly viral pneumonia; trauma; and cancer. Pulmonary hemorrhage is frequently associated with kidney disease, especially uremia, glomerulonephritis, or Goodpasture's syndrome. Goodpasture's syndrome often affects young males and is characterized by linear deposits of immunoglobulins on the renal basement membranes that can be demonstrated by immunofluorescent studies of a kidney biopsy. Circulating antiglomerular basement membrane antibodies can also be demonstrated, and in patients with pulmonary hemorrhage these immunoglobulins are also deposited on the basement membranes of the alveolar septal walls. Such findings are not present in IPH. Many patients at first thought to have IPH turn out to have Goodpasture's syndrome.

X-ray evidence of pulmonary hemorrhage is seen as widespread patchy alveolar densities. They often have a grainy or "ground glass" appearance and tend to involve the perihilar and lower lung areas. These densities clear rather slowly and frequently leave a background haze due to a large number of very small densities, which can resemble miliary tuberculosis. Total clearing usually occurs within 2 weeks. Pleural effusion is rare unless there is superimposed heart failure or infection. A pulmonary density that is sharply limited by a fissure or involves an apex or a cardiophrenic angle is suggestive of infection. The same is true if there is loss of definition of either the cardiac or diaphragmatic silhouettes. Repeated bleeds usually lead to pulmonary scarring and fibrosis. X-ray evidence of cor pulmonale may be seen when pulmonary function tests show severe restrictive disease.

Source Materials

1. Beckerman RC, Taussig LM, Pinnas JL. Familial idiopathic pulmonary hemosiderosis. Am J Dis Child 133:609, 1979.
2. Case records of the Massachusetts General Hospital. Case 30-1979. N Engl J Med 301:201, 1979.
3. Seltzer SE, Herman PG. Pulmonary hemorrhage and renal disease. JCE Radiol 1:11, 1979.
4. Turner-Warwick M, Dewar A. Pulmonary haemorrhage and pulmonary haemosiderosis. Clin Radiol 33:361, 1982.

Case 67

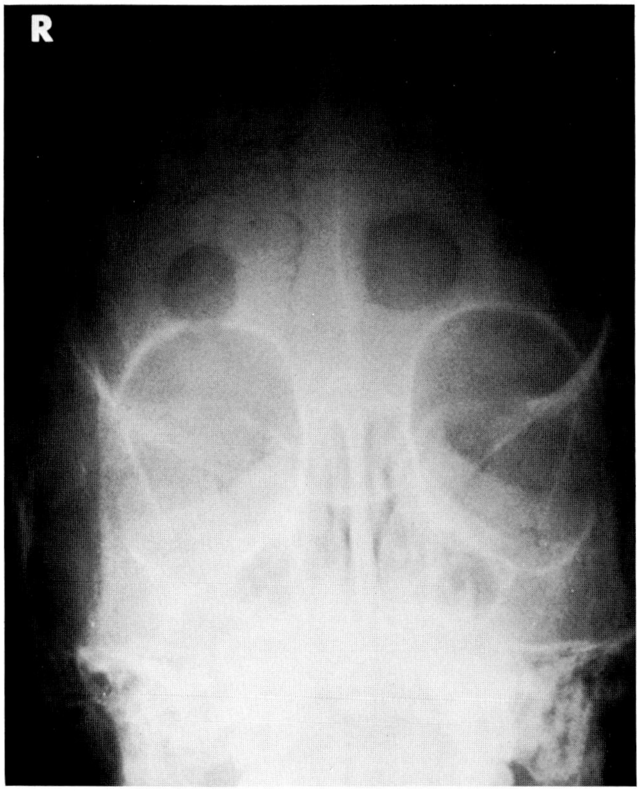

A

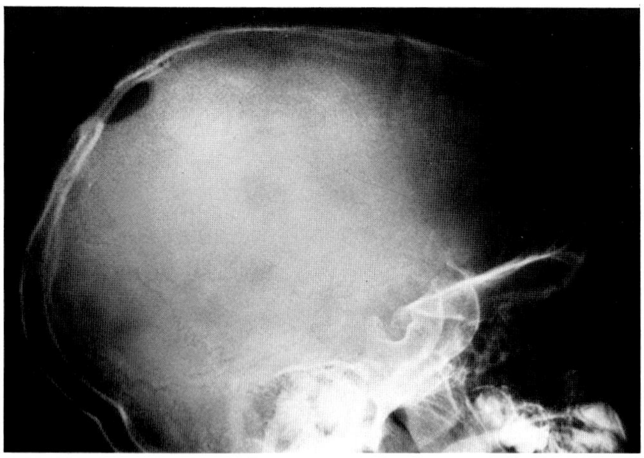

B

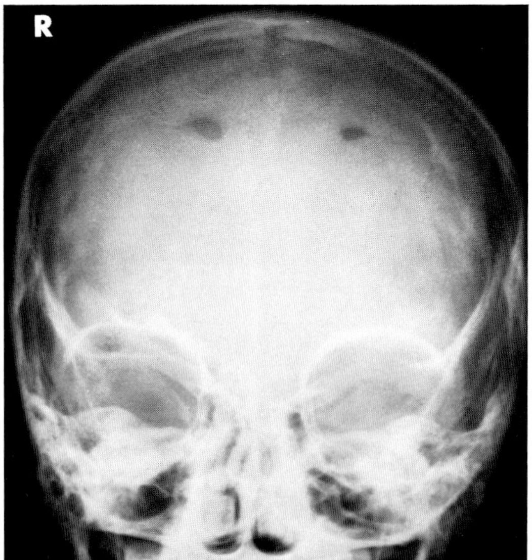

C (another patient)

Parietal Foramina

Clinical Information

Films of the skull were obtained on this 3½-year-old black female following a deep laceration above the right eye that was sustained from a fall on a concrete porch. She was otherwise completely normal.

Roentgen Findings

No fractures are seen. Rounded bilateral bony deficiencies, slightly larger on the left, which measure about 2 cm in diameter are present in the posterosuperior portion of each parietal bone (A, B). The margins of these defects are smooth and bevelled outwardly. The appearance is typical of parietal foramina.

Comments

Parietal foramina are round or oval defects in the posterosuperior portion of the parietal bones. The edges of these defects are smooth. They are often bevelled outwardly with the outer edge inscribing a slightly larger opening than does the inner edge. The foramina can be very small (see film C from another patient) or quite large, even reaching 50 mm in diameter. They are always located about 4 cm in front of the lambdoid suture and 1–2 cm from the midline. The defect is closed by a fibrous membrane which is common to both the dura and the pericranium. Very rarely there is a thin shell of bone over the defect, and the overlying scalp is occasionally hairless. Parietal foramina result from failure of mineralization in the area of bony deficiency. Total mineralization of this portion of the skull normally is not present at birth. It becomes completely ossified in the second year of life. Parietal foramina that are present at the end of the third year do not get smaller with the passage of time. These characteristic bony defects may be associated with various other anomalies, although they frequently are isolated and cause no symptoms. Inheritance is dominant (2, 3). Parietal foramina was described over 60 years ago in many members of a family named Catlin in Iowa. This led to the condition sometimes being known as the "Catlin mark."

Parietal foramina are but one of several variations seen in this region of the skull, called the obelion possibly for this very reason, since the word is derived from obelisk, an ancient symbol to indicate an abnormal passage. These variations include tiny openings called small parietal foramina or emissary parietal foramina. These transmit the vein of Santorini, which connects epicranial occipital veins with the superior sagittal sinus. A small branch of the occipital artery occasionally passes through these foramina, which are 1–2 mm in diameter, usually bilateral, and are present in about half of the population. There may be no bone in the midline, which leads to a persistent midline foramen. Multiple fenestrations are occasionally seen in the bone that forms the obelion. There may also be bone thinning in this region as well as encephaloceles, in addition to the relatively frequent large parietal foramina (1).

It is important not to confuse parietal foramina with burr holes, which are usually more posterior and farther lateral. Epidermoid cysts and syphilitic lesions usually are not situated in this location. Conditions such as histiocytosis x and metastatic disease are more likely to cause irregular bony defects.

Source Materials

1. Currarino G. Normal variants and congenital anomalies in the region of the obelion. AJR 127:487, 1976.
2. Fein JM, Brinker RA. Evolution and significance of giant parietal foramina: Report of five cases in one family. J Neurosurg 37:487, 1972.
3. Goldsmith WM. The Catlin mark: The inheritance of an unusual opening in the parietal bones. J Hered 13:69, 1922.
4. Murphy J. Gooding CA. Evolution of persistently enlarged parietal foramina. Radiology 97:391, 1970.

Case 68

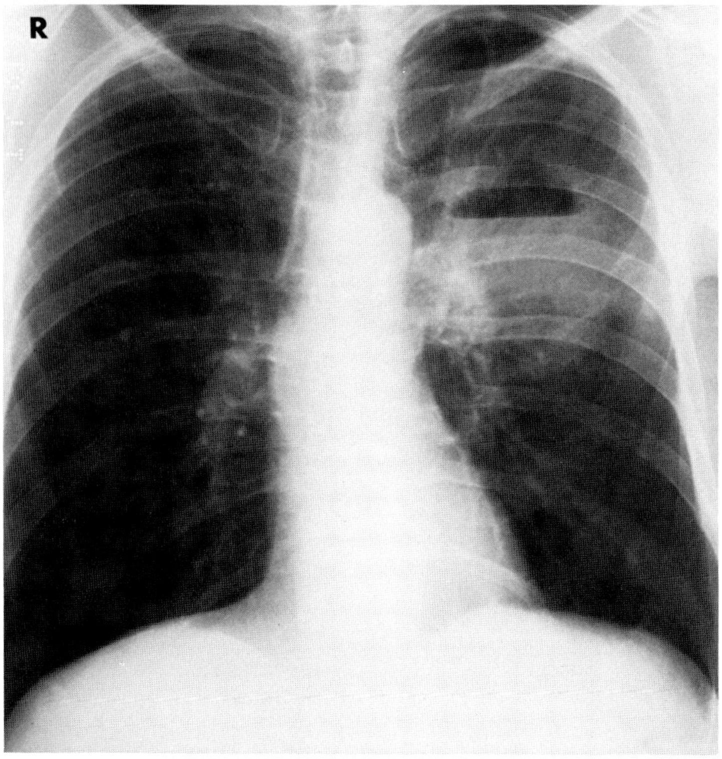

A

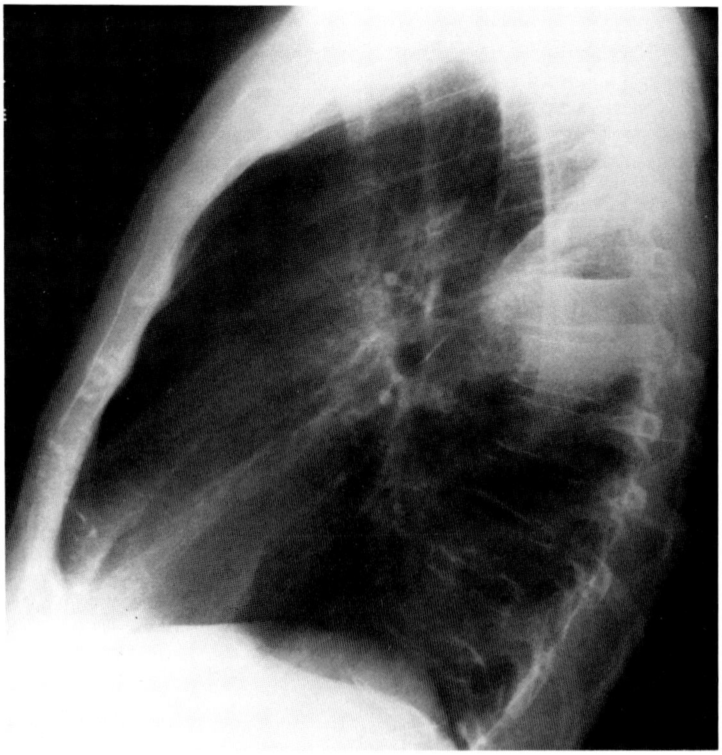

B

Lung Abscess

Clinical Information

This 52-year-old chronic alcoholic male had a normal chest film until 3 weeks before these films were taken, when he developed a cough, fever, foul-smelling sputum, and weight loss. His lung abscess closed after 4 months of antibiotic therapy.

Roentgen Findings

A fluid level of approximately equal length on the posteroanterior (A) and lateral (B) chest films is seen within a large, rounded parenchymal density in the superior segment of the left lower lobe. The wall of the cavity is smooth and measures about 4 mm in its thickest portion.

Comments

A lung abscess results from infectious necrosis of pulmonary tissue. Almost any organism, aerobic or anaerobic, can cause a lung abscess, but it is more likely to be Gram-negative than Gram-positive in a ratio of about 3:2. The flora of a lung abscess usually is mixed. Many conditions predispose a patient to develop a lung abscess. These include seizures, alcoholic abuse, general or topical anesthesia, sinusitis, and poor dental hygiene. All can lead to aspiration. Debilitation is commonly present. Septic emboli can cause multiple small abscesses. The source of septic emboli is usually thrombophlebitis or bacterial endocarditis of the tricuspid valve. The latter is most often encountered in drug addicts. Cancer can obstruct a bronchus and lead to an abscess in the distal atelectatic and consolidated pulmonary tissue. No antecedent cause is found in 15–20% of lung abscesses.

Lung abscesses tend to be segmental and peripheral. They are usually located in dependent pulmonary segments, namely, the posterior segments of the upper lobes and the superior segments of the lower lobes. A lung abscess is more likely to occur in the right lung because of its straighter main bronchus. Patients with a lung abscess often raise large amounts of foul-smelling, purulent sputum, which is sometimes bloody. The coughing often occurs in paroxysms precipitated by a change in position that effects a sudden drainage of the abscess. Clubbing may develop rapidly. About 25% of lung abscesses heal without treatment. In the absence of therapy, the remainder usually go progressively downhill with death from infection or complications such as a brain abscess or meningitis. Treatment is primarily medical. It is possible to drain the abscess surgically, at bronchoscopy, or even percutaneously (1, 2). Pneumothorax and empyema are possible complications. Improvements in treatment have reduced the mortality rate from near 50% to under 5%.

Chest films show excavation of an area of pulmonary infiltration as a lung abscess develops. Adjacent pleural reaction, including effusion, may be present. Hilar and mediastinal adenopathy are seen in about half of lung abscesses, even though the offending organism usually is not commonly thought of as causing lymphadenopathy. The thickness of the wall of a pulmonary cavity is diagnostically important (3, 4). A solitary pulmonary cavity with a wall that is no more than 4 mm at its thickest part is almost invariably benign, whereas 95% of cavities with a wall thickness of over 15 mm are malignant. Cavities with a wall that measures between 5 and 15 mm are about evenly divided between malignant and benign lesions. A smooth cavity lining is more likely to be benign in a ratio of about 2:1. An irregular lining of a cavity tends to be a malignant lesion in a ratio of about 4:1. Lung abscesses usually have thicker walls and more irregular shapes than do empyemas. The length of a fluid level in an empyema cavity may be different on the posteroanterior film from its length on the lateral film. This is in contrast to a lung abscess, which shows similar lengths in all projections because the lesion is relatively spherical. Septic emboli appear as multiple smaller abscess cavities scattered throughout the lungs.

Source Materials

1. Aronberg DJ, Sagel SS, Jost RG, Lee JI. Percutaneous drainage of lung abscess. AJR 132:282, 1979.
2. Estrera AS, Platt MR, Mills LJ, Shaw RR. Primary lung abscess. J Thorac Cardiovasc Surg 79:275, 1980.
3. Woodring JH, Fried AM, Chuang VP. Solitary cavities of the lung: Diagnostic implications of cavity wall thickness. AJR 135:1269, 1980.
4. Woodring JH, Fried AM. Significance of wall thickness in solitary cavities of the lung: A follow-up study. AJR 140:473, 1983.

Case 69

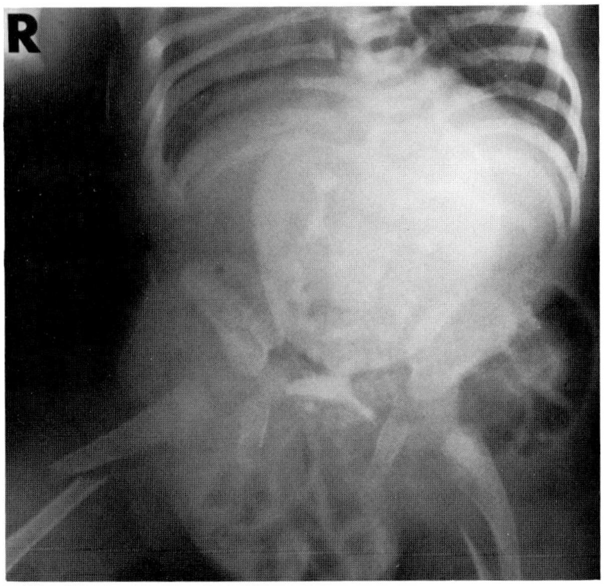

A

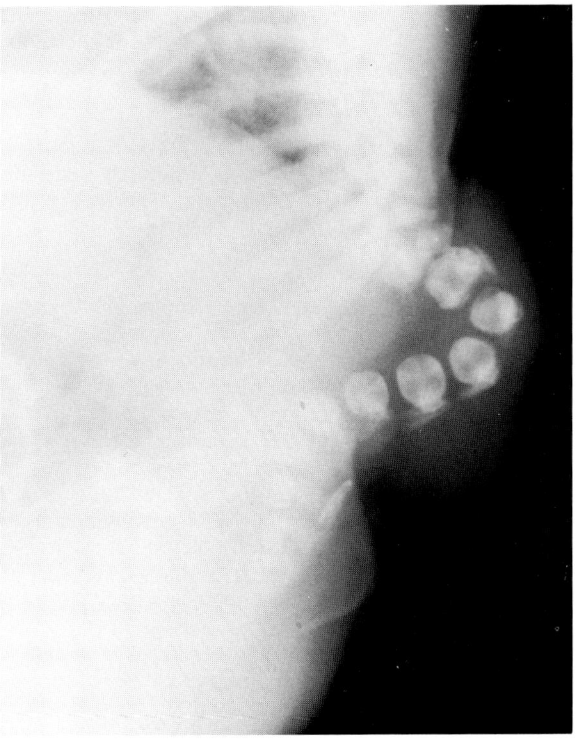

B

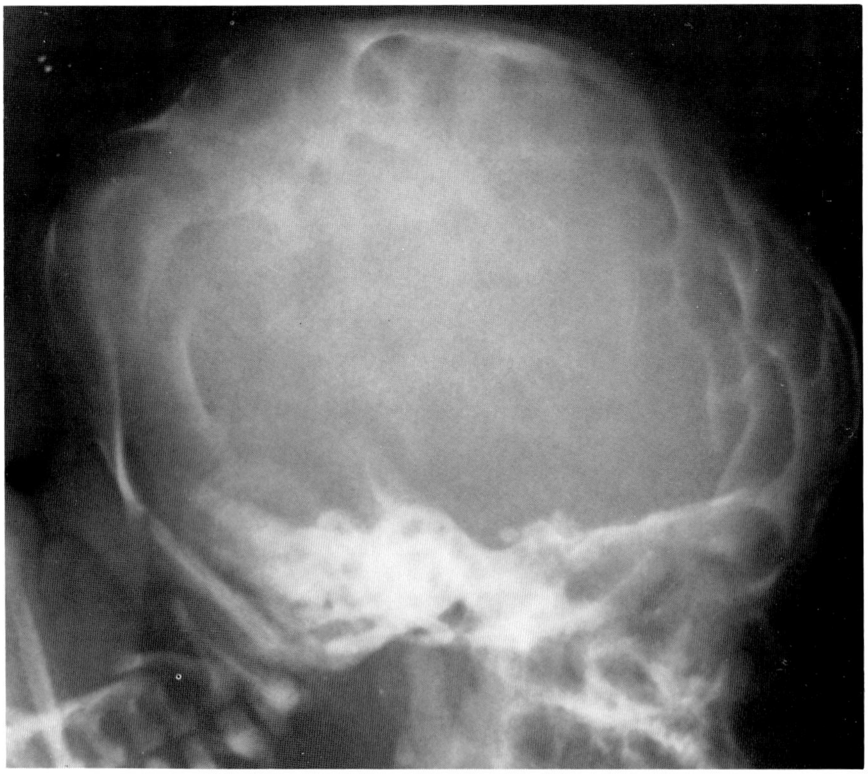

C

Myelomeningocele

Clinical Information

Nothing is known concerning the prenatal history or birth of this newborn male, who appeared to be paraplegic. Both feet were clubbed. Irreducible bilateral inguinal hernias were present. There was a weeping soft tissue mass on the lower back.

Roentgen Findings

An anteroposterior babygram (A) after injection of an intravenous contrast agent shows a large, sharply outlined midline soft tissue density in the lumbar region, which surrounds several markedly widened vertebrae. Hemivertebrae and other congenital spinal anomalies are evident. The lateral film (B) shows a sharp kyphosis within the soft tissue density. Both kidneys function adequately. The bladder is incompletely shown. A lateral skull film (C) shows craniolacunia. Unexplained femoral fractures are present.

Comments

Incomplete closure of the spinal canal takes many forms. There may be isolated lack of fusion of the posterior elements (spina bifida occulta). At times only meninges herniate through the spinal defect (meningocele). Inclusion of spinal cord parenchyma within the herniate tissue (myelomeningocele) is nine times more common than a meningocele. There is a considerable difference in the frequency of spina bifida cystica throughout the world. It varies between 0.2 per thousand in Japan to 4.2 per thousand in Ireland. The underlying embryologic pathogenesis is unknown, but developmental arrest or rupture of the neural tube is probably involved. Eighty percent of myelomeningoceles affect the lumbosacral region. Symptoms depend upon the neural damage and can vary from complete flaccid paralysis to no functional deficiency. There often are many associated anomalies. All of these patients have an Arnold-Chiari malformation. Associated hydrocephalus is extremely common and, along with hydromelia, may lead to increasing symptoms in patients who survive. Shunting may be beneficial. These patients often have a symptomatic tethered cord, which at times can be surgically divided with resulting clinical improvement. Half of untreated myelomeningocele patients die by 3 months of age, usually from hydrocephalus or central nervous system infection. Urinary tract disorders are very common. These patients often have a neurogenic bladder. Renal failure is the most common cause of death beyond 2 years of age.

No difficulty is encountered in reaching a clinical and radiologic diagnosis. Since treatment is usually unsatisfactory, one major consideration is directed toward an early intrauterine diagnosis to permit an abortion (3, 4). Intrauterine surgery may become available (2). Monitoring for abnormal levels of alpha-fetoprotein in either the mother's serum or the amniotic fluid can select patients for more definitive studies. Although only 1 of 10 children with a myelomeningocele is delivered from a mother who has had a previous baby with dysraphia, the probability of a second child being affected is 1 in 20. Two affected children increase the likelihood to 1 in 10. Elevation of amniotic alpha-fetoprotein to three times normal is associated with a tenfold increase in the likelihood of an abnormal baby. Although alpha-fetoprotein determinations may be either falsely negative or falsely positive, an abnormally elevated level most commonly indicates an open neural tube. Other conditions that can cause increased values include intestinal obstruction and Turner's syndrome. Ultrasound, an effective noninvasive method to search for a prenatal myelomeningocele, does not always demonstrate the abnormality, particularly when it is small (3). Fetoscopy or amniography may be used. Careful amniography is usually diagnostic if the fetal back is viewed in profile, unless the myelomeningocele does not bulge (4). This procedure is not without some risk of inducing labor or causing fetal injury. It is impossible to distinguish an intrauterine meningocele from a myelomeningocele.

Source Materials

1. Griscom NT, Frigoletto FD, Harris GBG. Amniography in second trimester diagnosis of myelomeningocele. AJR 133:1151, 1979.
2. Hodgen GD. Antenatal diagnosis and treatment of fetal skeletal malformations with emphasis on in utero surgery for neural tube defects and limb bud regeneration. JAMA 246:1079, 1981.
3. Miskin M, Baim RS, Allen LC, Benzie RJ. Ultrasonic assessment of fetal spine before 20 weeks' gestation. Radiology 132:131, 1979.
4. Probst FP, Sigurd J. Prenatal radiographic diagnosis of alpha-fetoprotein. Positive malformations in early infancy. Acta Radiol (D) 21:667, 1980.

Case 70

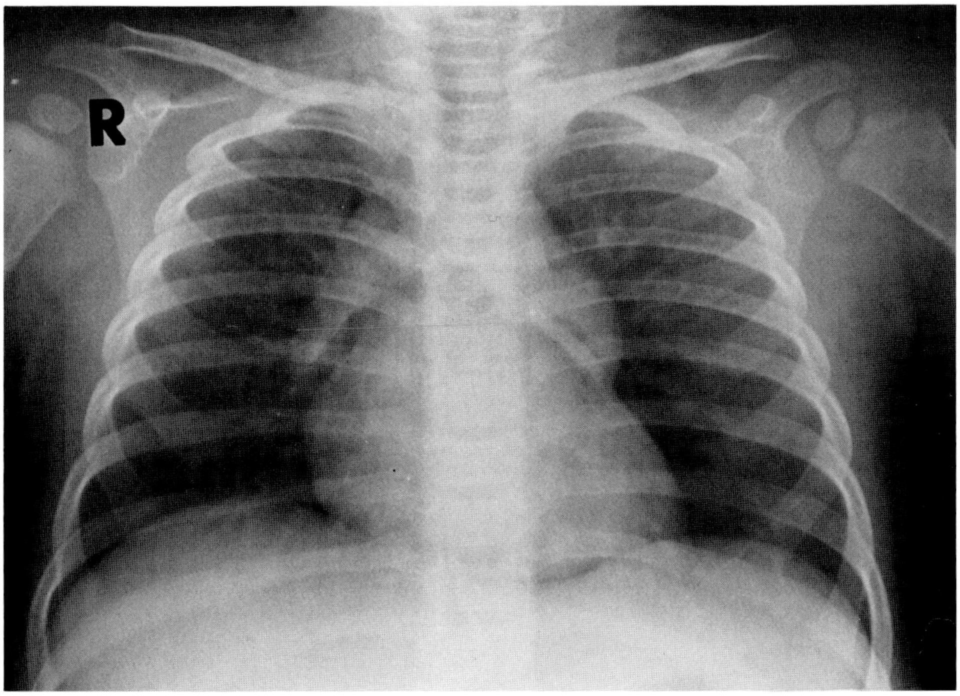

A

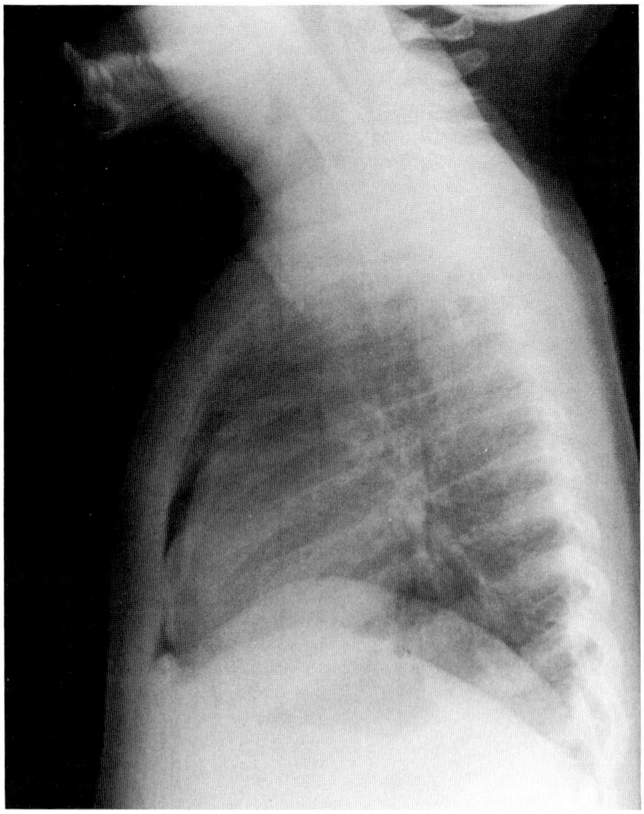

B

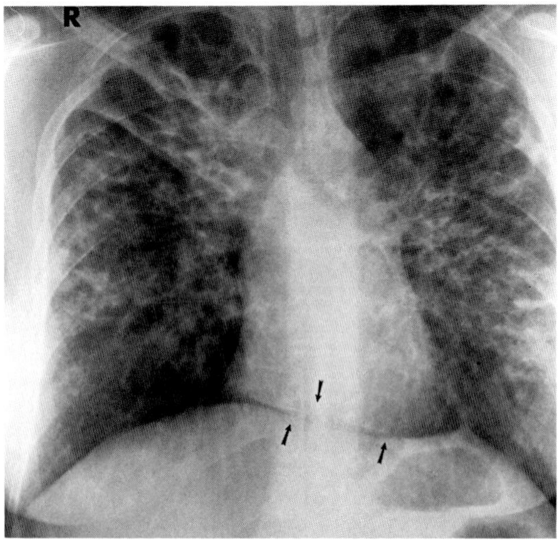

C (another patient)

Pneumomediastinum

Clinical Information

This 21-month-old infant had been coughing and strangling since aspiration of a peanut 10 hours earlier. The peanut was removed and the symptomatology disappeared, as did the x-ray findings.

Roentgen Findings

Posteroanterior (A) and lateral (B) films of the chest show the lung fields to be clear. Both lobes of the thymus are sharply outlined by surrounding air on the posteroanterior film. The appearance is a typical "spinnaker sail" or "angel wing" sign of air in the mediastinum. A thin zone of radiolucency is also visible behind the sternum on the lateral view. Air between the diaphragm and the heart, a "continuous diaphragm" sign also indicative of this condition, is barely discernible. A patient with cystic fibrosis (C) shows this sign better (arrows).

Comments

Pneumomediastinum, frequently called mediastinal emphysema, is due to an abnormal accumulation of air or gas in the mediastinum. It is of little importance in most cases but at times can be of great moment. Air most commonly reaches the mediastinum following alveolar rupture. The air that escapes from the alveoli dissects through the interstitial spaces along the pulmonary vessels to reach the mediastinum. Pneumomediastinum occasioned by this mechanism is particularly common during assisted ventilation. Infection with gas-forming bacillus can very rarely lead to mediastinal air. Air reaches the mediastinum more often from the neck, usually following a surgical procedure such as a tracheostomy. Air can also originate from a ruptured esophagus, trachea, or bronchus. A pneumoperitoneum may lead to mediastinal emphysema, although this is very unusual (4).

Mediastinal air can rupture into the pleural space and cause a pneumothorax. It can also dissect out through the thoracic inlet and lead to subcutaneous emphysema, an unusual event in newborns and infants. Another possible route is for the air to pass below the diaphragm and become retroperitoneal emphysema or, in some cases, it can rupture into the peritoneal cavity and cause a pneumoperitoneum. Mediastinal emphysema associated with extensive subcutaneous emphysema most often has its origin from the lungs, because the bellows action of the diaphragm can pump large quantities of air into abnormal locations. Air in the mediastinum can collect under pressure (tension pneumomediastinum) and obstruct venous blood flow to the heart. This is unusual. Ordinary pneumomediastinum requires no treatment other than stopping its cause. Tension requires prompt aspiration of the mediastinal air.

The x-ray findings of pneumomediastinum are usually characteristic (3). The posteroanterior projection shows the mediastinal pleura displaced laterally by a central shadow of air density. The radiolucency is often better seen just behind the sternum of the lateral film. A small pneumomediastinum may only outline a fine line of density, the mediastinal pleurae, which runs parallel to the left heart margin on the posteroanterior film. This line usually reaches to or above the aortic knob, thus distinguishing it from a pneumopericardium, which does not reach this far superiorly (1). Air may be present between the heart and diaphragm, where it must be distinguished from pneumothorax or pneumoperitoneum. The air in both of the latter conditions moves when the patient is placed in a lateral decubitus position, which also differentiates mediastinal air from a medial pneumothorax. Mediastinal air often causes a very characteristic "spinnaker sail" ("angel wing") or "rocker bottom" appearance of the thymus (2). The latter is said to simulate the rockers of a cradle.

Source Materials

1. Friedman AC, Lautin EM, Rothenberg L. Mach bands and pneumomediastinum. J Can Assoc Radiol 32:232, 1981.
2. Kogutt MS. "Rocker-bottom thymus." A new sign of pneumomediastinum in the neonate. JAMA 246:770, 1981.
3. Quattromani FL, Foley LC, Bowen A'D, et al. Fascial relationship of the thymus: Radiologic-pathologic correlation in neonatal pneumomediastinum. AJR 137:1209, 1981.
4. Schulman A, Fataar S, Van Der Spuy JW, et al. Air in unusual places: Some causes and ramifications of pneumomediastinum. Clin Radiol 33:301, 1982.

Case 71

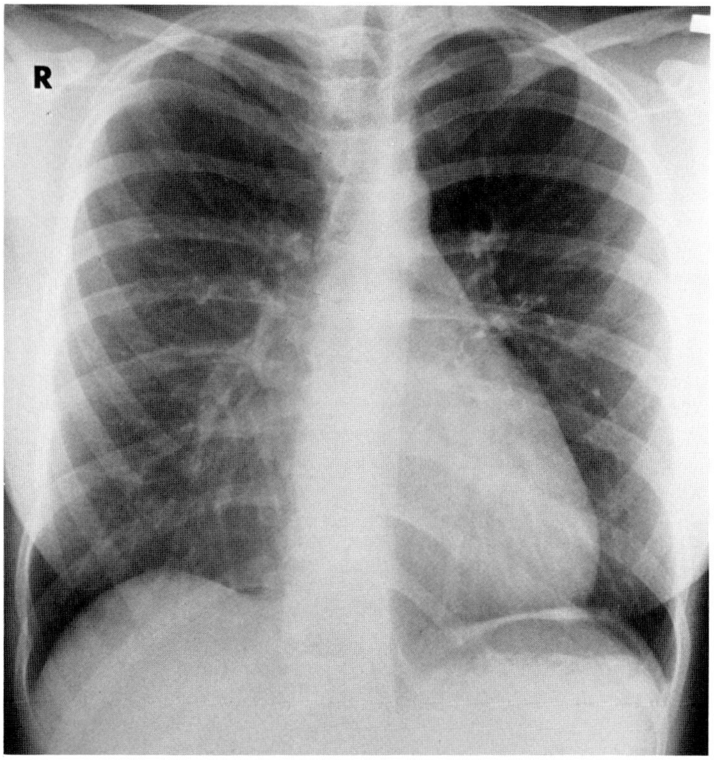

A

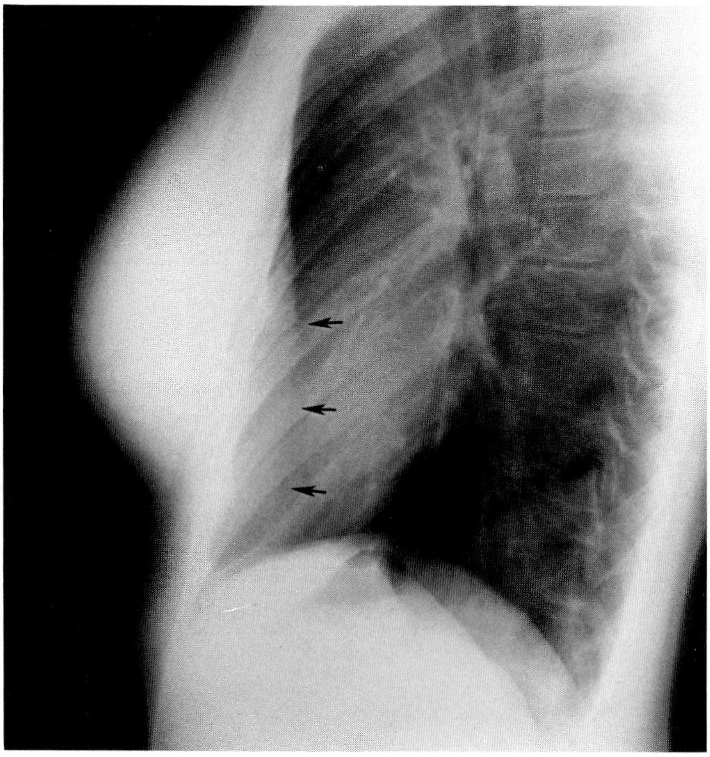

B

Pectus Excavatum

Clinical Information

This 14-year-old white female was admitted for removal of a fibroadenoma of the right breast. She had a grade I apical systolic murmur.

Roentgen Findings

A posteroanterior (A) chest film shows anterior ribs that sharply slope downward. The heart does not extend to the right of the mediastinum and appears displaced toward the left. A mild prominence of the middle left cardiac segment suggests an enlarged left atrial appendage. The right lower medial lung field is less lucent than usual, suggesting middle lobe disease. This is not borne out on the lateral film (B), which shows typical pectus excavatum.

Comments

Pectus excavatum, also called funnel chest, is characterized by a depression of the lower sternum, which when extreme may approach the anterior margins of the dorsal vertebrae. The condition can be minor in degree or extreme. The apex of the depression is at the xiphosternal junction. The upper sternum and manubrium are normal. This condition is probably due to a congenitally short central tendon of the diaphragm which pulls on the lower end of the sternum during inspiration. Its exact incidence is debated. The condition is said to occur in between 0.13 and 7.9 individuals per thousand. Males are affected twice as often as females. Pectus excavatum can run in families, is usually asymptomatic, but can have significant psychologic impact due to its cosmetic effect. There can be associated electrocardiographic changes and cardiac murmurs. Patients with pectus excavatum show large swings in the negative intrapleural pressure with respiration, which can deform the compliant chest of the newborn. Severe upper airway obstruction early in life from enlarged adenoids and tonsils can lead to pectus excavatum, which disappears when the obstruction is relieved (2).

The inward retraction on the lower sternum that occurs on inspiration pulls the anterior chest wall posteriorly. This can compress the heart and cause a decrease in its anteroposterior diameter. This relative flattening of the heart can lead to a paradoxical increase in its transverse diameter during inspiration (1). The opposite occurs in expiration. Expansion of the lungs in patients with severe pectus excavatum is largely in a lateral direction. The downward pull of the diaphragm causes the anteroposterior diameter of the lower chest to narrow. This results in a reduced quantity of pulmonary parenchyma relative to bone and soft tissues, which can cause the lung fields to appear less well aerated on inspiration than on expiration. This appearance is amplified by the associated increased transverse diameter of the heart. A lateral film is valuable in documenting the abnormal diaphragmatic motion, which is more fixed anteriorly than posteriorly. Surgery for pectus excavatum is only relatively successful.

The diagnosis of pectus excavatum is easy with a lateral film, which shows the lower sternum depressed posteriorly. The sharp downward inclination of the anterior rib ends on the posteroanterior film is also diagnostic. Further confirmation comes from displacement of the cardiac silhouette toward the left, sometimes with clockwise rotation, which can produce a prominence along the left heart border not unlike that seen in mitral disease. The right heart border may be indistinct or invisible, and there often is decreased lucency of the lower medial right lung, which simulates a positive silhouette sign of right middle lobe density. This appearance results from displacement of the heart, mediastinal density, and the narrow anteroposterior diameter of the thorax at this point. Pectus excavatum can mimic mediastinal and hilar masses, a situation that can be clarified with computed tomography (3).

Source Materials

1. Ben-Menachem Y, O'Hara AE, Kane HA. Paradoxical cardiac enlargement during inspiration in children with pectus excavatum: A new observation. Br J Radiol 46:38, 1973.
2. Fan L, Murphy S. Pectus excavatum from chronic upper airway obstruction. Am J Dis Child 135:550, 1981.
3. Soteropoulos GC, Cigtay OS, Schellinger D. Pectus excavatum deformities simulating mediastinal masses. J Comput Assist Tomogr 3:596, 1979.

Case 72

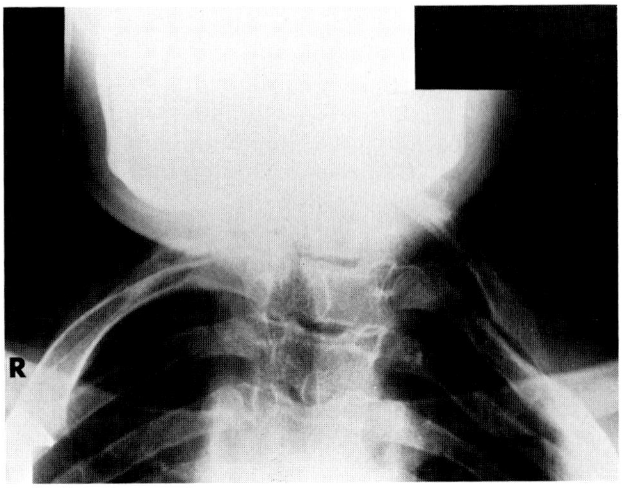

A

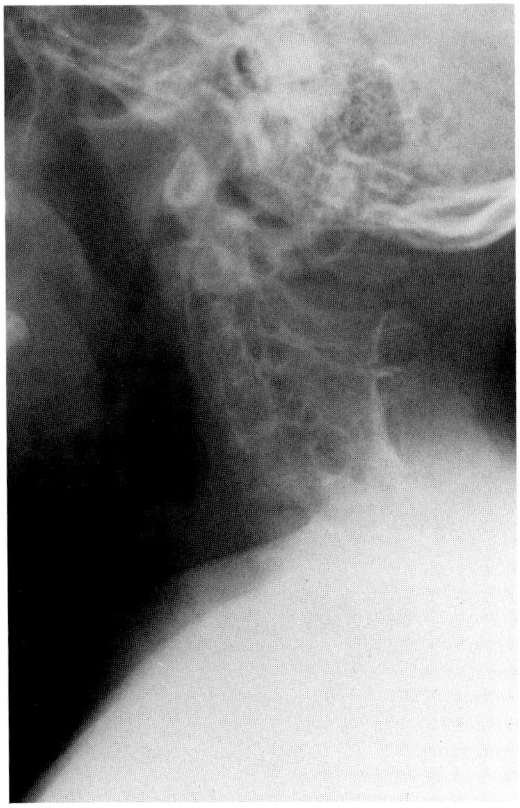

B

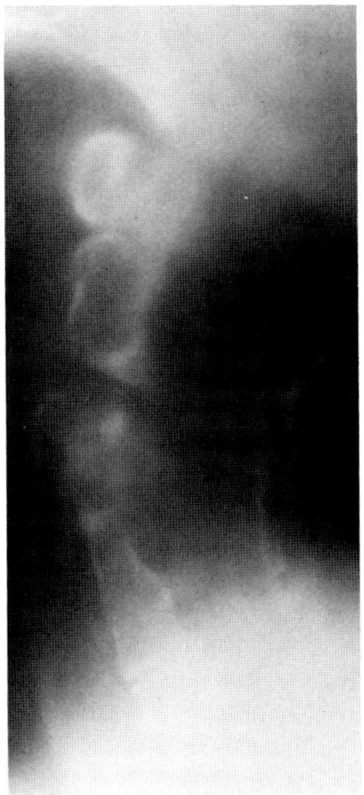

C

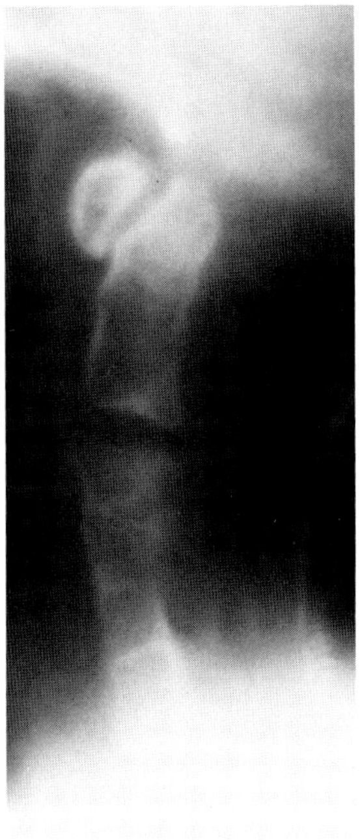

D

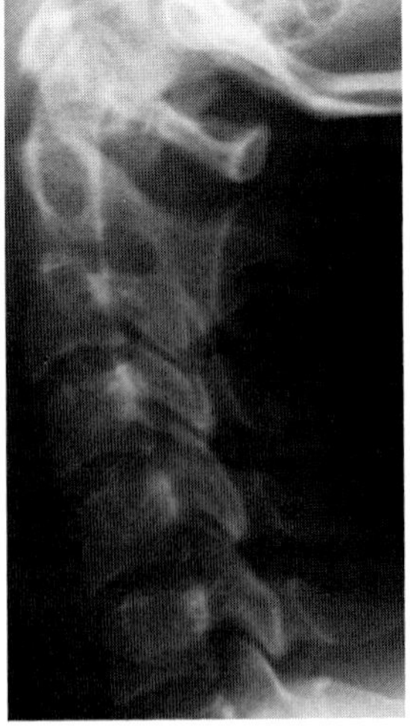

E (another patient)

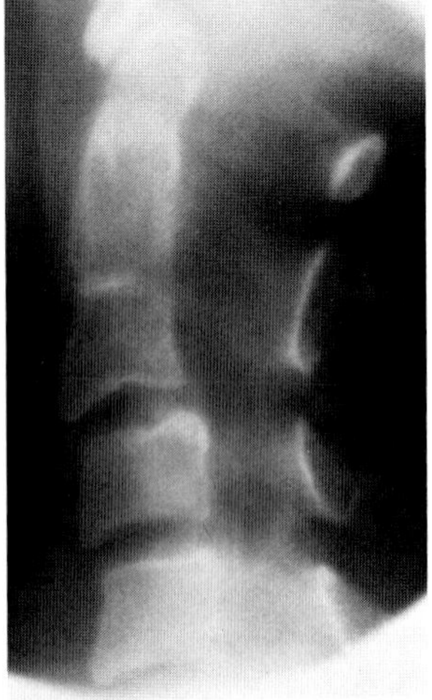

F (same patient as in E)

Klippel-Feil Syndrome

Clinical Information

This 14-year-old female complained of some weakness in her arms.

Roentgen Findings

Anteroposterior (A) and lateral (B) films of the cervical spine as well as lateral laminagrams (C, D) show an extremely short neck. There is fusion of the vertebral bodies and posterior elements from C3 through C7 with an abortive intervertebral space between C5 and C6. The spinal canal appears to be enlarged. Some of the vertebral bodies and posterior elements are malformed. This appearance is typical of the Klippel-Feil syndrome.

Comments

The Klippel-Feil syndrome is characterized by the triad of a low occipital hairline, fusion of the cervical vertebrae, and restricted motion of the neck, particularly rotation. This condition has been noted in prehistoric bodies found at excavations and was described in early anatomical dissections. The underlying cause of this anomaly is unknown. These patients often have no symptoms. The Klippel-Feil syndrome has been categorized into three types (1). In type I, the most common form, there is extensive fusion with associated anomalies of the cervical vertebrae. Many vertebral bodies, including portions of their neural arches, are involved. There may be no intervening disc spaces, although a few small remnants usually remain. Spina bifida occulta, cervical ribs, and hemivertebrae are often associated. Type II Klippel-Feil syndrome is characterized by segmental involvement of only one or two pairs of vertebrae. It is the type least frequently encountered. Some would prefer to designate the case shown in films E and F as fused vertebrae rather than type II Klippel-Feil syndrome. Type III Klippel-Feil syndrome is present when there are associated anomalies of the thoracic and lumbar vertebrae. Scoliosis is an additional abnormality in about 20% of all patients with Klippel-Feil syndrome. Basilar invagination is also quite common. Various genitourinary anomalies are present in two-thirds of these patients (3). About 30% suffer from deafness (4). Sprengel's deformity, often with an associated omovertebral bone, is present in a third of these patients. Synkinesia occurs in about a fifth of individuals with Klippel-Feil syndrome. Cardiac anomalies coexist in about 4%.

Radiographic studies show the expected findings of a short neck marked by fusions and irregularly shaped and anomalous vertebrae. Degenerative hypertrophic lipping is frequently present around the margins of unfused segments. Some individuals differentiate Klippel-Feil syndrome from block vertebrae by holding that the height of a pair of block vertebrae is equal to their combined heights less the intervening disc space. They also hold that the height of the fused mass in Klippel-Feil syndrome is somewhat less than the sum of the heights of the affected vertebrae. It is also suggested that posterior element fusion is more common in Klippel-Feil syndrome. The distinction, even if accurate, appears to have little significance.

Source Materials

1. Dolan KD. Developmental abnormalities of the cervical spine below the axis. Radiol Clin North Am 15:167, 1977.
2. McElfresh E, Winter R. Klippel-Feil syndrome. Minn Med 56:353, 1973.
3. Moore WB, Matthews TJ, Rabinowitz R. Genitourinary anomalies associated with Klippel-Feil syndrome. J Bone Joint Surg 57A:355, 1975.
4. Windle-Taylor PC, Emery PJ, Phelps PD. Ear deformities associated with the Klippel-Feil syndrome. Ann Otol Rhinol Laryngol 90:210, 1981.

Case 73

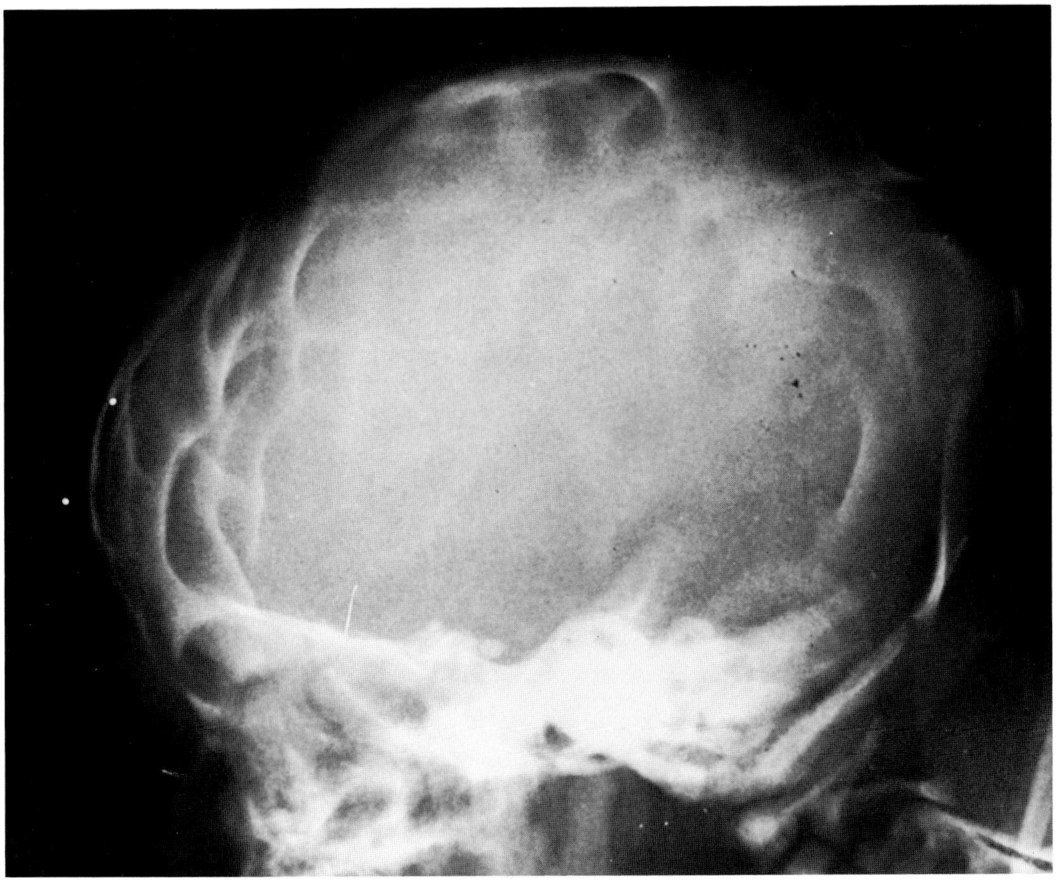

Lacunar Skull

Clinical Information

This newborn male had a large lumbar myelomeningocele.

Roentgen Findings

A lateral film of the skull shows the face and calvaria to be normal in size and shape. There are numerous oval, smoothly outlined radiolucencies throughout the cranial vault. These lucencies are most prominent near the summit of the skull. They tend to have their long diameter directed relatively anteroposteriorly. The anterior fontanelle does not bulge, nor is there other evidence of increased intracranial pressure.

Comments

Lacunar skull, also called lückenschädel or craniolacunia, is an abnormality of osseous development of the calvaria characterized by round, oval, or finger-shaped depressions on the inner surface of the cranial vault. These depressions are separated by smooth, dense ridges of bone to form a weblike pattern. The condition is present at birth and is almost invariably associated with severe central nervous system abnormalities, the most common of which are meningoceles, meningomyeloceles, encephaloceles, and the Arnold-Chiari malformation. The defects will disappear within 3–12 months if the patient survives. Only the inner table and diploë are involved in a typical patient. On rare occasions the bony defects extend through the outer table and create a hole or holes in the skull, a situation called craniofenestria. The radiolucencies are most prominent in the parietal, frontal, and occipital bones, especially toward the upper portion of the head. Abnormal ossification may affect other portions of the skull and can lead to widening of the cranial sutures. This can cause a striking midline frontal separation called cranium bifidum, which must not be mistaken for an encephalocele or increased intracranial pressure.

The etiology of a lacunar skull is unknown, although it most surely is not the result of increased intracranial pressure as was previously thought. The gyri of the brain do not correspond in position to the rounded areas of radiolucency. In fact, the frontal and occipital gyri may be hypoplastic with a lacunar skull. The open sutures of the newborn bulge with increased intracranial pressure, thereby decompressing the underlying brain and avoiding gyral pressure against the inner table.

A lacunar skull must be differentiated from normal digital markings. This differentiation is relatively easy, since normal digital markings do not appear until 6–12 months of age. They are not prominent until 3–15 years of age and are more evident in lower portions of the skull. These normal depressions correspond to the convolutions of the brain. It is also necessary to distinguish craniolacunia from craniosynostosis. The exaggerated radiolucencies in craniosynostosis also correspond to the gyri of the brain but are most prominent near the closed sutures. These depressions, like normal digital markings and the "beaten silver" appearance of increased intracranial pressure, are never present at birth when a lacunar skull is most striking. In fact, a lacunar skull has been noted in utero on several occasions. The "beaten silver" appearance of increased intracranial pressure is usually associated with widened, fuzzy sutures and other characteristic radiologic abnormalities.

It is evident that no real differential diagnostic possibilities exist for a lacunar skull, a condition that alone has no inherent significance. Its only importance is that a lacunar skull virtually always is associated with severe central nervous system abnormalities. It is true, however, that patients with a lacunar skull have a lower intelligence than patients without this disorder, although no relationship is said to exist between the degree of lowered intelligence and the severity of the x-ray changes (1). This may not be a significant finding, because age at the time of the observation is very important, since the changes of a lacunar skull rapidly disappear in all patients who survive.

Source Materials

1. Fishman MA, Palkes HS, Shackelford GD, McAlister WH. Lacunar skull deformity and intelligence. Pediatrics 59:296, 1977.
2. McRae DL. Observations on craniolacunia. Acta Radiol 5:55, 1966.
3. Shopfner CE, Jabbour JT, Vallion RM. Craniolacunia. AJR 93:343, 1965.

Case 74

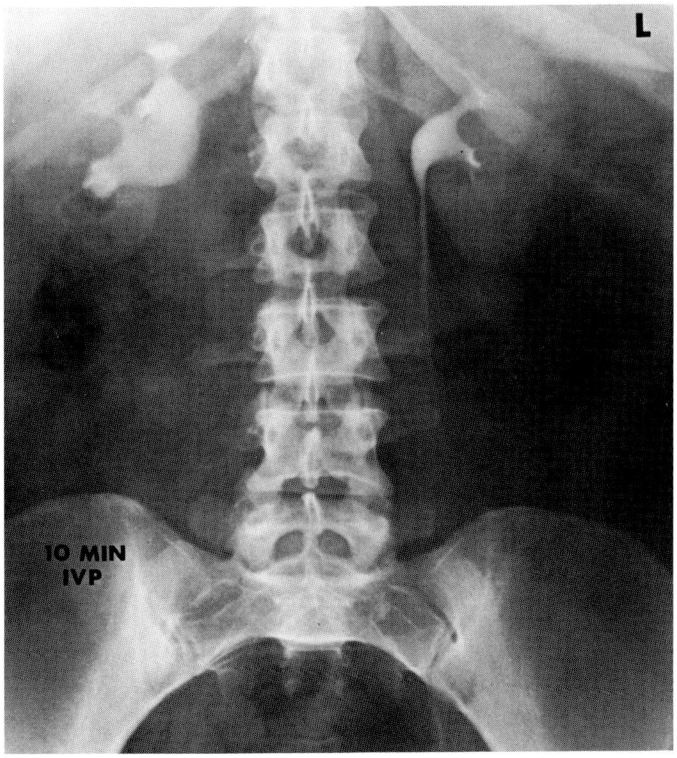

A

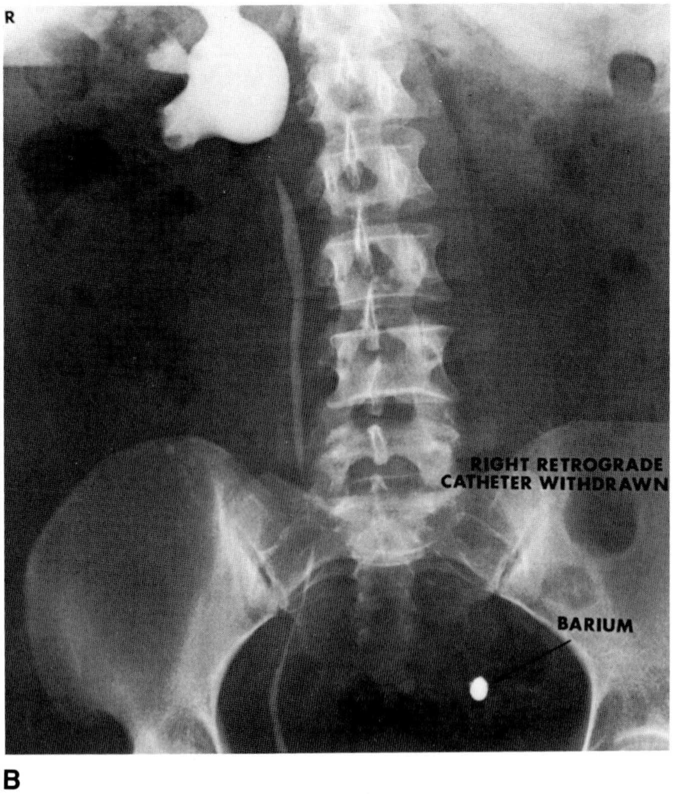

B

Ureteropelvic Junction Obstruction

Clinical Information

This 43-year-old white multigravida was admitted because of urinary stress incontinence. She was found to have a third-degree cystocele and first-degree rectocele but refused surgical therapy. Her blood urea nitrogen was normal. The ureteropelvic junction obstruction had not led to massive destruction of renal tissue and apparently was causing no symptoms.

Roentgen Findings

A 10-minute intravenous urogram (A) shows a normal left drainage system. The right renal pelvis is dilated, the right renal calyces less so. A normal amount of renal cortex remains. None of the right ureter is visible. A retrograde right pyelogram after catheter withdrawal (B) shows a tulip-shaped pelvis with ureteropelvic junction narrowing.

Comments

Ureteropelvic junction obstruction is a common congenital anomaly of the urinary tract. It is the most frequent cause of hydronephrosis in a neonate, being present in about 22% of these patients (3). There is a male predominance of about 2:1. The etiology of this condition is debated. It is most often considered to be congenital narrowing at the ureteropelvic junction caused by excessive replacement of muscle by collagen and fibrosis. An intraluminal valve has been discovered on rare occasions. Some feel the basic disturbance is neuromuscular dysfunction. Aberrant renal vessels may seem to be obstructive, but this appearance is probably secondary to the pelvic dilatation that has overlapped the vessels.

Ureteropelvic junction obstruction has occasionally been first discovered in adults, sometimes in individuals who have previously had a normal intravenous urogram (1). There may be marginal or borderline ureteropelvic junction obstruction, which only becomes evident radiologically or causes symptoms after overhydration. Excessive beer drinking is a common cause of symptoms in these patients. Ureteropelvic junction obstruction is commonly first diagnosed in early life, particularly during the first year (4). A urinary tract infection usually precipitates its discovery. The amount of renal damage varies. Occasionally the kidneys are totally destroyed when the condition is first diagnosed. Presenting symptoms are pain, which is often periumbilical, or a palpable mass frequently accompanied by vomiting and other gastrointestinal complaints. About 25–50% of patients with ureteropelvic junction obstruction have bilateral disease. Mild obstruction needs no treatment. Several types of surgical and interventional treatment have been recommended for patients with severe symptoms and renal drainage (2).

An abdominal film in a patient with ureteropelvic junction obstruction is normal or only reveals a flank mass without calcification. Excretory urograms usually show delayed function on the affected side. At times pools of opaque medium within dilated calyces are seen. Later films outline a dilated, tulip-shaped renal pelvis. The degree of dilatation varies. Function may be too poor to outline the drainage system. In such cases antegrade studies and ultrasound are very helpful. The renal pelvis does not gradually taper to form the upper ureter as is seen when the ureteropelvic junction is normal. The ureter exits from the renal pelvis at a higher level than normal. The ureter should exit from the most dependent portion of the renal pelvis. The ureteropelvic junction is narrowed and usually forms a rather acute angle. The proximal ureter is often also narrowed and usually poorly seen with excretory studies. Details are best depicted in retrograde examinations, although these studies should be avoided when possible to reduce the likelihood of infection.

Source Materials

1. Jacobs JA, Berger BW, Goldman SM, et al. Ureteropelvic obstruction in adults with previously normal pyelograms: A report of 5 cases. J Urol 121:242, 1979.
2. Kadir S, White RI Jr, Engel R. Balloon dilatation of a ureteropelvic junction obstruction. Radiology 143:263, 1982.
3. Kirks DR, Merten DF, Grossman H, Bowie JD. Diagnostic imaging of pediatric abdominal masses: An overview. Radiol Clin North Am 19:527, 1981.
4. Lees RF. Pelvic-ureteric obstruction in children. Australas Radiol 20:138, 1976.

Case 75

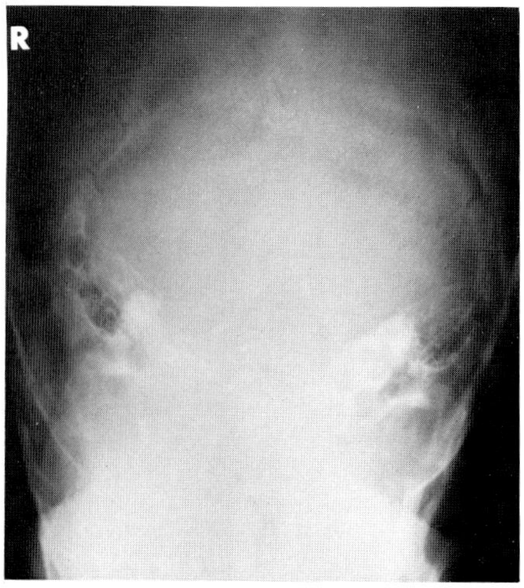

A

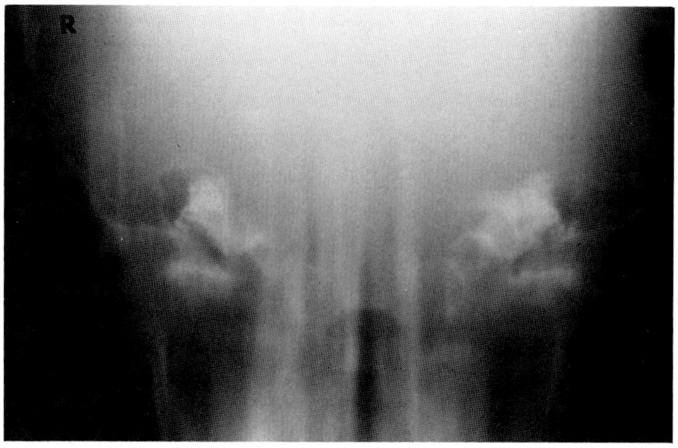

B

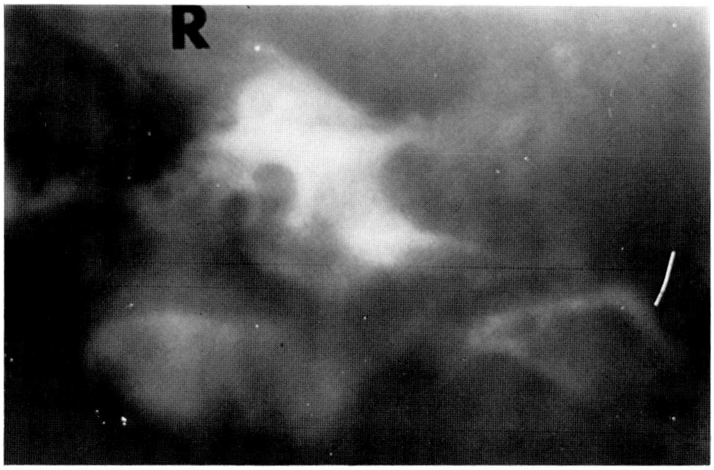

C (another patient)

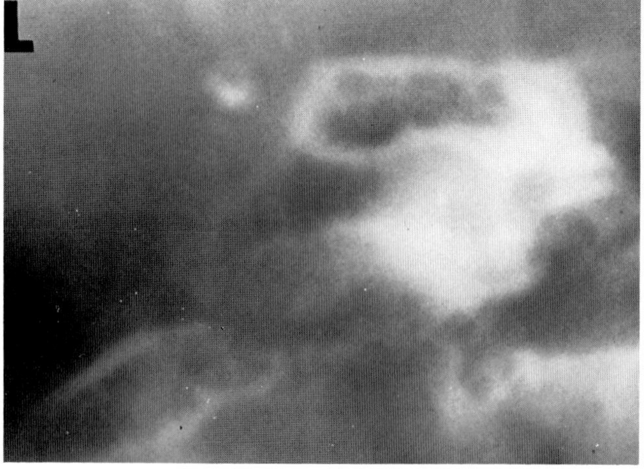

D (same patient as in C)

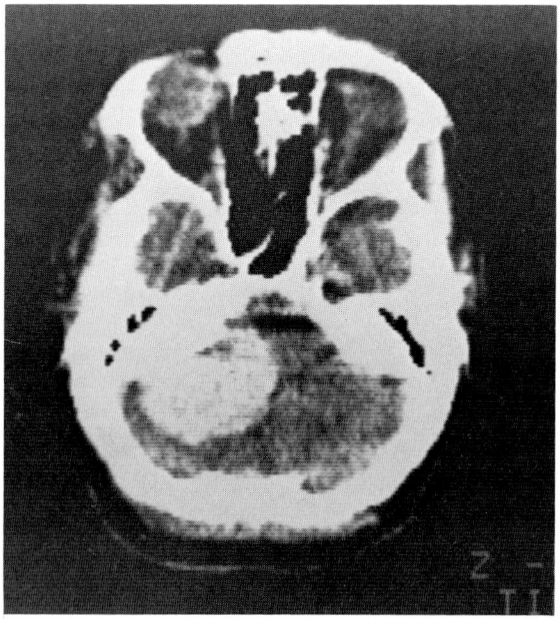

E (a third patient)

Acoustic Neuroma

Clinical Information

This patient's acoustic neuroma caused headaches and dizziness.

Roentgen Findings

The Towne's view of the skull (A) and a laminagram (B) show extensive erosion of the petrous portion of the right temporal bone with marked shortening of the right internal auditory canal. Complex motion tomography of another patient (C, D) also shows shortening and expansion of the right internal auditory canal. An enhanced computed tomographic scan of still another patient (E) shows a right acoustic neuroma.

Comments

An acoustic neuroma is a schwannoma of the sheath of the eighth cranial nerve. This lesion accounts for about 7% of all intracranial tumors. It is rare in early life, is most commonly encountered in the middle years, and accounts for the vast majority of cerebellopontine angle tumors. It is twice as frequent in females as in males and is usually unilateral. Bilateral acoustic neuromas are almost invariably associated with neurofibromatosis. The usual symptoms are gradual loss of hearing and tinnitus due to involvement of the acoustic and vestibular branches of the eighth nerve. These tumors vary in size between about 1 and 4 or more cm in diameter. A large tumor can obstruct the cerebrospinal fluid pathways with predictable results. The only effective treatment is surgical excision. Favorable results vary inversely with the size of the tumor. Since growth is slow and the lesion usually discovered late in its course, this tumor frequently cannot be totally removed. The recurrence rate is relatively high. From 30% to 50% of these patients succumb within 3 years, often due to a recurrence.

Years ago the diagnosis of an acoustic neuroma was made by clinical means, usually caloric evaluation of the vestibular function of the eighth nerve. It was subsequently shown that up to 75% of these patients may show visible changes in the internal auditory canal on plain films. Erosion and shortening of its posterior wall are particularly diagnostic. Minor enlargement of the internal auditory meatus can occur normally. Width of an internal auditory canal of 2 mm more than the opposite side is significant, as is shortening of 3 mm. Very small tumors do not cause visible changes on plain films. Cisternography with a radiopaque contrast agent may reveal these smaller tumors. Many acoustic neuromas stain by angiography. About 90% enhance.

CT studies will show most acoustic neuromas but can miss very small lesions. The most definitive diagnostic study for an acoustic neuroma at present is air-CT cisternography (1, 2). Thin sections are obtained by CT after a small amount of air or carbon dioxide is introduced into the intrathecal space and positioned within the cerebellopontine angle cistern. Tumors that are less than 1 cm in diameter can be shown. Failure of the air to enter the internal auditory canal is evidence of a tumor. This examination avoids the pitfalls and hazards of Pantopaque and metrizamide studies. It is indicated if clinical evaluation, skull films, complex motion tomography, and enhanced CT fail to provide definitive information. Some would eliminate complex motion tomography. Nuclear magnetic resonance promises to be of great value in the diagnosis of acoustic neuromas, because this examination is not hampered by bone artifacts (3).

Source Materials

1. Pinto RS, Kricheff II, Bergeron RT, Cohen N. Small acoustic neuromas: Detection by high resolution gas CT cisternography. AJR 139:129, 1982.
2. Valavanis A, Dabir K, Hamdi R, et al. The current state of the radiological diagnosis of acoustic neuroma. Neuroradiology 23:7, 1982.
3. Young IR, Bydder GM, Hall AS, et al. The role of NMR imaging in the diagnosis and management of acoustic neuroma. AJNR 4:223, 1983.

Case 76

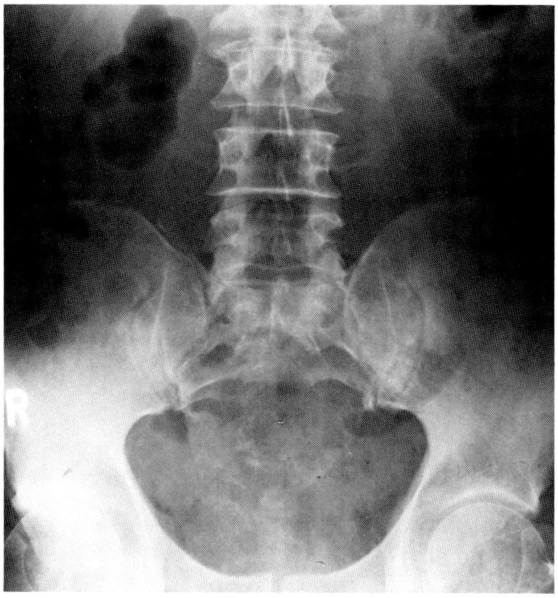

A

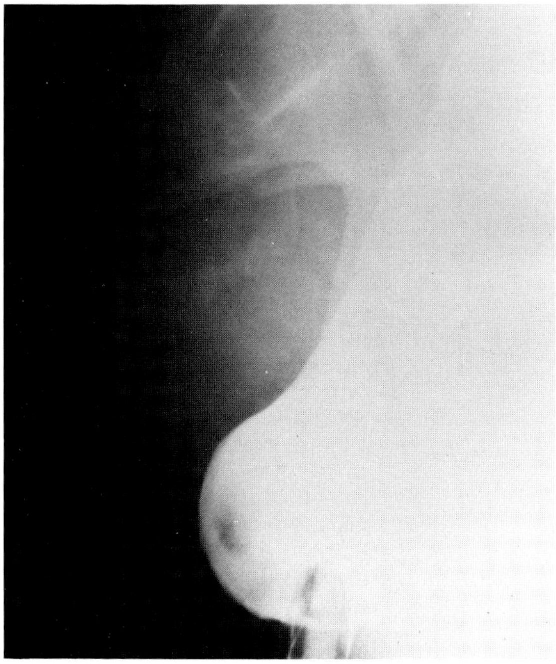

B

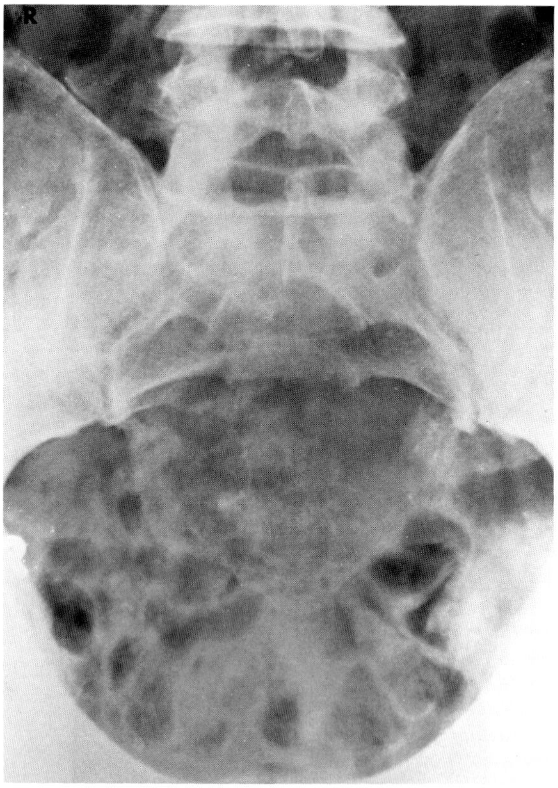

C

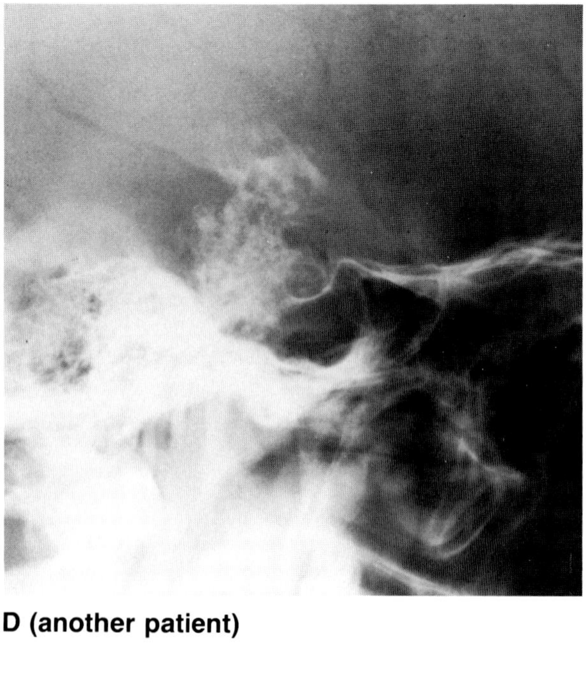

D (another patient)

Chordoma

Clinical Information

This 65-year-old white male developed rectal pain and fecal incontinence following drainage of a perirectal abscess. Subsequent studies revealed a sacral chordoma.

Roentgen Findings

Films of the abdomen (A) and sacrum (C) and a lateral film of the rectum obtained during a barium enema (B) show a large area of bony destruction in the lower sacrum. The destruction appears to be primarily in the midline, is not sharply limited in its extent, contains irregular calcification, and displaces the rectum anteriorly. Extensive midline calcification and erosion of the clivus in a 22-year-old male with an intracranial chordoma are shown in D.

Comments

Chordomas account for fewer than 1% of all tumors. The most common location for a chordoma is in the sacrococcygeal region, followed relatively closely by the base of the skull near the clivus. The remainder are scattered along the cervical and thoracic spine. Chordomas develop from heterotopic notochord remnants. There is a 2:1 male predominance. Sacral chordomas are usually discovered rather late in life, since they grow very slowly and do not cause early symptoms, but may be seen in young adults (1). Intracranial chordomas are manifested at an earlier age and lead to death more rapidly (2). Twenty percent of all types of chordomas survive 10 years, although intracranial tumors usually survive less than 6 years. Reported metastases are relatively uncommon and are virtually always associated with a chordoma located outside the cranial cavity. Sacral chordomas lead to slowly progressive pain, sciatica, difficulty in walking, and problems with urination or defecation. All forms of therapy are unsatisfactory. Radiation may give temporary relief. Chemotherapy does not seem to be useful. The only possible treatment for cure is surgical resection, but it usually is not possible to remove all of the tumor (4). The strut of the S1 and the sciatic nerves must be preserved if the patient is to function adequately after an operative excision.

About half of intracranial chordomas are located on the midline. An equal number contain calcification and involve the clivus. The vast majority of intracranial chordomas cause bony erosions in the base of the skull or in portions of the sphenoid bone. The area of destruction may show a sclerotic rim. A chordoma often affects the sella, which may be eroded but is rarely expanded. A nasopharyngeal mass is present in about a third of patients with an intracranial chordoma. Cervical or thoracic vertebrae affected by a chordoma often show involvement of the intervertebral spaces. This occurs more commonly with a chordoma than any other neoplasm, although the intervertebral spaces are often spared by this tumor.

The soft tissue mass of sacral chordomas is always larger than the visible bony destruction. A chordoma occasionally enhances with contrast. A sacral chordoma is characterized by midline bony destruction, which most commonly is located anterior to the sacrum and displaces the rectum. The involved bone is expanded and destroyed. The margins of the lesion are often sclerotic. Calcification or bony fragments within the tumor are less frequent than with an intracranial chordoma. Angiography may show abnormal vessels. A chordoma does not encase normal blood vessels but can displace them. There may be increased uptake of technetium-99m by a chordoma. Computed tomography is very useful to show the extent of the tumor (3).

Source Materials

1. Hertzanu Y, Glass RBJ, Mendelsohn DB. Sacrococcygeal chordoma in young adults. Clin Radiol 34:327, 1983.
2. Kendall BE, Lee BCP. Cranial chordomas. Br J Radiol 50:687, 1977.
3. Krol G, Sundaresan N, Deck M. Computed tomography of axial chordomas. J Comput Assist Tomogr 7:286, 1983.
4. Saxton JP. Chordoma. Int J Radiat Oncol Biol Phys 7:913, 1981.

Case 77

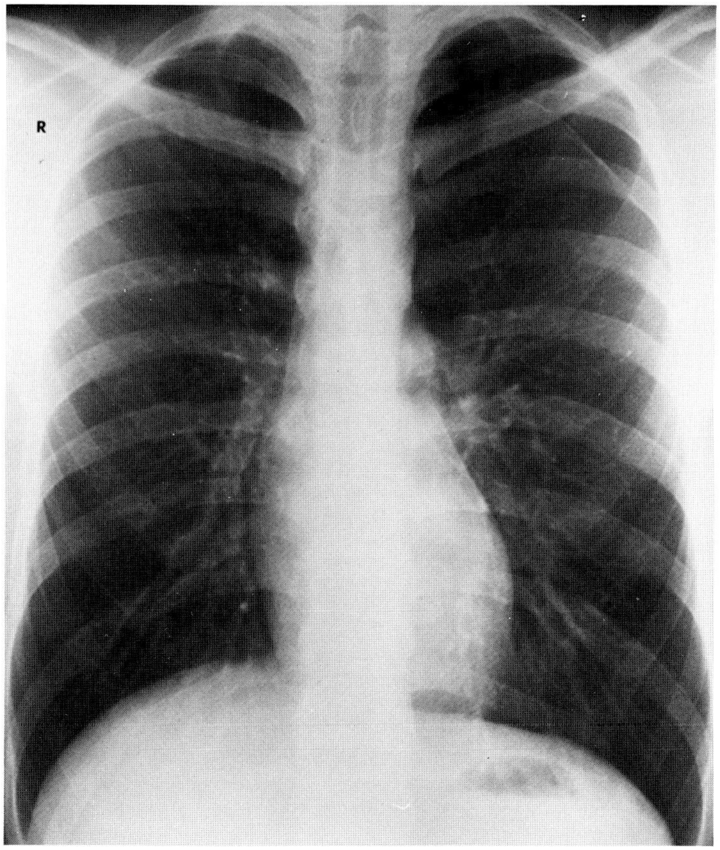

A

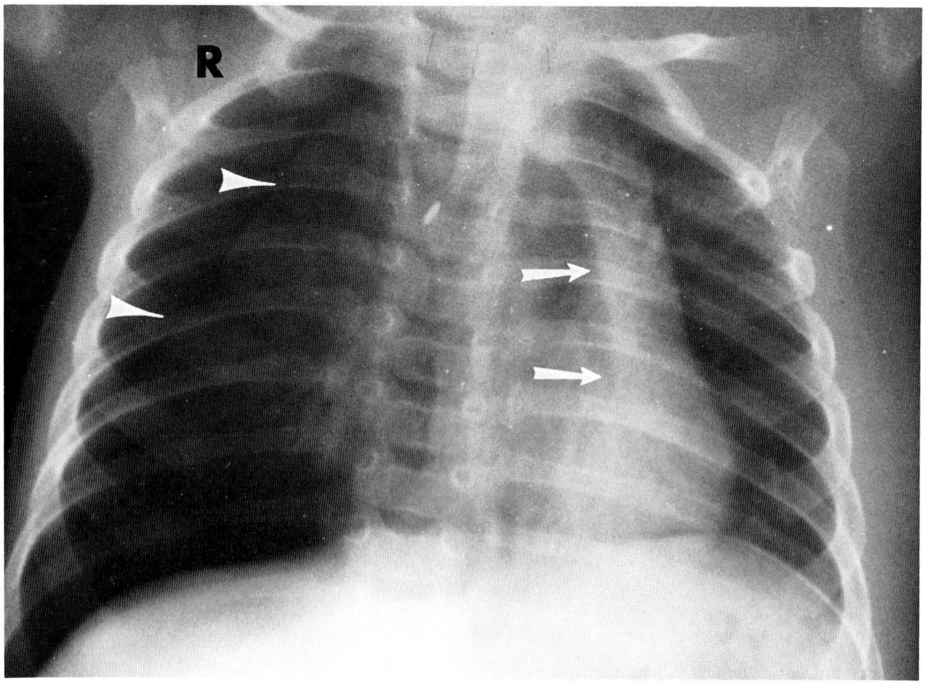

B (another patient)

Pneumothorax

Clinical Information

This 19-year-old male experienced a sudden onset of left chest pain and mild dyspnea. The spontaneous pneumothorax resolved without specific therapy.

Roentgen Findings

A posteroanterior chest film (A) reveals a small pneumothorax surmounting the left lung. No vascular markings extend beyond the lung edge marked by the visceral pleura.

Comments

A pneumothorax can result when either the visceral or the parietal pleura is interrupted and the intervening pleural space is exposed to positive atmospheric pressure. This permits the ingress of air. Pneumothorax most commonly is a spontaneous event in an otherwise normal individual (2). It results most frequently from rupture of a subpleural bleb, which creates a pathway through which air can reach the pleural space. Many diseases such as emphysema, sarcoidosis, and histiocytosis X predispose to bleb formation. Air that escapes following rupture of distended alveoli can dissect along the sheaths of the pulmonary vessels and bronchi to reach the mediastinum and subsequently break into the pleural space. This series of events is abetted by assisted respiration, bronchial asthma, injury, or bronchial obstruction by mucus or a tumor. Penetrating trauma, or even nonpenetrating injury as can occur from a rib fracture or rupture of the esophagus or a bronchus, can create a communication between the atmosphere and the pleural space. Although 5% of patients with a pneumothorax have no symptoms, there usually is some shortness of breath and chest pain. The distress is not proportional to the size of the pneumothorax (3). Pneumothorax frequently recurs. Treatment can consist of watchful waiting if the pneumothorax is small, although resolution is hastened by the introduction of a chest tube.

A tension pneumothorax results from a check valve mechanism, which allows air to enter the pleural space but prevents its escape—a serious situation that demands immediate attention. A tension pneumothorax complicating a ventriculoatrial shunt, the tip of which is visible in the superior vena cava, is shown in B. It has led to a low right diaphragm and widened intercostal spaces, and has displaced the heart and mediastinum to the left. Occasionally the lung will not reexpand after a pneumothorax, due to occlusion of the ipsilateral main bronchus, a persistent air leak, a defective drainage system, or acute depletion of surfactant (1).

The x-ray diagnosis of pneumothorax is usually easy. The thin line of the visceral pleura is displaced from and parallels the chest wall. It usually is easily seen and marks the peripheral edge of the pulmonary vascular markings. A pleural line is confined within the chest cavity, which distinguishes it from a skin fold. A skin fold can be identified because it, unlike a pleural line, is not sharply outlined along both its margins. Air in the pleural space tends to collect anteriorly if the patient is supine, particularly in children. A cross-table lateral film can be of value in reaching a definitive diagnosis. A lateral decubitus film can also be helpful, because it will show movement of pleural air to the lateral chest wall. An expiratory film exaggerates a pneumothorax, since the chest cavity, unlike the pleural air, is reduced in size on expiration. It rarely, if ever, shows a pneumothorax that is not visible on an inspiratory film. The lung beneath a pneumothorax does not increase in density until it is fairly well collapsed, since blood is shunted to the opposite lung. Adhesions can cause a pneumothorax to be localized. Too rapid reexpansion of a pneumothorax may lead to unilateral pulmonary edema. Fluid, which often is blood due to ruptured vascular adhesions, may accumulate along with air. This creates a fluid level, which can be a sensitive indicator of a minimal pneumothorax.

Source Materials

1. Galvis AG, Bowen A'D, Oh KS. Nonexpandable lung after drainage of pneumothorax. AJR 136:1224, 1981.
2. Melton LJ, Hepper NGG, Offord KP. Influence of height on the risk of spontaneous pneumothorax. Mayo Clin Proc 56:678, 1981.
3. Rhea JT, De Luca SA, Greene RE. Determining the size of pneumothorax in the upright patient. Radiology 144:733, 1982.
4. Ziter FMH Jr, Westcott JL. Supine subpulmonary pneumothorax. AJR 137:699, 1981.

Case 78

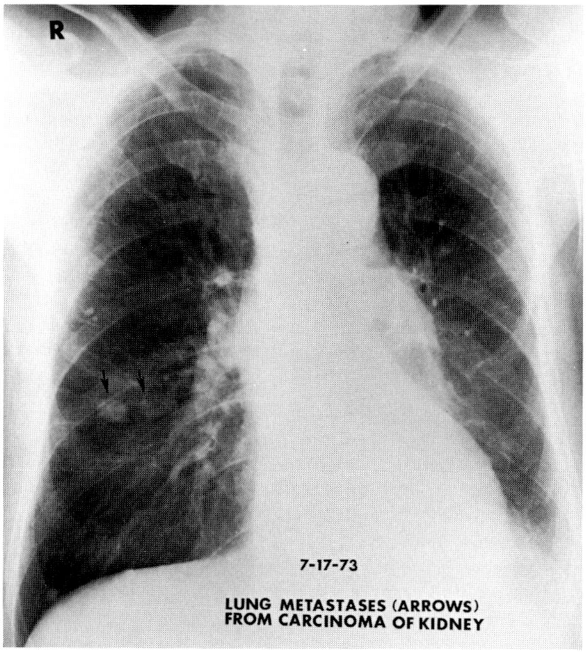
R
7-17-73
LUNG METASTASES (ARROWS)
FROM CARCINOMA OF KIDNEY

A

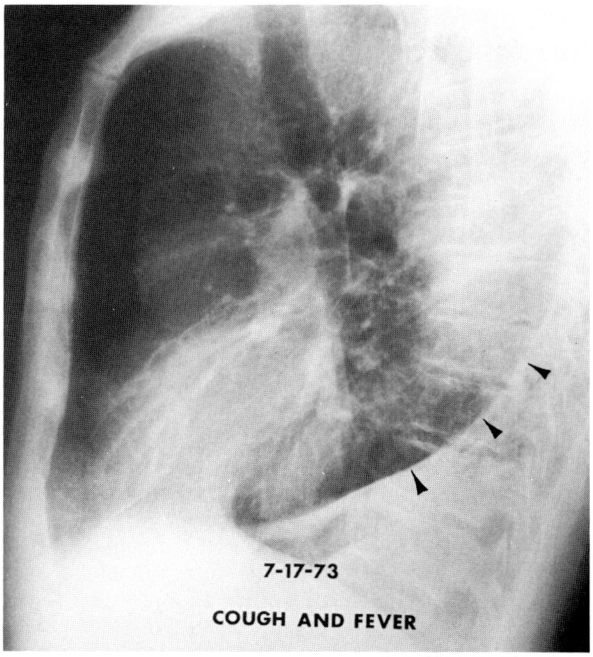
7-17-73
COUGH AND FEVER

B

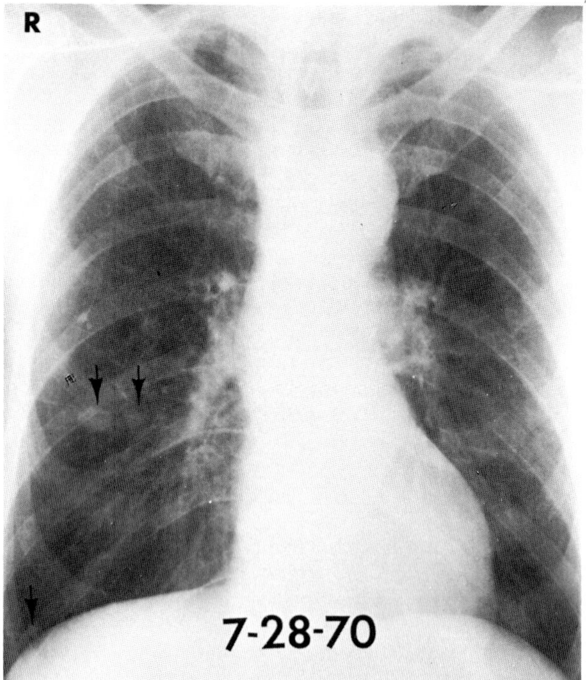
R
7-28-70

C

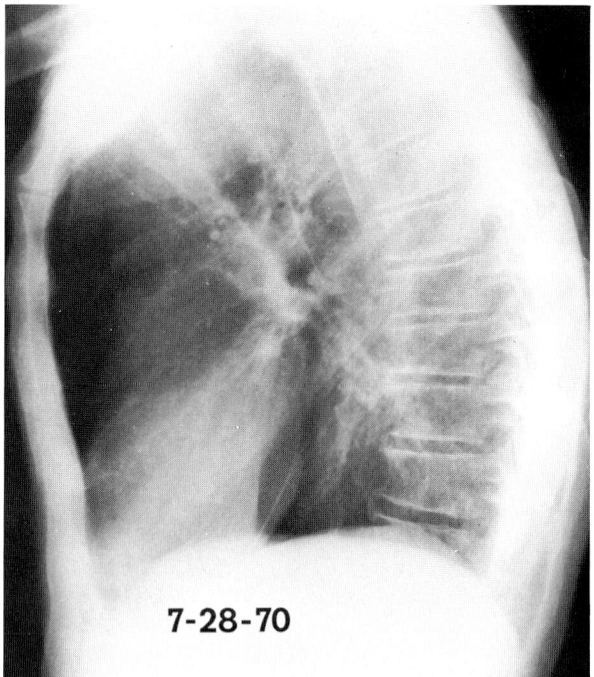
7-28-70

D

Lower Lobe Collapse

Clinical Information

This 69-year-old white male with known pulmonary metastases from a kidney carcinoma was admitted with a 3-day history of cough, fever, and left chest pain. A mucous plug was bronchoscopically removed from the left lower lobe bronchus with clearing of the left lower lobe collapse.

Roentgen Findings

Posteroanterior (A) and lateral (B) chest films show metastases in the right lung (arrows). The left diaphragmatic leaf is obscured on both films. The collapsed left lower lobe is seen as a sharply outlined semilunar density on the lateral film (arrowheads). Films taken 11 days later (C, D) show the collapse to have cleared.

Comments

Although there are many radiologic signs of extensive lower lobe atelectasis or collapse, only a limited number are seen in any specific patient. At times only loss of the interface with the diaphragm is evident. The direct x-ray signs are an increase in density localized to a lower lobe and displacement of the major fissure. The former may not be apparent. Fissural displacement, best seen on the lateral film, tends to be in a downward, backward, and medial direction. The frontal film may show the lower portion of the major fissure to have become oriented into an anteroposterior plane. Indirect signs of extensive atelectasis or collapse of a lower lobe include elevation of the hemidiaphragm and displacement of the mediastinum. Both are variable in occurrence. Downward displacement of the hilum is more common. Compensatory overinflation of unaffected lobes may not be evident, and narrowing of the ipsilateral costal interspaces may not exist. Crowding of the bronchovascular markings is not clearly discernible without a bronchogram.

The x-ray appearance of complete lower lobe collapse is similar on both sides and appears as a triangular density in the lower lung fields medially, with its apex at the hilum (4). The wedge shape may not be present in left lower lobe collapse if the pulmonary ligament is absent (1). Peripheral segments lying along the margin of the thorax are more evident in incomplete collapse than their narrow hilar connection. Round atelectasis is almost always, if not always, in a lower lobe (2).

Some difficulty can be experienced in differentiating involvement of only the right lower lobe from collapse of both the right lower and middle lobes. In the latter instance the right heart border is obscured and the density is much more likely to extend to the lateral costophrenic sinus on the posteroanterior film (4). Extensive right lower lobe atelectasis may lead to the upper triangle sign; collapse of the left lower lobe to the flat waist sign and obliteration of the top of the aortic knob (3). The upper triangle sign is a wedge of paramediastinal density extending upward with its apex at the hilum. It results from a shift of the upper portion of the mediastinum secondary to the lower lung collapse. The flat waist sign results from relative clockwise rotation of the heart, which straightens the normal cardiac contour near the pulmonary outflow tract. The heart looks as if it is slightly rotated into the right anterior oblique position.

Source Materials

1. Glay J, Palayew MJ. Unusual pattern of left lower lobe atelectasis. Radiology 141:331, 1981.
2. Hanke R, Kretzschmar R. Round atelectasis. Semin Roentgenol 15:174, 1980.
3. Kattan KR. Upper mediastinal changes in lower lobe collapse. Semin Roentgenol 15:183, 1980.
4. Proto AV, Tocino I. Radiographic manifestations of lobar collapse. Semin Roentgenol 15:117, 1980.

Case 79

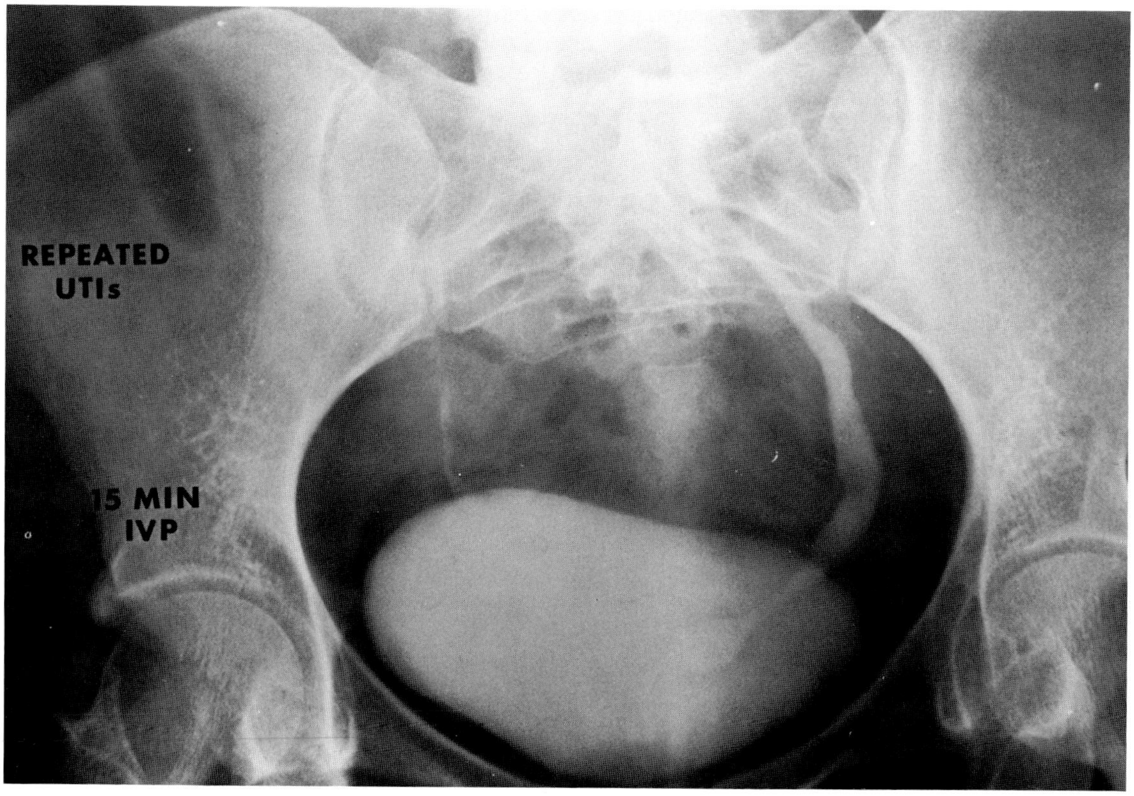

A

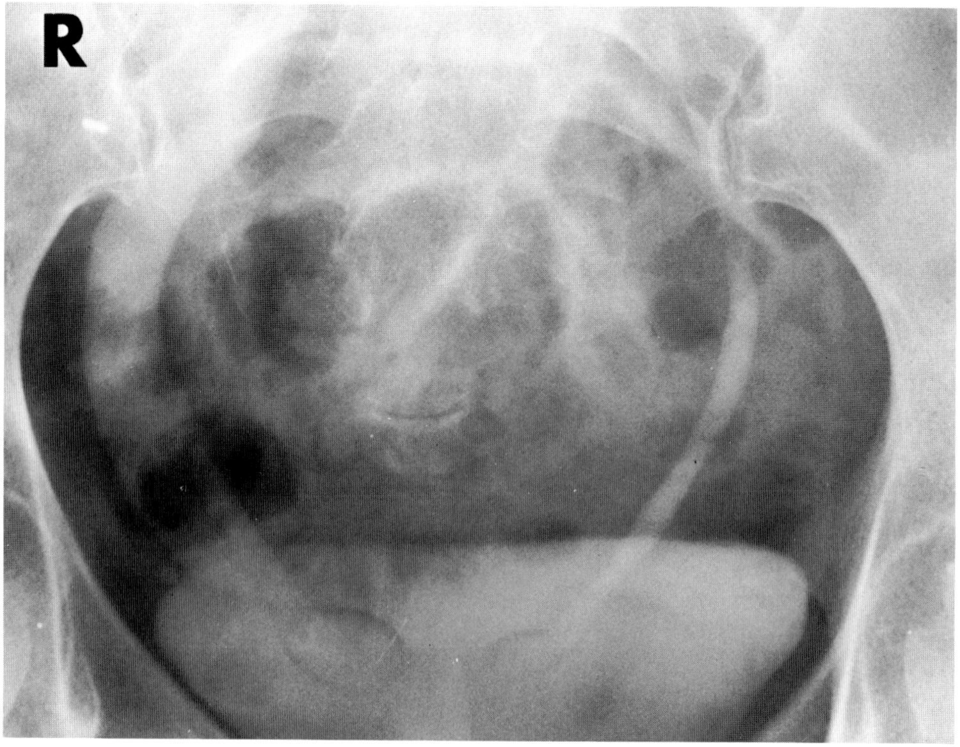

B (another patient)

Simple Ureterocele

Clinical Information

This 25-year-old black female had experienced repeated episodes of urinary tract infection since childhood. Urine culture revealed an *E. coli* infection, which cleared with appropriate therapy.

Roentgen Findings

A 15-minute intravenous urogram showed normal upper urinary tracts. The distal end of the left ureter is bulbous and presents a "cobra head" appearance with a surrounding radiolucent halo (A) that is typical of a simple ureterocele.

Comments

A ureterocele represents a localized dilatation of the distal end of a ureter. A simple or orthotopic ureterocele occurs in a normally positioned ureter. An ectopic ureterocele empties at an abnormal location and usually is associated with duplication of the ipsilateral upper urinary tract. Ectopic ureteroceles are more common in females, are usually discovered in childhood, and are more likely to cause obstruction and symptomatology (3).

Simple ureteroceles have no sexual predilection. They usually are asymptomatic and generally discovered in adults. Symptoms, when present, commonly relate to urinary tract infection, although stones and milk of calcium have been discovered in simple ureteroceles (2). They usually are unilateral but can be bilateral, as seen in film B from a patient with long-standing severe right pyelonephritis and right ureteral dilatation. A ureterocele results from stenosis of the distal ureteral orifice associated with a deficiency of the connective tissue attachment of the ureter to the bladder wall. The dilatation protrudes into the bladder lumen due to the ureter's deficient attachment to the bladder wall. The stenosis causes the distal ureter to dilate. Lack of support by a surrounding bladder wall abets and helps localize the dilatation of the ureterocele and accounts for its radiologic appearance. Mild dilatation may extend to the intramural portion of the ureter and sometimes even to the distal third of the ureter. Complications are rare in simple ureteroceles. Patients with symptoms can be treated successfully with a simple ureteroneocystostomy.

A ureterocele presents a diagnostic x-ray appearance. It assumes the shape of a "cobra head" or "spring onion." The ureterocele fills with contrast agent on intravenous urography. It is surrounded by a thin radiolucent halo, which represents the ureteral wall. A retrograde study will show the ureterocele as a filling defect. The filling defect must be distinguished from a tumor, a stone, or even rectal gas. Both simple and ectopic ureteroceles can be identified with ultrasonography (1). An ectopic ureterocele is easily distinguished from a simple ureterocele by its abnormal location and lack of a halo. It is important to distinguish a simple ureterocele from a pseudoureterocele (4). The latter is an acquired dilatation of the distal ureter most commonly due to a stone or neoplasm, more often the latter. Although it can mimic a benign simple ureterocele, a pseudoureterocele usually shows some asymmetry of the dilated distal ureter. Either can have a halo. The dilatation in a pseudoureterocele also involves the distal submucosal segment of the ureter. The halo in a pseudoureterocele is usually thicker and tends to be somewhat irregular, because it often represents a portion of the pathologic process that has led to the dilatation. The obstruction of a pseudoureterocele is more severe and involves a larger portion of the ureter. The upper urinary tract is often dilated. There usually is evidence of the obstructing lesion.

Source Materials

1. Griffin J, Jennings C, MacErlean D. Ultrasonic evaluation of simple and ectopic ureteroceles. Clin Radiol 34:55, 1983.
2. Poulos A, Fried AM, Woodring JH, et al. Milk of calcium ureterocele. South Med J 75:1012, 1982.
3. Shapiro SR. Ectopic and orthotopic ureteroceles. Radiological case of the month. Am J Dis Child 131:707, 1977.
4. Thornbury JR, Silver TM, Vinson RK. Ureteroceles vs pseudoureteroceles in adults. Urographic diagnosis. Radiology 122:81, 1977.

Case 80

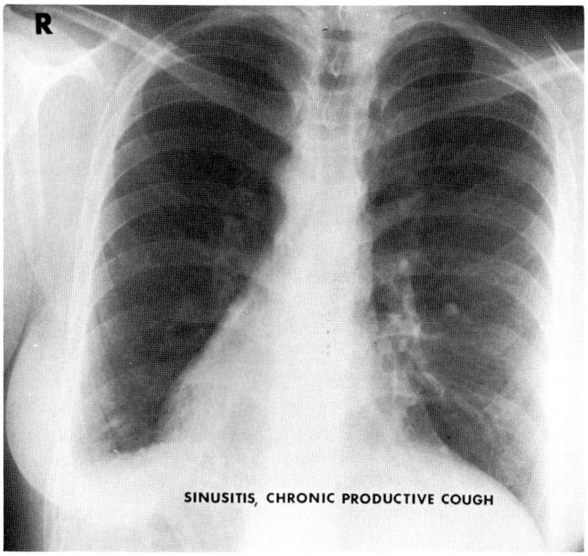

A

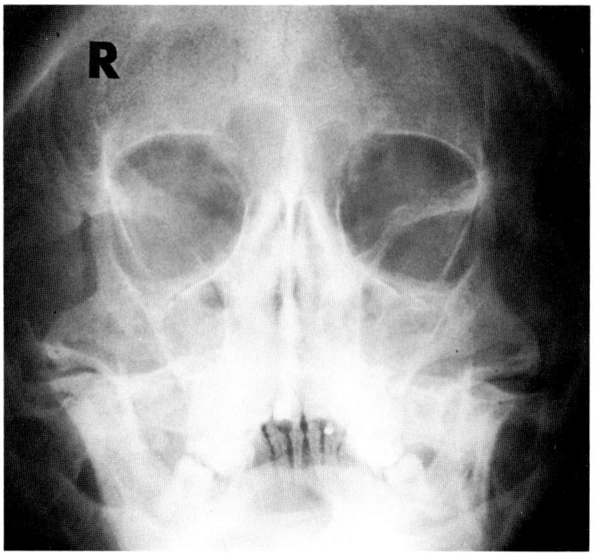

B

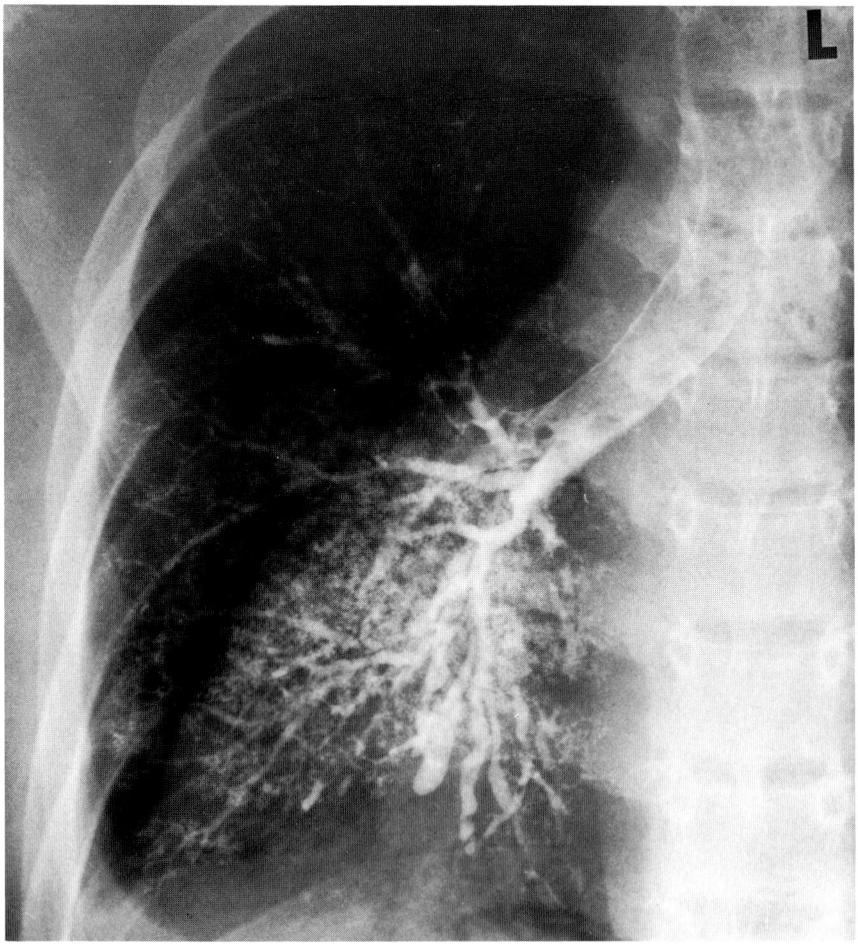

C

Kartagener's Syndrome

Clinical Information

This 18-year-old white female was evaluated for dextrocardia, sinusitis, and a chronic productive cough. Bronchoscopy revealed a bilobed right-sided lung and a trilobed left-sided lung. Electron microscopy of a tracheal biopsy showed absence of dynein arms indicative of immotile cilia thought to be characteristic of Kartagener's syndrome (2–4).

Roentgen Findings

A posteroanterior film of the chest (A) shows situs inversus with the cardiac apex directed toward the right and the stomach bubble in the right upper quadrant. A patch of density in the right lower lung field and blunting of the right costophrenic angle are evident. A Waters view of the paranasal sinuses (B) shows all the visible sinuses to be clouded. There is a questionable fluid level in the left maxillary antrum. A subsequent bronchogram (C) shows bronchiectasis of the basal segments of the lower lobe of the right-sided lung. The arrangement of the bronchi in the right-sided lung is that usually seen in a left lung.

Comments

Kartagener's syndrome is characterized by situs inversus, chronic paranasal sinusitis, and bronchiectasis. Although the association between bronchiectasis and situs inversus was first noted in 1904, the syndrome has carried Kartagener's name since his report in 1933. The incidence of bronchiectasis in the general population is only 0.2–0.5%, but it is approximately 20% in patients with situs inversus. Kartagener's syndrome is found in about one of every 40,000 individuals. The condition has a strong familial tendency but usually appears in only one generation, with many siblings being involved. There often is consanguinity. The parents are normal. These circumstances indicate a recessive mode of inheritance, possibly involving several genes. Relative sterility of the males with Kartagener's syndrome helps explain involvement of a single generation.

Patients with Kartagener's syndrome rarely have significant heart disease. Their main symptoms center around sinopulmonary disease. Complaints usually appear in early childhood. The symptoms and x-ray findings are similar to those in situs solitus patients with the same conditions. All aspects of the syndrome may not be present. Some may have only one clinical manifestation. Sinus involvement is the least distinctive aspect. Occasionally the only abnormality is hypoplasia or polyps rather than frank sinusitis.

The etiology of Kartagener's syndrome is somewhat unclear. No association has been shown with sex, blood groups, or hypersensitivity states. These and similar patients have been noted to have immotile sperms and a deficiency of normal mucociliary transport, with immotile cilia on the respiratory epithelium. The respiratory cilia often are unable to utilize energy and produce motility. Consequently, they may be unable to clear the paranasal sinuses and bronchi of bacteria. This abets infection. More than one type of electron microscopic abnormality has been associated with sperm and cilial immotility. A spectrum of these conditions probably exists (1, 2). It has been suggested that they be called the "immotile cilia syndrome" (2, 3). The relationships between the immotile cilia and situs inversus are speculative.

Source Materials

1. Jonsson MS, McCormick JR, Gillies CG, Gondos B. Kartagener's syndrome with motile spermatozoa. N Engl J Med 307:1131, 1982.
2. Rossman CM, Forrest JB, Ruffin RE, Newhouse MT. Immotile cilia syndrome in persons with and without Kartagener's syndrome. Am Rev Resp Dis 121:1011, 1980.
3. Whitelaw A, Evans A, Corrin B. Immotile cilia syndrome: A new cause of neonatal respiratory distress. Arch Dis Child 56:432, 1981.
4. Woodring JH, Royer JM, McDonagh D. Kartagener's syndrome. JAMA 247:2814, 1982.

Case 81

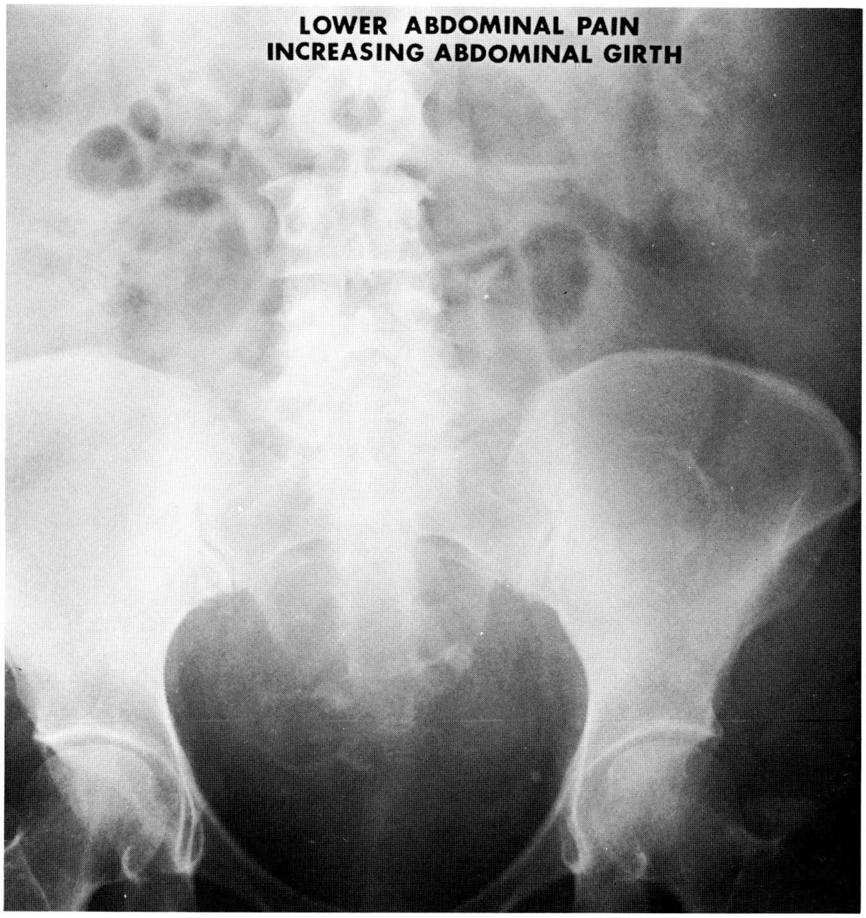

A

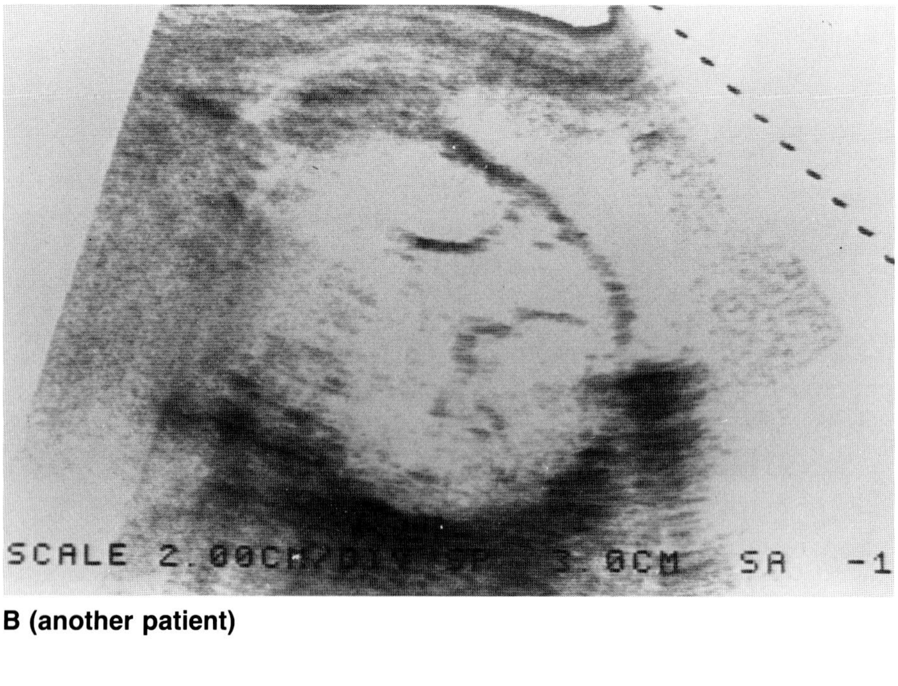

B (another patient)

Ovarian Serous Cystadenocarcinoma

Clinical Information

This 54-year-old woman complained of increasing abdominal girth and lower abdominal pain. A papillary serous cystadenocarcinoma of the right ovary was completely removed at surgery.

Roentgen Findings

A film of the abdomen (A) shows mild haziness of the entire abdomen. A central location of gas-filled intestinal loops suggests the possibility of ascites. There is evidence of a sizable pelvic mass with ill-defined edges and containing irregular areas of calcification. This calcification is streaky in appearance and somewhat horizonal in orientation. Close inspection vaguely suggests a granular composition of these calcifications, which occupy most of the true pelvis and extend upward over the left iliac bone.

Comments

Ovarian neoplasm, although the third most prevalent gynecologic tumor, is said to be the most common cause of death from malignancy of the female genital tract. This unfortunate outcome occurs because the tumor is often far advanced when a diagnosis is confirmed. Patients with a malignant ovarian tumor average about 50 years of age. This contrasts to 34 years of age for females with benign ovarian tumors. Up to 20% of malignant ovarian tumors are bilateral. This contrasts with only a 5% bilaterality of benign tumors of this organ. The usual initial symptom is lower abdominal pain and increasing girth. Gastrointestinal and urinary complaints, weight loss, and ascites are common.

Most ovarian tumors, whether benign or malignant, are cystic in nature. The cysts contain either mucinous or serous material, which accounts for the names of mucinous or pseudomucinous and serous cystadenoma and cystadenocarcinoma, respectively. Mucinous tumors comprise about 20% of all ovarian neoplasms. The serous form is more frequent. The mucinous form is benign in a ratio of 7:1, whereas the serous form is malignant in a ratio of 9:1. Pseudomucinous cystadenocarcinomas of an ovary tend to be larger than serous tumors. One has been said to weigh as much as 328 pounds. The descriptive term "papillary" refers to a morphologic appearance that is almost exclusively seen in the serous type. Rupture of a malignant ovarian cyst can lead to numerous tumor implants upon the serosal surfaces of the peritoneal cavity. Rupture of the mucinous form can cause the abdomen to become filled with material much like the pseudomyxoma peritonei seen following rupture of a mucocele of the appendix.

The most common x-ray finding of an ovarian carcinoma is a mass in the pelvis. Pseudomucinous ovarian tumors may contain curvilinear calcifications, whereas the calcifications in serous tumors are likely to be fine, more faint, or amorphous (2). The calcifications in a serous tumor can be very compact and collect into more or less discrete masses. The appearance may suggest residual barium in the gastrointestinal tract (4). The calcification in the serous form is psammomatous in nature and can be closely mimicked by the very rare gonadoblastoma. Ultrasonic findings are highly characteristic with ovarian cystadenomas and cystadenocarcinomas (1). An irregular cystic ovarian mass that contains solid areas of echogenicity suggests malignancy (A sonogram of a complex cystic adnexal mass, which represented an ovarian cystadenocarcinoma, is shown in B.) Some feel that a cystic mass in the pelvis that contains papillary projections is virtually diagnostic of an ovarian cystadenocarcinoma (3).

Source Materials

1. Deland M, Fried AM, Van Nagell JR, Donaldson ES. Ultrasonography in the diagnosis of ovarian tumors. Surg Gynecol Obstet 148:346, 1979.
2. Moncada R, Cooper RA, Garces M, Badrinath K. Calcified metastases from malignant ovarian neoplasm. Radiology 113:31, 1974.
3. Requard CK, Mettler RA Jr, Wicks JD. Preoperative sonography of malignant ovarian neoplasms. AJR 137:79, 1981.
4. Teplick JG, Haskins ME, Alavi A. Calcified intraperitoneal metastases from ovarian carcinoma. AJR 127:1003, 1976.

Case 82

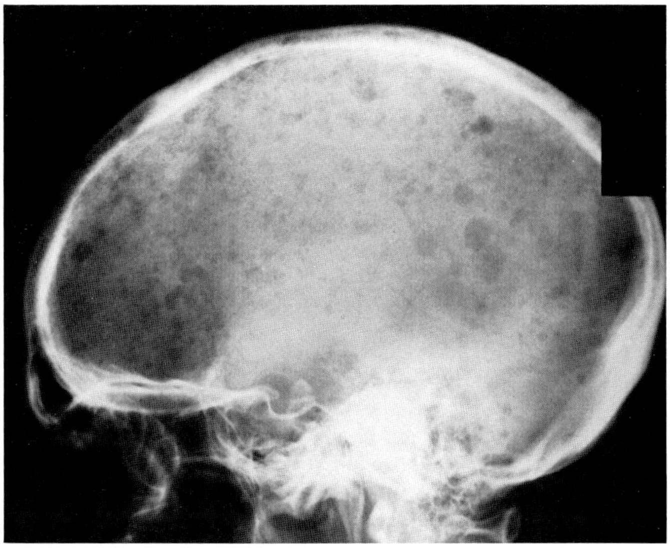

A

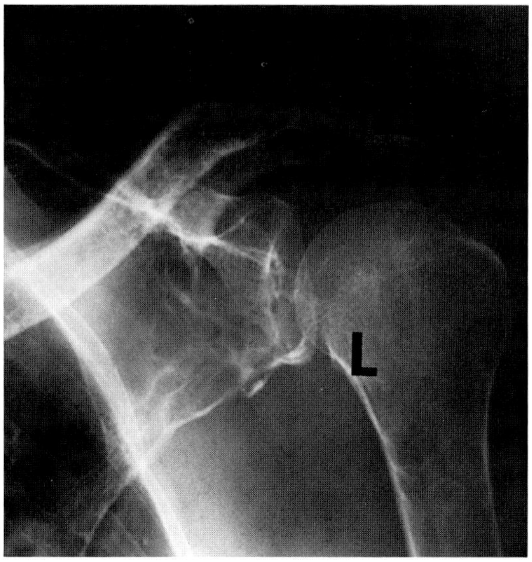

B

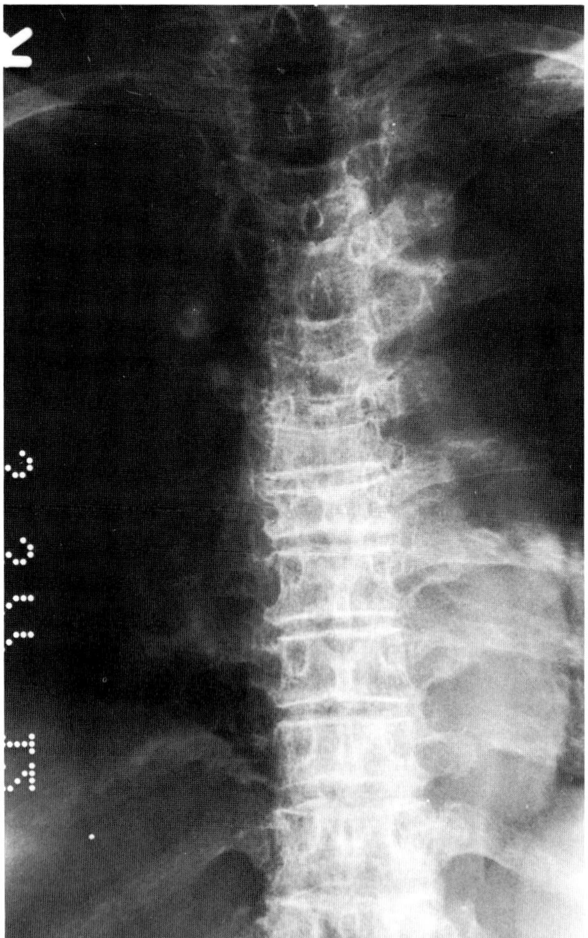

C

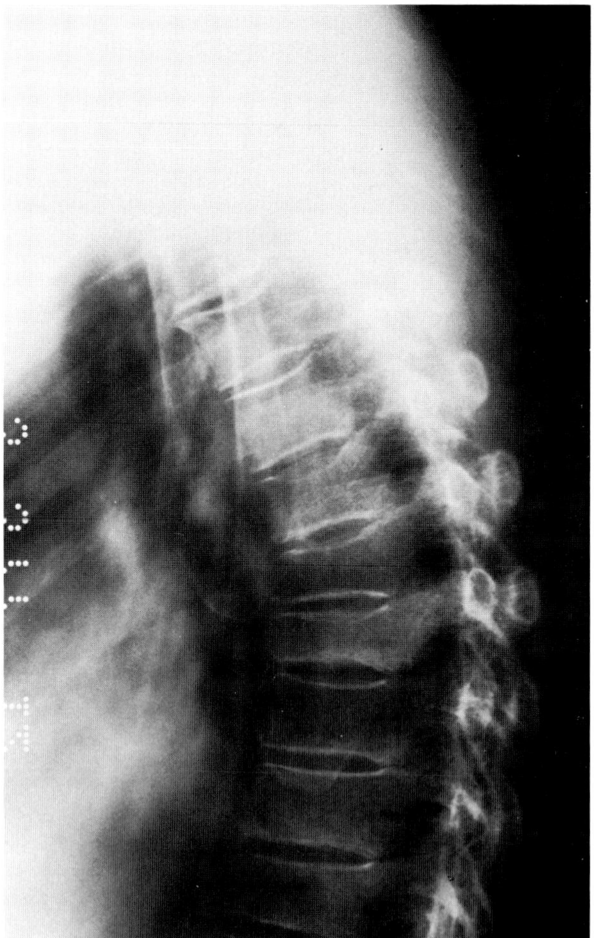

D

Multiple Myeloma

Clinical Information

This 61-year-old black female had noted increasing pain in her back and left shoulder as well as progressive weakness for the past year. Her serum calcium, total proteins, and alkaline phosphatase were elevated. Serum electrophoresis showed an M-type spike. Bone marrow biopsy confirmed the diagnosis of multiple myeloma.

Roentgen Findings

A lateral view of the skull (A) shows multiple punched-out lesions characteristic of multiple myeloma. A film on the left shoulder (B) reveals a large multilocular area of destruction in the scapula near the glenoid fossa as well as destruction in the humeral shaft and left clavicle. The dorsal spine (C, D) is markedly osteoporotic. Several vertebrae have collapsed. The posterior ribs also show considerable destruction.

Comments

Multiple myeloma, often called plasma cell myeloma, is the most common malignant tumor of bone. It apparently arises from the plasma cell series of the bone marrow. The disease is most frequently seen between the ages of 40 and 70 years and is slightly more common in males. The outstanding symptom is vague bone pain, which most often affects the axial skeleton, especially the sternum, vertebrae, and ribs. The pain becomes severe following a pathologic fracture. Low-grade fever is common. Renal insufficiency, hypertension, generalized lymphadenopathy, and splenomegaly are fairly frequent. Amyloidosis, which may appear before or after the multiple myeloma, is an associated condition in about 15% of these patients. The relationship between the two is obscure. Anemia is often present and probably results from marrow replacement and myelofibrosis as well as hypersplenism. Hypercalcemia, thought to be due to bone destruction, occurs in over 50% of patients with multiple myeloma. Hyperglobulinemia with reversal of the albumin-globulin ratio is seen in approximately 60% of cases. Plasma electrophoresis shows a characteristic M-type peak. There often are abnormal Bence Jones proteins in the urine. Bence Jones proteinuria may be present for many years before the development of a myelomatous process (1). Treatment involves chemotherapy and radiation.

The most common x-ray abnormality in plasma cell myeloma is diffuse osteoporosis. The presence of osteoporosis without a local bony lesion is sometimes called myelomatosis. Destructive lesions are often present. They are most commonly found in the spine, ribs, and skull as well as the proximal ends of the humeri and femurs. Typical punched-out lesions indicate classical multiple myeloma, although a few other malignancies can present a similar appearance. A single bone may be involved for a long period before the disease disseminates. Since there is no bone production, radionuclide studies are usually negative unless there is a fracture (4). Sclerosis is uncommon without therapy. Care must be exercised in performing an intravenous urogram in the presence of multiple myeloma, because acute precipitation of protein in the renal tubules may occur. Patients with plasma cell myeloma who require an intravenous urogram should be well hydrated.

The most difficult differential diagnostic consideration is metastatic carcinoma. A biopsy may be required. Bone marrow biopsy sites have been mistaken for multiple myeloma (2). It has been said that destruction of the vertebral pedicles is more indicative of metastatic carcinoma than myeloma, because there is a very small amount of bone marrow, if any, in the pedicles. Myeloma must be distinguished from other plasma cell dyscrasias such as Waldenström's macroglobulinemia and the POEMS syndrome (3).

Source Materials

1. Kyle RA, Greipp PR. "Idiopathic" Bence Jones proteinuria. Long-term follow-up in seven patients. N Engl J Med 306:564, 1982.
2. O'Gara CM, Cigtay OS. Iliac marrow biopsy sites in adults. J Can Assoc Radiol 30:230, 1979.
3. Resnick D, Greenway GD, Bardwirk PA, et al. Plasma-cell dyscrasia with polyneuropathy, organomegaly, endocrinopathy, M-protein, and skin changes: The POEMS syndrome. Radiology 140:17, 1981.
4. Wahner HW, Kyle RA, Beabout JW. Scintigraphic evaluation of the skeleton in multiple myeloma. Mayo Clin Proc 55:739, 1980.

Case 83

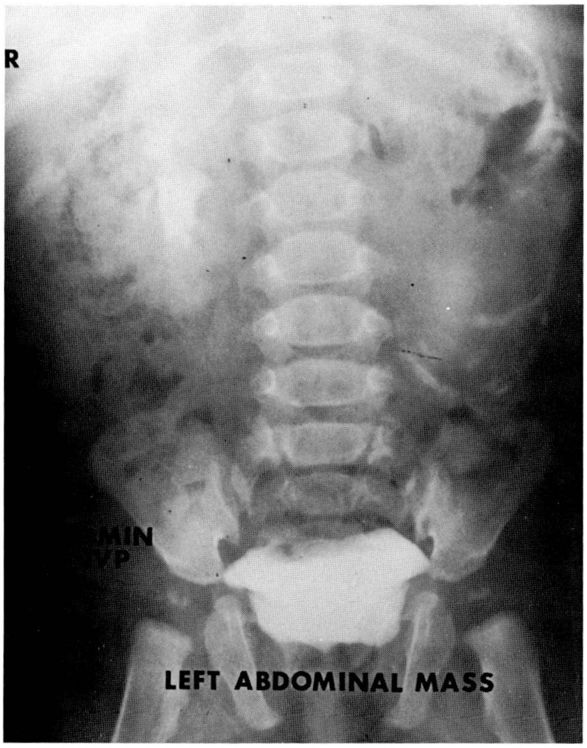

A

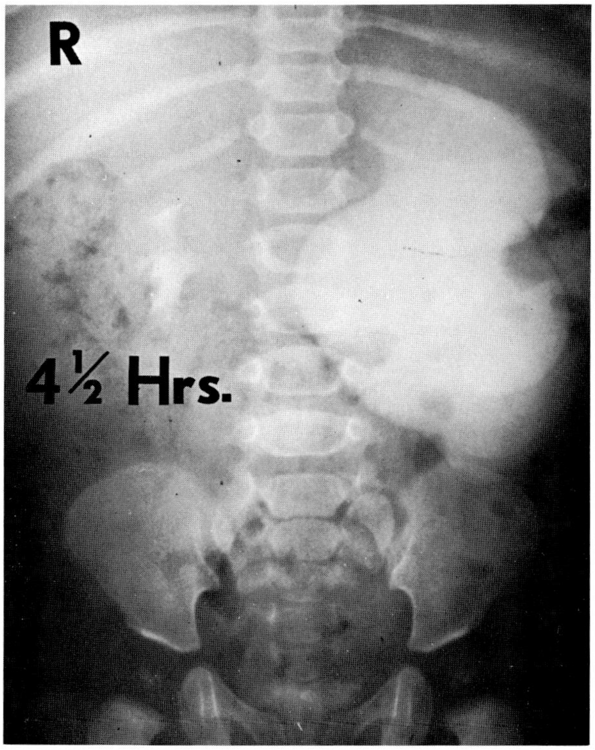

B

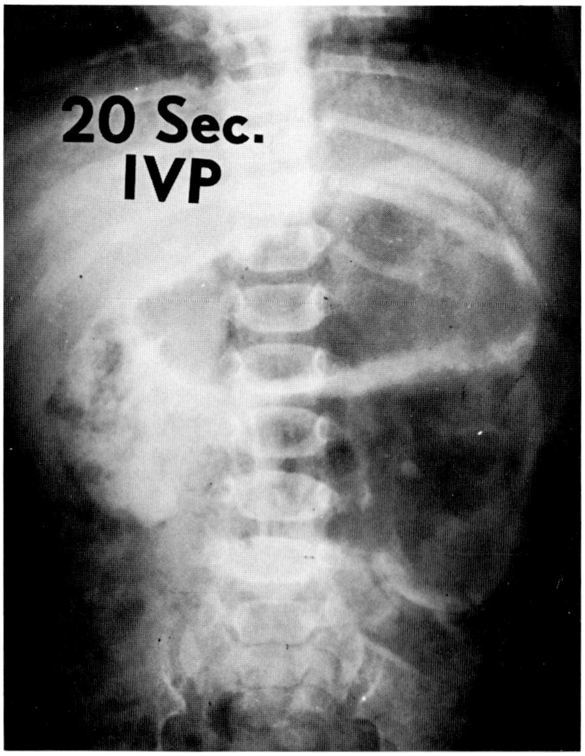

C (another patient)

Crescent (Calyceal) Sign of Hydronephrosis

Clinical Information

This 10-month-old female presented with a left-sided abdominal mass. A subsequent left nephrectomy revealed a massively hydronephrotic left kidney secondary to ureteropelvic junction obstruction.

Roentgen Findings

The 10-minute film of an intravenous urogram (A) shows a normal drainage system on the right. Curvilinear streaks of radiodensity are present in the left side of the abdomen. They appear to be located along the periphery of an enlarged reniform soft tissue structure. Small bilateral bladder ears are visible. The 4½-hour film (B) shows a massive left hydronephrosis secondary to ureteropelvic junction obstruction.

Comments

The crescentic densities represent an accumulation of contrast medium in the distal collecting ducts. A rim of recognizable renal tissue usually remains between the crescents and the renal margin. The calyceal crescent sign is diagnostic of hydronephrosis (1). Increasing pressure in the drainage system from chronic obstruction, whatever the cause, will eventually flatten the papillae and reorient the collecting ducts until the latter come to lie tangential to the surface of the calyces. This distortion of the ducts augments the obstruction. The obstruction causes relative stasis, which permits the opaque medium within these ducts to become more concentrated and radiopaque due to continued reabsorption of water.

The crescents of hydronephrosis disappear with relief of the obstruction. The crescent sign is uncommon in adults. In less severe obstruction the opaque medium can sometimes be seen in distal portions of the individual ducts (ducts of Bellini) as specks of radiopacity surrounding dilated calyces. (2). It is these ducts that are displaced by more severe and prolonged chronic obstruction to form a large portion of the structures that create the densities in the calyceal crescent sign.

The calyceal crescent sign is only seen with chronic obstruction. It would not be expected in acute obstruction, since the calyces do not have time to dilate and displace the collecting ducts. The density of the opaque medium in the crescent sign is greater than the density of the rim sign (C, from another patient), which is seen much sooner after injection of the opaque medium (4). The calyceal crescent sign usually appears between 10–30 minutes after injection. The rim sign is in fact a nephrogram of the remaining renal parenchyma. Septations of increased density within the substance of an enlarged nonfunctioning kidney at this age can be seen on intravenous urography in a multicystic dysplastic kidney (3). They somewhat resemble the calyceal crescent sign but have a different orientation, are not located so peripherally, and are less dense. The margins of overlying gas shadows could be mistaken for calyceal crescents.

Source Materials

1. Dunbar JS, Nogrady MB. The calyceal crescent—A roentgenographic sign of obstructive hydronephrosis. AJR 110:520, 1970.
2. Griscom NT, Kroeker MA. Visualization of individual papillary ducts (ducts of Bellini) by excretory urography in childhood hydronephrosis. Radiology 106:385, 1973.
3. Lachman RS, Lindstrom RR, Hirose RM. The "septation sign" in multicystic dysplastic kidney. Pediatr Radiol 3:117, 1975.
4. Ransley PG. Opacification of the renal parenchyma in obstruction and reflux. Pediatr Radiol 4:226, 1976.

Case 84

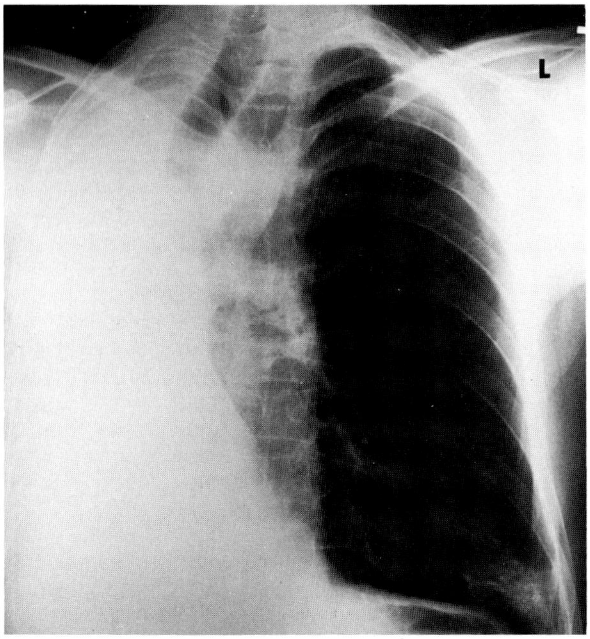

A

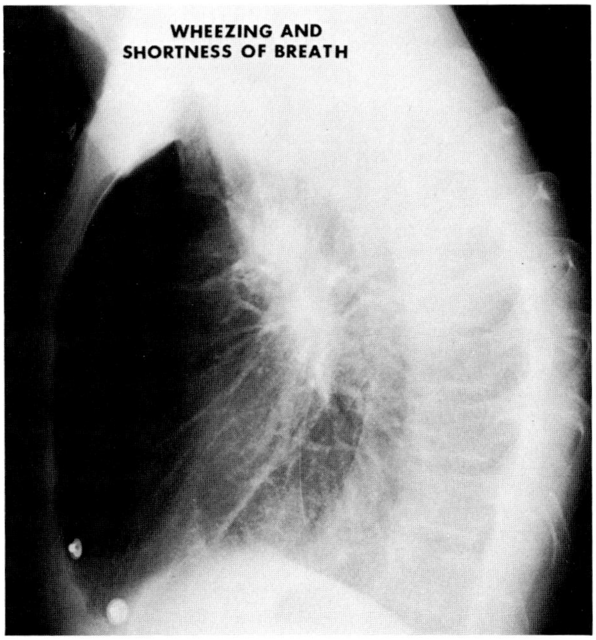

B

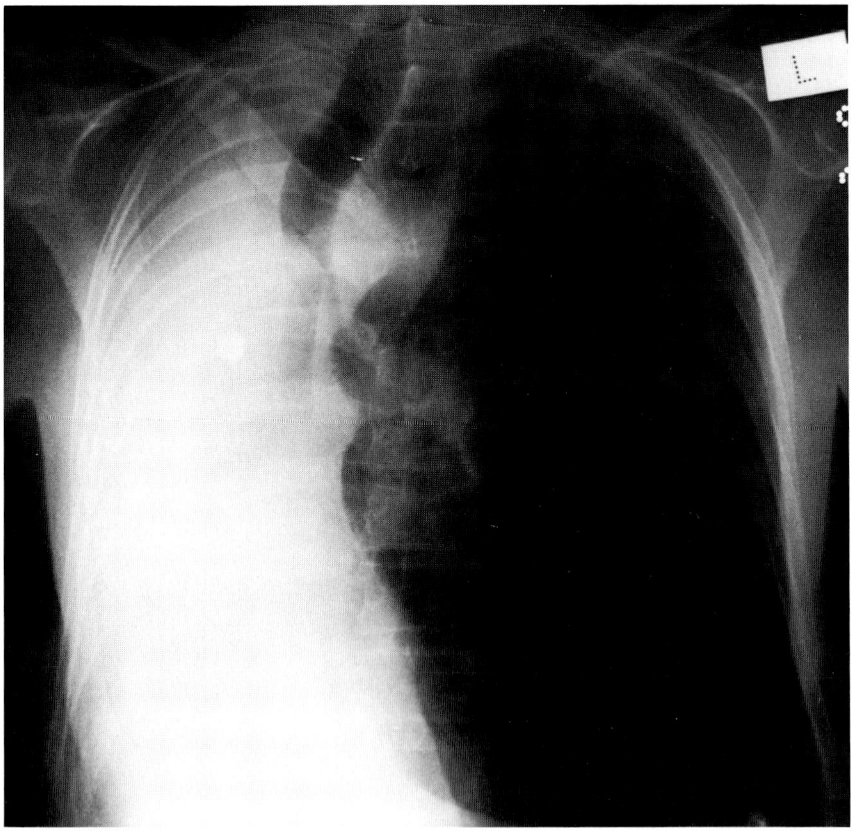

C

Total Collapse of One Lung

Clinical Information

This 60-year-old white man had complained of a wheezing sensation in his right chest and increasing shortness of breath for the preceding 3 months. Bronchoscopy revealed a squamous cell carcinoma near the carina, which had occluded his right mainstem bronchus and extended far into the left mainstem bronchus.

Roentgen Findings

Posteroanterior (A) and lateral (B) chest films show the right hemithorax to be opaque and the trachea, heart, and mediastinum displaced far to the right. The right heart margin is lost in the right-sided density. The left lung is herniated into the right hemithorax. There is a sharp cutoff of the right mainstem bronchus near the carina by a soft tissue mass, which encroaches upon the lumen of the left mainstem bronchus. A pneumonic infiltrate is noted in the extreme lower left lung field. The lateral film reveals only one diaphragmatic leaf with striking retrosternal radiolucency due to anterior herniation of the left lung across the midline. An overpenetrated film (C) shows the opacity in the lateral and lower portion of the right hemithorax to be sharply demarcated medially and superiorly by the herniated left lung.

Comments

The most frequent etiology for collapse of an entire lung is bronchial obstruction due to an intrinsic mass, which most commonly is a bronchogenic carcinoma. A mucous plug, foreign body, or inflammatory stenosis that has progressed to total occlusion of a mainstem bronchus are less frequent causes. Collapse can also result from extrinsic pressure by an aneurysm, mediastinal tumor, or enlarged lymph nodes.

The posteroanterior chest film in collapse of an entire lung presents a characteristic appearance (2, 3). It shows the atelectatic lung as a homogeneous density that is markedly reduced in size. The affected lung collapses posteriorly, inferiorly, and laterally. The diaphragm on the affected side is elevated and the rib spaces are narrowed. The trachea, heart, and mediastinum are displaced toward the affected side. The opposite lung compensatorily overinflates and usually herniates across the midline. The herniation occurs anterior and superior to the heart and great vessels. This accounts for the striking retrosternal radiolucency of the lateral chest film, which contrasts with the much greater radiodensity posteriorly and inferiorly, in the location of the collapsed lung.

Differential diagnostic considerations include extensive pneumonia, pleural effusion, and previous pneumonectomy. Surgical deformities such as resected ribs and metallic clips or sutures usually betray a previous pneumonectomy. The surgically amputated bronchus is often apparent. Massive unilateral pleural effusion consumes space and, in contrast to collapse or a pneumonectomy, usually produces a dense hemithorax that is as large if not larger than normal. There also is no relative increase in retrosternal radiolucency on the lateral film with a massive pleural effusion, since there is no lung herniation. The fluid acts as a generalized filter of all the opposite normal air-containing lung (1). A combination of effusion and collapse is relatively common, particularly in the presence of bronchogenic carcinoma. The lateral film suggests effusion rather than collapse. The same is true if massive effusion occurs with extensive pneumonia. Pneumonia involving all the lobes of one lung is rarely so homogeneously dense as either pleural effusion or total collapse. It will not increase the size of the affected hemithorax. There usually is some reduction due to associated peripheral atelectasis. When pneumonia of an entire lung is associated with extensive collapse, the lateral film is suggestive of collapse but the area of density is larger than with collapse alone.

Source Materials

1. Lubert M, Krause GR. Total unilateral pulmonary collapse. A study of the roentgen appearance in the lateral view. Radiology 67:175, 1956.
2. Proto AV, Tocino I. Radiographic manifestations of lobar collapse. Semin Roentgenol 15:117, 1980.
3. Robbins LL, Hale CH. The roentgen appearance of lobar and segmental collapse of the lung. III. Collapse of an entire lung or major part thereof. Radiology 45:23, 1945.

Case 85

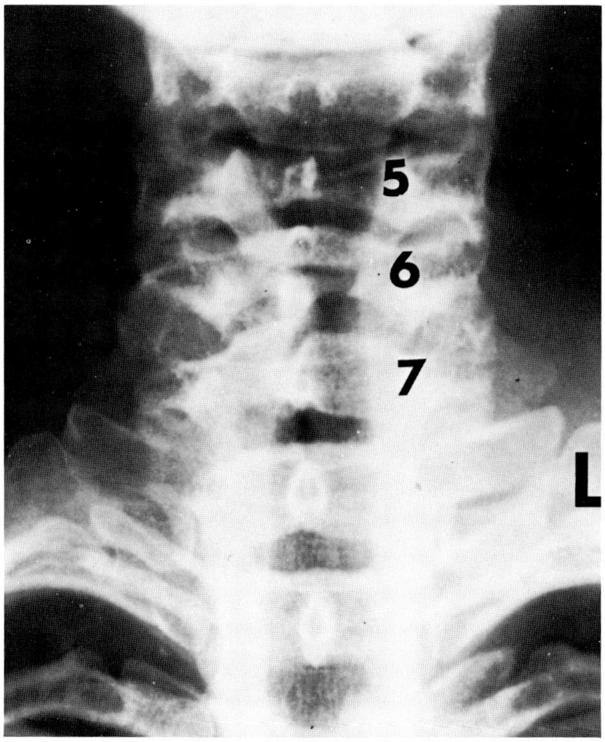

A

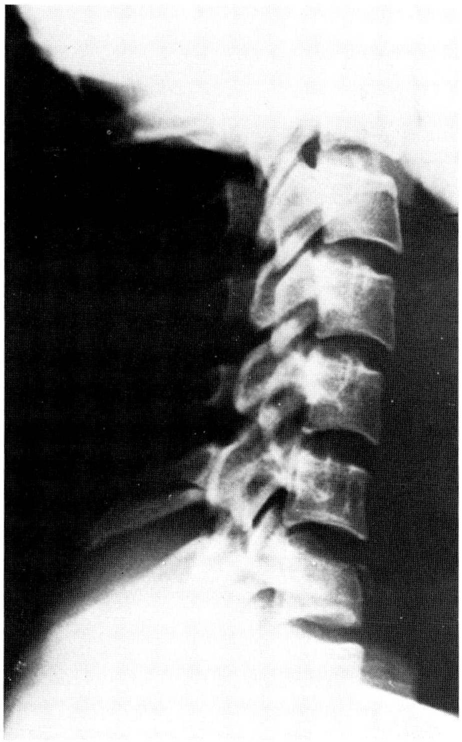

B

Clay Shoveler's Fracture

Clinical Information

This 21-year-old white male was involved in an automobile accident 9 hours before these films were obtained. He complained of cervical pain without radiation, which cleared with symptomatic therapy.

Roentgen Findings

Anteroposterior (A) and lateral (B) films of the neck show an oblique fracture through the spinous process of C6. A small fragment has been fractured from the anterosuperior margin of the body of C7. The anteroposterior film reveals a radiolucent defect through the spinous process of C6.

Comments

Most of the recently reported cases of clay shoveler's fracture, sometimes called root puller's fracture, have resulted from automobile or football injuries. This injury may also result from persistent repetitive trauma that eventually leads to a stress fracture (3). C7 is most commonly involved, although this type of injury can affect any spinous process from C6 to T3. This type of fracture was common among construction workers who built the first German autobahn in 1936 (2). Many additional cases were seen in ditchdiggers in southwestern Australia. The clay they were digging was unusually sticky and required considerable effort to disengage the clay from the shovel. The condition is also seen in hay pitchers, individuals who dip molten magnesium, and cricket players. A clay shoveler's fracture that occurs in an automobile accident is often associated, as in this case, with other spinal column injuries.

A clay shoveler's fracture is particularly frequent in individuals who previously had sedentary occupations. The complaints usually develop after some 20 or more days of the new activities. This suggests the injury is a stress fracture. The patient experiences a "pop" in the neck with resultant interscapular pain. There is local tenderness, which clears with symptomatic therapy. The avulsed fragment usually does not unite and eventually presents eburnated margins. The loose fragment has been resected in some patients. This treatment may be followed after work is resumed by a fracture of the next caudal spinous process. Symptomatic therapy is all that is usually needed. Healing occurs without significant disability.

The fracture tends to occur at the narrowest point of the spinous process, which is about 2 cm from its tip. There usually is caudal displacement of the avulsed fragment, which probably is the result of strong ligamentous pull. The fracture line is more or less perpendicular to the orientation of the interspinous ligaments. A clay shoveler's fracture and the bony displacement are clearly visible on a lateral film of the cervical spine. The anteroposterior film shows a double density at the location of the affected spinous process (1). The differential diagnosis includes calcification in the nuchal ligament. Such calcification is usually aligned perpendicular to the spinous processes and does not display a trabecular pattern. It is important not to confuse a duplicated spinous process with a clay shoveler's fracture. In duplication the bifid spinous process is seen on an anteroposterior film as two densities located in the same horizontal plane. With a clay shoveler's fracture, the fragments are located at different levels. The apophysis for the spinous processes at C6 and C7 should be fused by 20 or 25 years. Only rarely do they fail to fuse. Schmitt's disease, sometimes called clay shoveler's fracture of the adolescent, is usually seen in teenage males following exertional stress or trauma (4). This injury is apparently an avulsion of the apophysis of the spinous process.

Source Materials

1. Cancelmo JJ Jr. Clay shoveler's fracture. AJR 115:540, 1972.
2. Matthes HG. Unsere Erfahrungen bei der Schipperkrankheit. Arch Orthop Unfallchir 37:232, 1937.
3. Venable JR, Flake RE, Kilian DJ. Stress fracture of the spinous process. JAMA 190:103, 1964.
4. Weston WJ. Clay shoveler's disease in adolescent (Schmitt's disease). A report of two cases. Br J Radiol 30:378, 1957.

Case 86

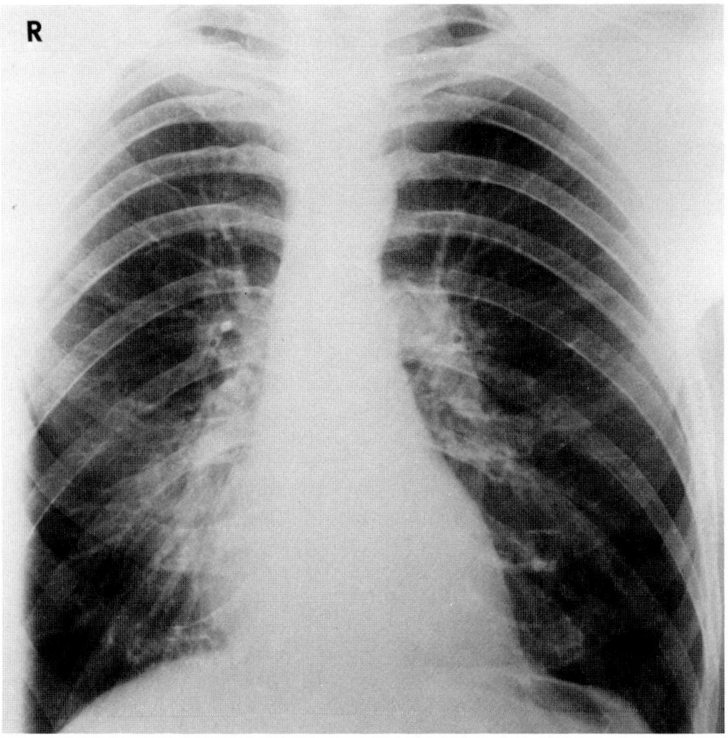

A

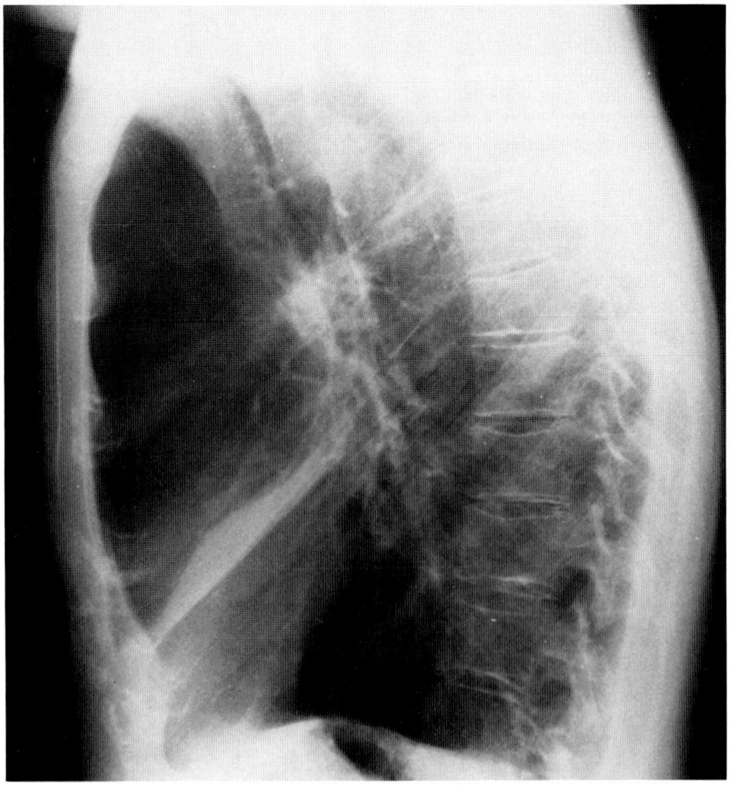

B

Middle Lobe Collapse

Clinical Information

This 35-year-old febrile white male had a long history of bronchial asthma. Expectoration of a large mucous plug was followed by expansion of the right middle lobe.

Roentgen Findings

The posteroanterior chest film (A) shows a vague density obscuring a bit of the right heart border. The lateral film (B) reveals a sharply demarcated narrow density running from the hilum to the lower anterior chest wall. This appearance is typical of right middle lobe collapse.

Comments

Right middle lobe collapse is relatively common for several reasons. First, the middle lobe bronchus has quite a long course before it divides into its medial and lateral branches. This obviously increases the likelihood for both intrinsic and extrinsic processes to affect this bronchus. Second, the caliber of the middle lobe bronchus is smaller than other bronchi that serve lung segments of comparable volume. Third, the right middle lobe bronchus branches from the bronchus intermedius at an acute angle. This arrangement encourages the accumulation of secretions that can obstruct the lumen. Last, and most important, this bronchus is surrounded by many lymph nodes. These lymph nodes may become enlarged in response to inflammatory disease. Enlarged lymph nodes can exert extrinsic pressure, which may occlude or at least narrow the middle lobe bronchus. Bronchial stenosis abets the retention of secretions, chronic infection, and eventually atelectasis and collapse. The right middle lobe is a common site of bronchiectasis. The medial and lateral segments of the right middle lobe may collapse simultaneously or individually, more often the latter. The medial segment, which lies anteromedially and inferiorly, approximates the right heart border. It collapses more frequently than the lateral segment, which is situated posterolaterally along the minor fissure. The lateral segment does not touch the right heart border. Middle lobe atelectasis and infection have often been designated as the "middle lobe syndrome" (1).

The right middle lobe is bounded anteriorly and anterolaterally by the chest wall, medially by the mediastinum, superiorly by the minor fissure, and posteroinferiorly by the anterior portion of the major fissure. The minor and major fissures move toward each other as the lobe collapses. This causes the lobe to collapse in an inferomedial direction and creates a tapering wedge that is widest at its medial and anterior extremities.

It can be difficult to diagnose right middle lobe collapse from a posteroanterior film, which may only show blurring of the right heart border. The diagnosis is clearly apparent on a lateral film. The lateral film reveals right middle lobe collapse as a triangular density with its base against the anterior chest wall and diaphragm or, at times, only the inferior aspect of the anterior chest wall. The apex of the triangle is located centrally in the hilar region just beneath the right pulmonary artery in the region of the right middle lobe bronchus. At times the collapse is sufficiently complete, as in this case, to appear as a rectangular band of density. An abnormal bulge of the collapsed lobe seen on the lateral view in the hilum indicates a mass has caused collapse. A collapsed middle lobe is evident on a lordotic view as a triangle of density along the right heart border. The base of the triangle in this projection is located medially in contrast to the appearance seen on a lateral film. The anteromedial location of the maximal width of the wedge caused by right middle lobe collapse accounts for the base of the triangular density being anterior on the lateral film and medial on the lordotic view. On the lordotic view the posterior portion of the wedge can sometimes be seen through the anterior portion, creating a so-called "wedge-within-a-wedge" appearance. Right middle lobe infiltration without collapse may present a density with convex margins. This contrasts to the sometimes concave borders of right middle lobe collapse. Fluid in the anterior end of the major fissure also produces convex margins, but this density almost invariably terminates against the right hemidiaphragm.

Source Materials

1. Albo RJ, Grimes OF. The middle lobe syndrome: A clinical study. Dis Chest 50:509, 1966.
2. Proto A, Tocino I. Radiographic manifestations of lobar collapse. Semin Roentgenol 15:117, 1980.

Case 87

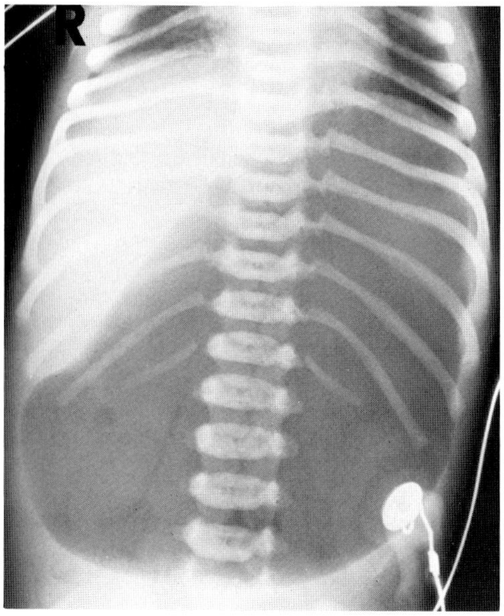

A

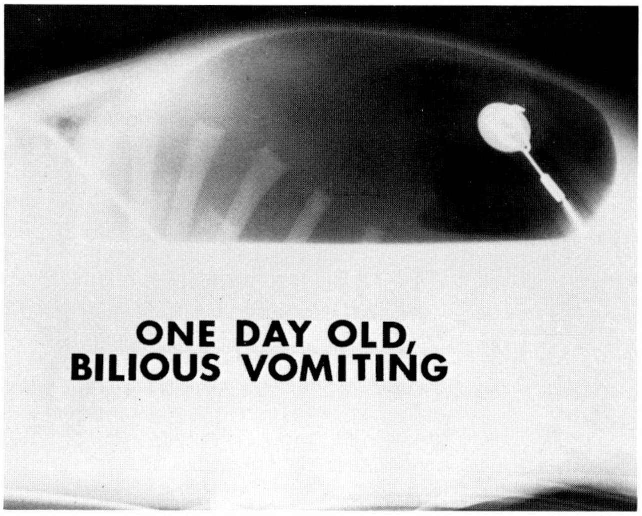

B

Duodenal Atresia

Clinical Information

This 1-day-old infant was examined because of bilious vomiting since birth. Exploratory laparotomy revealed a membrane that totally occluded the duodenum just below the ampulla of Vater.

Roentgen Findings

Supine anteroposterior (A) and cross-table lateral (B) films of the abdomen show a hugely dilated stomach. The cross-table lateral film reveals a fluid level in the stomach. A gas-containing duodenal bulb is visible as a second radiolucency superimposed upon the dilated stomach. No gas is noted distal to the duodenal bulb. The lung fields are clear.

Comments

Duodenal atresia occurs once in approximately 2000 live births and accounts for about 25% of alimentary tract obstructions in the newborn. It is the third most common form of intestinal obstruction in the neonate, being exceeded only by esophageal atresia and an imperforate anus. The atretic segment is usually situated just below the ampulla of Vater. This location accounts for the bile-stained vomitus (4). The obstructing lesion is often intrinsic and varies from a thin membrane to a blindly ending duodenal segment connected by a fibrous cord to more distal portions of the small bowel. An intrinsic obstructing lesion leads more often to atresia than to stenosis. The pathogenesis of the obstructing lesion is debated. Failure of recanalization is a favored explanation. Less common causes of obstruction are usually extrinsic. Obstructing peritoneal (Ladd's) bands are associated with colonic malrotation and commonly affect the third portion of the duodenal loop. A less frequently encountered etiology of partial duodenal obstruction is an annular pancreas, which affects the second portion. An annular pancreas may not cause symptoms until adulthood. Choledochal cyst and duodenal duplication are rare causes of duodenal obstruction.

Associated anomalies are frequent and include anomalies of the esophagus, anus, lumbosacral spine, limbs, and heart. About 30% of these patients have congenital cardiac defects. A third have Down's syndrome. Symptoms characteristically appear shortly after birth and consist of persistent vomiting, which usually is bile-stained. There occasionally is aspiration of the vomitus. Meconium may be passed during the first day of life. Treatment is surgical.

Duodenal atresia leads to diagnostic radiologic findings. Gas is visible in the stomach and duodenal bulb—the "double bubble" sign—which are either markedly dilated or of normal size if the patient is examined shortly after birth or vomits just prior to filming. Fluid levels are nearly always evident on upright films. The almost invariable presence of gas makes the introduction of an opaque medium unnecessary and inadvisable. Intestinal gas beyond the duodenum usually indicates stenosis rather than atresia, although a Y-shaped pancreatic duct has been present in a few of these patients (3). Insertion of one limb of the pancreatic duct above the atresia and another below provides a pathway for gas to pass from the dilated duodenum into the distal gut. Pregnant women who are bearing a fetus with this condition often have polyhydramnios. It is possible to diagnose duodenal atresia sonographically in utero (1). An incorrect ultrasonic diagnosis may be made if the incisura angularis of the stomach is prominent (2).

Source Materials

1. Gee H, Abdulla U. Antenatal diagnosis of fetal duodenal atresia by ultrasonic scan. Br Med J 2:1265, 1978.
2. Gross BH, Filly RA. Potential for a normal fetal stomach to simulate the sonographic "double bubble" sign. J Can Assoc Radiol 33:39, 1982.
3. Kassner EG, Sutton AL, de Groot TJ. Bile duct anomalies associated with duodenal atresia: Paradoxical presence of small bowel gas. AJR 116:577, 19872.
4. Salonen IS. Congenital duodenal obstruction. Acta Paediatr Scand [Suppl] 272:1, 1978.

Case 88

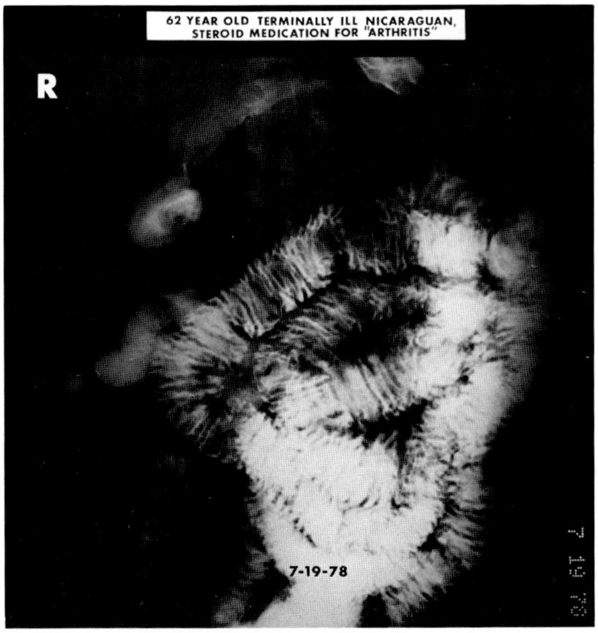
62 YEAR OLD TERMINALLY ILL NICARAGUAN,
STEROID MEDICATION FOR "ARTHRITIS"
R
7-19-78
7 19 78

A

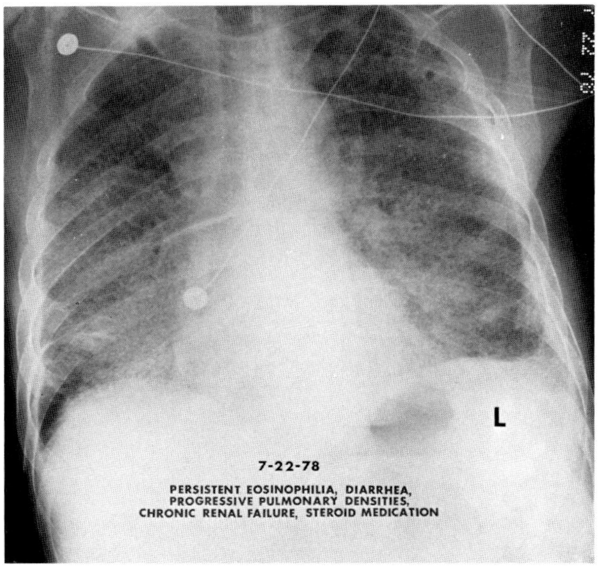
L
7-22-78
PERSISTENT EOSINOPHILIA, DIARRHEA,
PROGRESSIVE PULMONARY DENSITIES,
CHRONIC RENAL FAILURE, STEROID MEDICATION

B

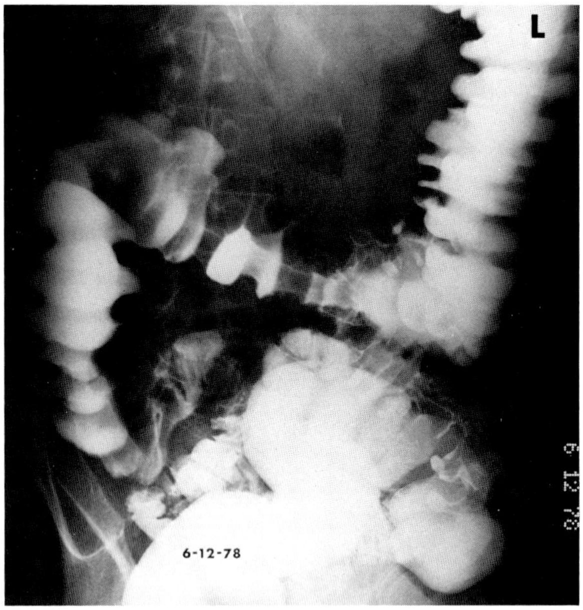
L
6-12-78
6 12 78

C

Strongyloidiasis

Clinical Information

This 62-year-old Nicaraguan died the day after the chest film (B) was obtained. He had chronic renal failure, diarrhea, and persistent eosinophilia. There had been prolonged treatment of his "arthritis" with steroids. Previous chest films had shown migratory densities, which steadily increased in size. The larvae of *Strongyloides stercoralis* were recovered from his stools the day before death. Medication with thiabendazole was begun shortly before he expired.

Roentgen Findings

Film A shows thickened jejunal mucosal folds. Occasional nodular filling defects are seen. The chest film reveals confluent alveolar densities throughout both lung fields. The appearance strongly suggests pulmonary edema, although the heart is not enlarged. There are bilateral pleural effusions. A barium enema (C) shows thickening of the bowel wall and questionable thumbprinting in the transverse colon.

Comments

Strongyloidiasis is caused by infestation with a nematode, *Strongyloides stercoralis.* The condition is very common in tropical climates. It is said that from 0.25% to 6% of the United States population are infected (2). Strongyloidiasis is more common in institutions and other situations associated with poor hygiene. Males are affected more often than females and adults more frequently than children (1, 2). An altered immune status abets hyperinfection, which may be fatal (3). Severe infestation can be complicated by *E. coli* septicemia. These bacteria apparently reach the bloodstream through the intestinal ulcers caused by the parasites.

Strongyloides are found in dogs, chimpanzees, and human beings. The parasite is initially contracted by human beings from the soil. A larval form burrows through the skin. A rash often develops at this time. Upon reaching the bloodstream the larvae travel to the lungs, where they become adult worms and move through the respiratory and alimentary passages to reach the large and small bowels. The adult female lays eggs in the gastrointestinal tract. Some hatch into infective larvae and pierce the mucosa or else burrow through the perianal skin. Strongyloidiasis is the only infestation that can be maintained without continued ingestion of contaminated material. Most patients with this infection have no symptoms. The passage of the parasites through the lungs can lead to hemorrhages and pneumonic infiltrates. The most common complaints are vomiting, abdominal pain, and diarrhea. Malabsorption, chest pain, cough, fever, and hemoptysis may occur. There almost always is a persistent eosinophilia. Therapy with thiabendazole is usually curative.

No x-ray abnormalities are seen in most people who harbor strongyloides. Duodenal and jejunal changes can occur with heavy infestation. The duodenum and jejunum may become dilated and exhibit prominent mucosal folds. A dilated atonic duodenum is especially common with severe infestation. Ulcerations and nodular intramural defects due to granuloma formations have been noted in both the small and the large intestines. The disease can eventually lead to fibrosis throughout the bowels (4). The resulting rigid colon can suggest ulcerative colitis. X-ray findings in the small bowel may mimic Crohn's disease. Migrating infiltrates are the most frequently encountered pulmonary abnormalities. Pulmonary edema and hemorrhage are especially likely to be seen in an immunosuppressed patient with hyperinfection.

Source Materials

1. Burke JA. Strongyloidiasis in childhood. Am J Dis Child 132:1130, 1978.
2. Drasin DF, Moss JP, Cheng SH. *Strongyloides stercoralis* colitis: Findings in four cases. Radiology 126:619, 1978.
3. Dwork KG, Jaffe JR, Lieberman HD. Strongyloidiasis with massive hyperinfection. NY State J Med 75:1230, 1975.
4. Louisy CL, Barton CJ. The radiological diagnosis of *Strongyloides stercoralis* enteritis. Radiology 98:535, 1971.

Case 89

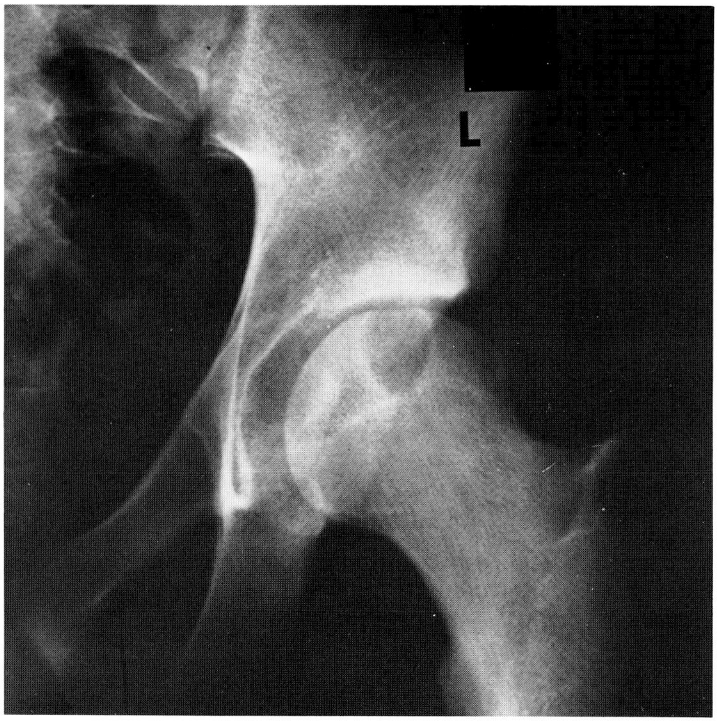

A

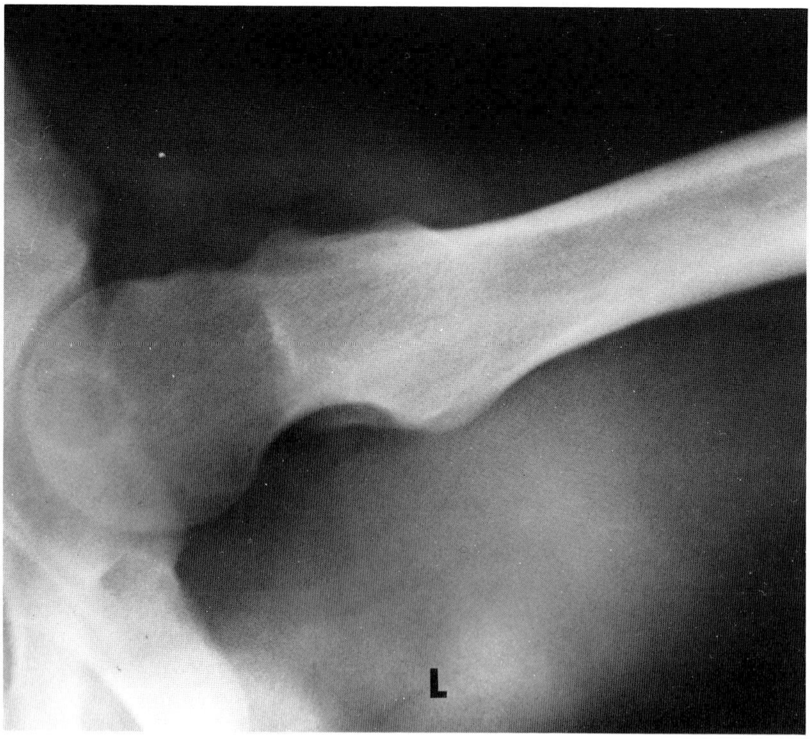

B

Chondroblastoma

Clinical Information

This 15-year-old male presented with a 6-month history of left hip pain. Subsequent surgery revealed the lesion in the left femoral head to be a chondroblastoma, which was thoroughly curettaged. Recovery was uneventful.

Roentgen Findings

Anteroposterior (A) and lateral (B) views of the left hip show a rounded radiolucency in the femoral head that measures about 2 cm in diameter. No calcification is seen within its matrix. The lesion demonstrates a sharply demarcated, narrow sclerotic rim. The history and x-ray changes are characteristic of chondroblastoma.

Comments

Chondroblastoma is a rare condition and accounts for no more than 1% of all bone tumors. There is a slight male predominance of patients with this tumor. Chondroblastoma is usually seen during the second decade of life. The tumor is most frequently located within the epiphysis of the femur, humerus, or tibia but has been seen in other locations such as the skull, patella, talus, pelvis, and calcaneus. Chondroblastomas are more likely to be seen in unusual locations if the patient is beyond 20 years of age.

The epiphyseal location and the patient's age are important diagnostic considerations. Chondroblastomas and giant cell tumors are the only bone tumors commonly seen in the epiphysis. It is theorized that a chondroblastoma arises from the epiphyseal line and grows into the epiphysis. On some occasions the tumor has been discovered in the metaphysis (1). This situation is felt to represent a chondroblastoma that has arisen from the epiphyseal line as usual, but for some unknown reason has grown into the metaphysis. Chondroblastomas have a cartilaginous matrix, which contains many multinucleated osteoclasts and may be partially calcified. It was previously thought to be a giant cell tumor variant. Patients with this condition usually have a history of rather prolonged but mild pain with some limitation of motion. Only rarely are there associated changes in the surrounding soft tissues. Chondroblastomas are usually successfully treated with conservative methods such as curettage. The tumor has recurred on rare occasions. A few chondroblastomas have multiple locations. The soft tissues very rarely have been invaded. Indeed, metastatic lung deposits have been seen in a few cases. Two patients have died from metastases. Many of the patients whose tumors demonstrated malignant behavior have had therapeutic irradiation.

The x-ray changes seen with chondroblastoma are characteristic (2, 4). The tumor appears as a round or oval radiolucency with a very thin sclerotic margin within an epiphysis. It rarely measures more than 3 cm in diameter. There may be mottled, stippled chondroid calcification within its matrix. The lucent area occasionally appears to be septated. Chondroblastomas that extend into the metaphysis frequently excite a periosteal reaction. The tumor rarely breaks through the cortex. Both standard and computed tomograms can provide helpful information. Nuclear medicine studies are of little value (3). Angiographic examinations have shown this tumor to be very vascular. The most significant differential diagnostic consideration is a giant cell tumor, since it too is found in the epiphysis. A giant cell tumor, however, characteristically appears at a later age. It nearly always extends to the articular surface and is rarely seen before the associated epiphyseal line closes. There is a larger number of differential possibilities with metaphyseal chondroblastomas.

Source Materials

1. Aronsohn RS, Hart WR, Martel W. Metaphyseal chondroblastoma of bone. AJR 127:686, 1976.
2. Hudson TM, Hawkins IF Jr. Radiological evaluation of chondroblastoma. Radiology 139:1, 1981.
3. Humphry A, Gilday DL, Brown RG. Bone scintigraphy in chondroblastoma. Radiology 137:497, 1980.
4. Nolan DJ, Middlemiss H. Chondroblastoma of bone. Clin Radiol 26:343, 1975.

Case 90

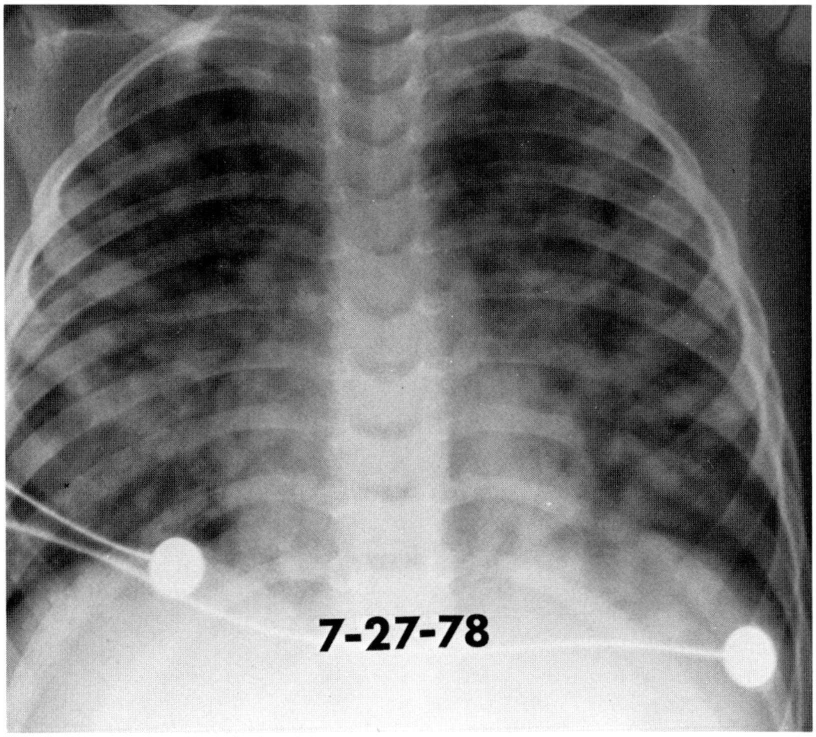

A

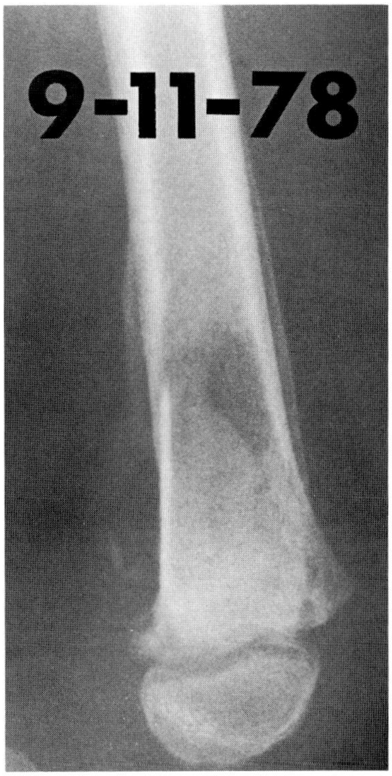

B

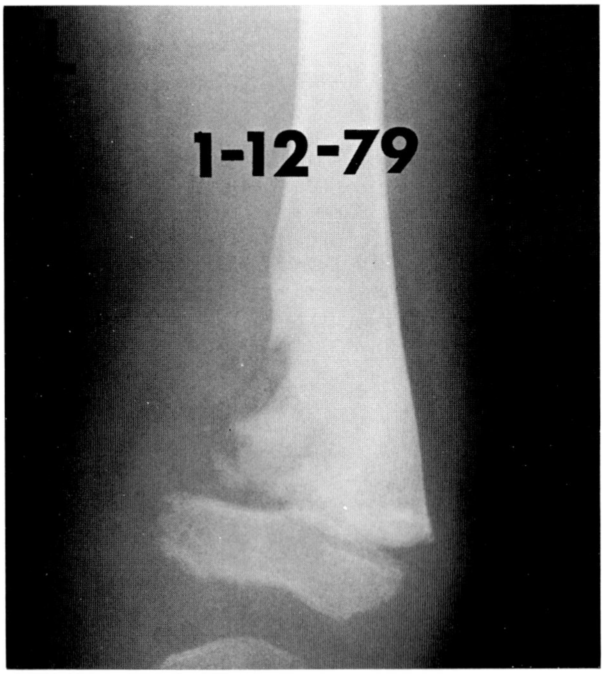

C

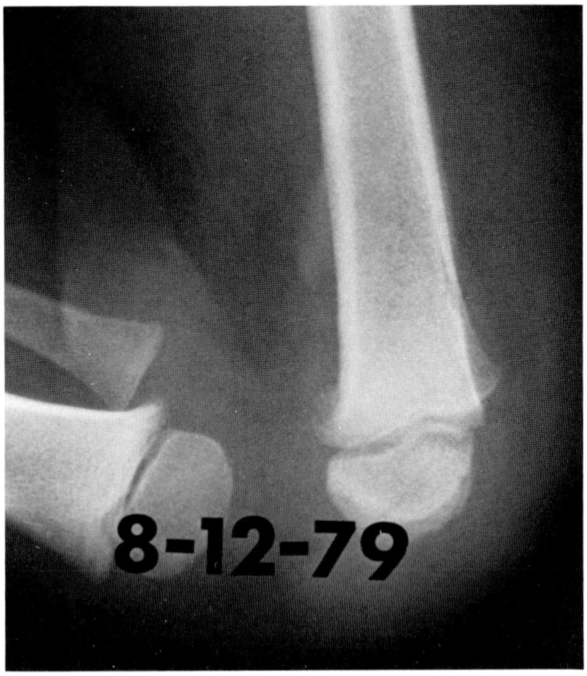

D

Chronic Granulomatous Disease of Childhood

Clinical Information

This 3-year-old white male developed lethargy, a high fever, and multiple skin pustules that rapidly became large ulcerations despite antibiotic therapy. He had episodes of cardiorespiratory arrest, pneumonia, and osteomyelitis before a slow recovery occurred. A nitroblue tetrazolium test revealed chronic granulomatous disease of childhood (CGDC).

Roentgen Findings

The chest film taken shortly after admission (A) shows numerous round infiltrates in both lungs. Some of these densities cavitated before they slowly cleared. During prolonged hospitalization the patient developed left thigh pain. A lateral film dated 9-11-78 (B) shows early destruction and periosteal reaction in the lower left femur, which was drained. It continued, however, to suppurate (C). The infection markedly improved by 8-12-79 (D).

Comments

CGDC is rare and results from "impotent" leukocytes that can phagocytize bacteria but cannot destroy them. These white blood cells become packed with organisms and have been characterized as "constipated" leukocytes. An enzyme deficiency of the leukocyte prevents the production of hydrogen peroxide, which is necessary for its lethal action on bacteria. Certain organisms such as *Streptococcus pneumoniae* rarely affect CGDC patients, because these bacteria lack the catalase needed to break down endogenously produced hydrogen peroxide. These bacteria apparently are killed by their own toxic metabolic byproducts. Catalase-positive organisms that are able to break down hydrogen peroxide, such as *Staphylococcus aureus, E. coli,* and nocardia, are common in CGDC patients (3). CGDC is usually thought to be an X-linked trait affecting males, although it has been said that Job's syndrome may be its counterpart in females. Some believe CGDC can be either sex-linked or an autosomal recessive. Others hold that females may have mild lupus-like symptoms from CGDC although most carriers are asymptomatic. The condition has been known by several names including fatal granulomatous disease, progressive septic granulomatosis, and congenital dysphagocytosis. The "childhood" portion of the name is not strictly correct. Although most of these patients have symptoms early in life and are dead in 7 or 8 years, a few live to adulthood. In fact, the disease occasionally does not appear until adult life.

CGDC is characterized by protracted febrile illnesses, frequent recurrences, and early death. Eczematoid skin reactions, lymph node swelling and suppuration, lung abscesses, and osteomyelitis are common. The x-ray changes reflect the chronic infection. There often is pneumonia, hilar and mediastinal lymphadenopathy, empyema, and hepatosplenomegaly. Resolution is very slow. Abscesses are also seen in the liver, spleen, brain, and skin. A liver abscess in an infant is CGDC until proved otherwise. Antibiotics that do not pass through the cell wall of the leukocytes are of no therapeutic value. Also, bacteria located within phagocytic vacuoles are usually protected from circulating antibodies. Chloramphenicol can penetrate the cell wall, as can rifampin. The latter causes the early development of resistance. Leukocyte transfusions, especially monocytes, may be of value (2). Operative intervention is not often required since healing usually eventually occurs with medical therapy.

X-ray findings of extensive bone destruction can be seen before the appearance of severe clinical signs and symptoms (3). The causative organism of osteomyelitis in CGDC may be of low virulence. Bone healing can occur with little sclerosis. The small bones of the hands and feet are often affected and may simulate tuberculous dactylitis. Osteomyelitis can develop in new areas despite continued therapy. Bone abscesses and sequestra are rarely seen.

Source Materials

1. Altman AR. Thoracic wall invasion secondary to pulmonary aspergillosis: A complication of chronic granulomatous disease of childhood. AJR 129:140, 1977.
2. Beuscher ES, Gallin JI. Leukocyte transfusions in chronic granulomatous disease. Persistence of transfused leukocytes in sputum. N Engl J Med 307:800, 1982.
3. Case Records of the Massachusetts General Hospital. Case 26-1981. N Engl J Med 304:1592, 1981.
4. Gaisie G, Bowen A'D, Quattromani FL, Oh KS. Chest wall invasion by *Aspergillus* in chronic granulomatous disease of childhood. Pediatr Radiol 11:203, 1981.

Case 91

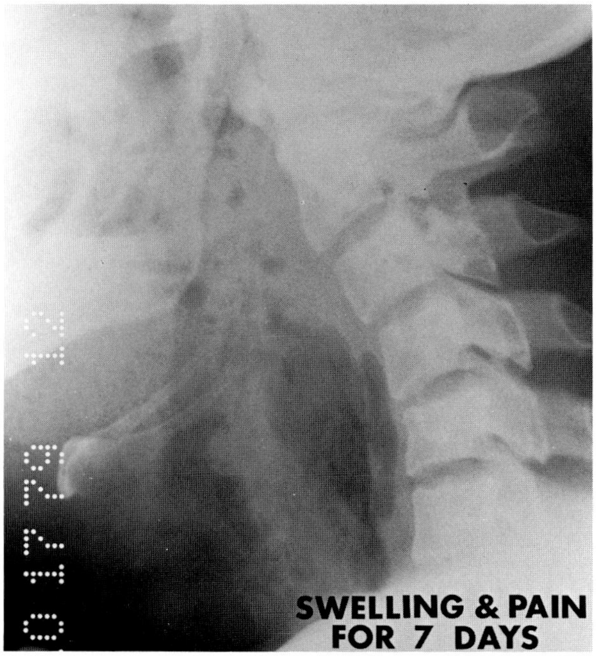

A

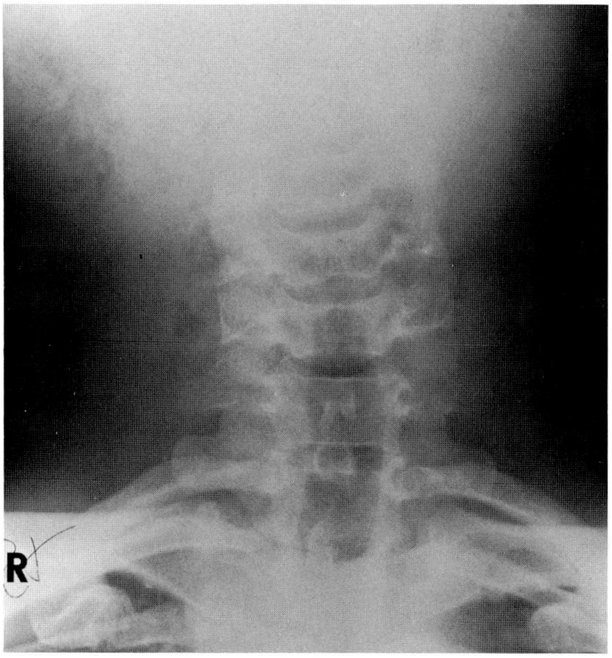

B

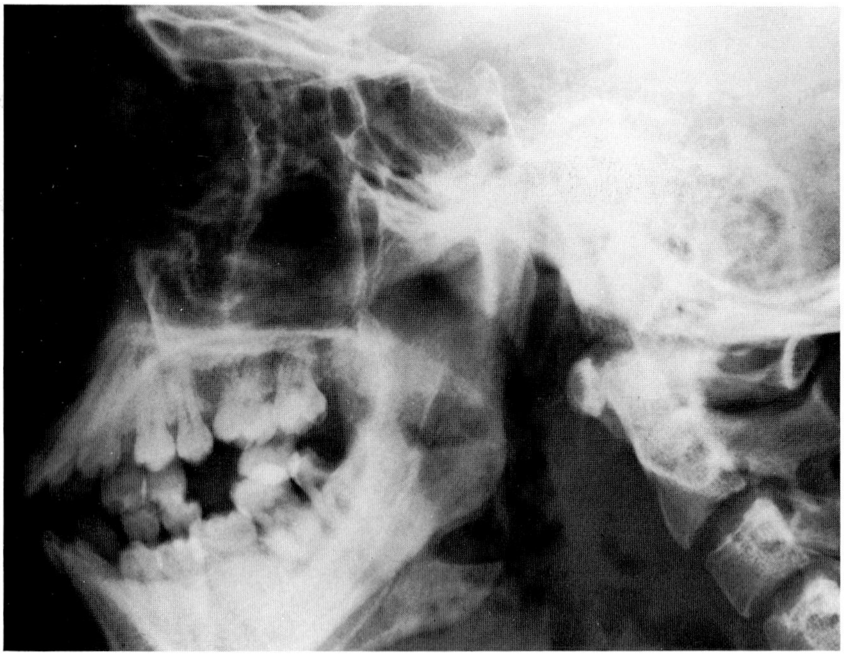

C

Retropharyngeal Abscess

Clinical Information

This 23-year-old black, febrile male had been treated at an outside hospital for an abscessed tooth. There was crepitation, swelling, and marked induration of the right side of his neck. Two abscessed teeth were removed. The retropharyngeal abscess was drained with release of 300 ml of pus. Mixed flora were cultured. Recovery was uneventful.

Roentgen Findings

Films of the neck (A–C) show swelling and extensive gas in the soft tissues. These changes are more marked on the right side. Gas is abundant in the retropharyngeal area where the prevertebral soft tissues are strikingly widened. Air-fluid levels are seen. The cervical spine is slightly kyphotic, but no intrinsic bony abnormality is seen.

Comments

An abscess in the retropharyngeal space has become relatively uncommon because of the widespread use of effective antibiotics. This space lies between the posterior pharyngeal wall and the prevertebral fascia and extends downward from the base of the skull to near the tracheal bifurcation. It contains lymph nodes and lymph channels, which drain the nasopharynx and posterior nasal passages. Retropharyngeal absesses are more common in infancy and early childhood. They apparently develop from the suppuration and breakdown of lymph nodes.

The most common offending organism is an alpha-hemolytic streptococcus. A retropharyngeal abscess is occasionally caused by a staphylococcus and sometimes results from extension of tuberculosis from the spine. The infection can follow trauma, especially from a swallowed fishbone or pin. Other etiologies include dental infection, trauma (from an endotracheal tube), and so forth. The clinical diagnosis is usually obvious. There is evidence of acute infection with fever, swelling, tenderness, and dysphagia. Infants tend to lie with their necks hyperextended and often have noisy, gurgling respiration. A neck mass is evident.

An x-ray examination of the neck shows widening of the cervical prevertebral soft tissues. There is argument concerning the normal widths of these structures at different levels, particularly in a child where change with flexion and extension is significant. In general, the anteroposterior diameter of these soft tissues should not exceed the anteroposterior diameter of the immediately posterior vertebral body. Some people feel the soft tissues can normally be somewhat wider than the vertebrae in an infant or a very young child. Older individuals do not normally have prevertebral soft tissues that exceed one-half the anteroposterior diameter of the underlying cervical vertebral body. The cervical vertebrae are usually straightened with loss of normal lordosis. Children may show flexion at the C2–3 level. The transverse ligament of the atlas is occasionally detached, especially in children. This permits atlantoaxial dislocation when the head is flexed. The underlying vertebrae and intervertebral discs should be studied carefully, since they may be the source of the infection (4). Air bubbles suggest infection with gas-forming bacteria. There are many conditions that can widen the retropharyngeal space, including tumors (most often cystic hygroma), hematoma, and myxedema (1, 2). An acute febrile history with appropriate clinical findings and distinct widening of the cervical prevertebral soft tissues, especially in the presence of gas bubbles, are diagnostic of a retropharyngeal abscess.

Source Materials

1. Hayden CK Jr, Swischuk LE. Retropharyngeal edema, airway obstruction, and caval thrombosis. AJR 138:757, 1982.
2. McCook TA, Felman AH. Retropharyngeal masses in infants and young children. Am J Dis Child 133:41, 1979.
3. Ramilo J, Harris VJ, White H. Empyema as a complication of retropharyngeal and neck abscesses in children. Radiology 126:743, 1978.
4. Seid AB, Dunbar JS, Cotton RT. Retropharyngeal abscesses in children revisited. Laryngoscope 89:1717, 1979.

Case 92

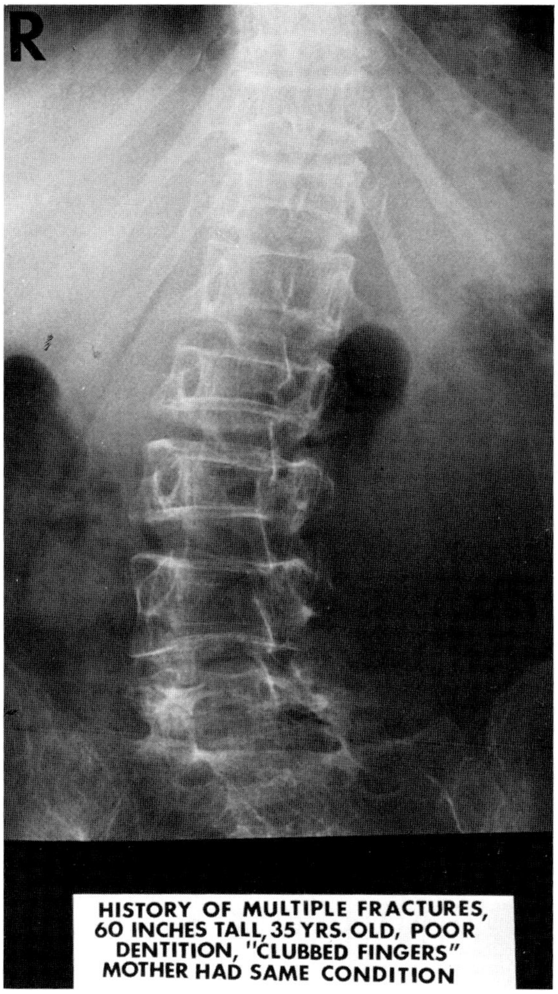
R
HISTORY OF MULTIPLE FRACTURES,
60 INCHES TALL, 35 YRS. OLD, POOR
DENTITION, "CLUBBED FINGERS"
MOTHER HAD SAME CONDITION

A

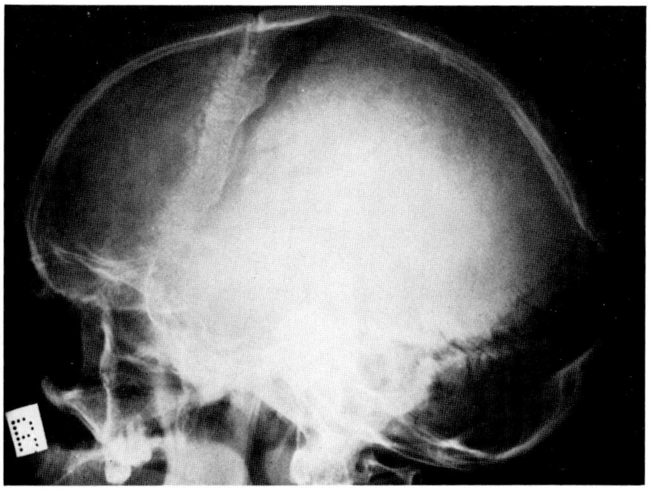

B

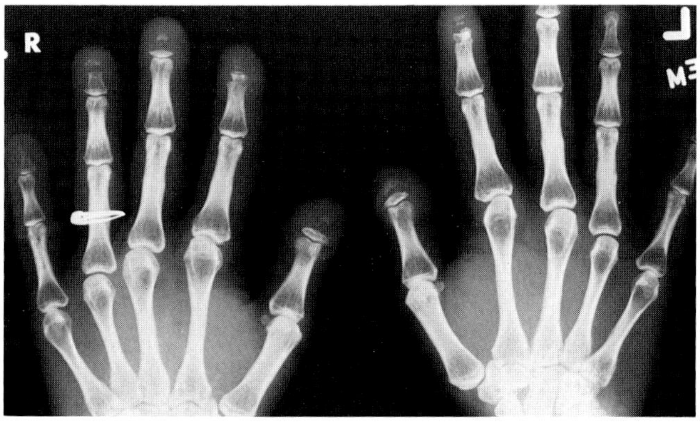
R
L

C

Hajdu-Cheney Syndrome

Clinical Information

This 35-year-old female considered herself to be in good health. There was a history of multiple fractures that had resulted from relatively minor trauma. She was 60 inches tall and had short fingers and toes that were "pseudoclubbed." Only a few abnormally appearing teeth were present. Her head was dolichocephalic. The patient's mother was of similar size and appearance.

Roentgen Findings

Rather poor mineral content is evident in the lumbar vertebrae (A), which show osteoporotic "picture framing." Biconcave collapse of several vertebral bodies can be seen. Mild scoliosis is present. Very few teeth are seen in the portion of the maxilla that is visible on the lateral film of the skull (B), which exhibits a prominent bathrocephalic deformity. Most of the terminal phalanges of the hands (C) exhibit a transverse linear band of bony deficiency.

Comments

The history and roentgen findings are diagnostic of Hajdu-Cheney syndrome. The disorder has been reported both as sporadic and as demonstrating dominant inheritance (1, 3). It is characterized by acro-osteolysis of the distal phalanges of the hands and feet, generalized loss of bone density, poor dentition, and bathrocephaly with late closures of the cranial sutures and fontanels. The patients are invariably short in stature, have pseudoclubbing of the digits, low set ears, a recessed mandible, and various other bony changes. Multiple fractures from minor trauma are characteristic. The fractures apparently reflect the reduced strength of osteoporotic bones. These patients often have lax joints. Kyphosis and scoliosis are common. The teeth are late to erupt, are frequently decayed, and usually are abnormal in appearance. The mandibular and maxillary alveolar processes may be resorbed. Hearing defects and speech impairment are common. Other bony abnormalities less consistently seen include poorly developed frontal sinuses, tubulation disturbances, and abnormalities of joint alignment. Renal function is normal. Laboratory studies are characteristically negative. Patients with Hajdu-Cheney syndrome rarely have symptoms or other indications of the disease in early childhood. The initial difficulties usually appear in the teens and are slowly progressive with increasing age. There occasionally are sensory disturbances with paresthesias in the fingers and toes.

The transverse band of bone loss in the terminal phalanges is very much like the occupational acro-osteolysis that occurred following exposure to polyvinyl chloride (4). Similar appearing acro-osteolysis has also been seen less frequently in conditions such as pyknodysostosis and Rothmund's syndrome. Osteolysis has been reported in Hajdu-Cheney syndrome to affect other bones such as the mandible and those that compose the acromioclavicular joints (2). The cause of this condition is unknown. It appears to be some type of osseous dysplasia. Several pathogenetic theories have been suggested.

The x-ray findings in Hajdu-Cheney syndrome are diagnostic when considered along with clinical information. The short height, bathrocephaly, dolichocephalic skull, biconcave osteoporotic vertebrae, and bandlike acro-osteolysis of the terminal phalanges of the hands and feet are virtually pathognomonic. It should be noted that the bands of bony deficiencies of the terminal tufts of the digits affect both the hands and the feet in Hajdu-Cheney syndrome. The feet are usually spared in polyvinyl chloride occupational acro-osteolysis.

Source Materials

1. Cheney WD. Acro-osteolysis. AJR 94:595, 1965.
2. Gilula LA, Bliznak J, Staple TW. Idiopathic nonfamilial acro-osteolysis with cortical defects and mandibular ramus osteolysis. Radiology 121:63, 1976.
3. Hajdu M, Jauntz R. Cranioskeletal dysplasia. Br J Radiol 21:42, 1948.
4. Kozlowski K, Barylak A, Eftekhari F, et al. Acroosteolysis. Problems of diagnosis—Report of four cases. Pediatr Radiol 8:79, 1979.

Case 93

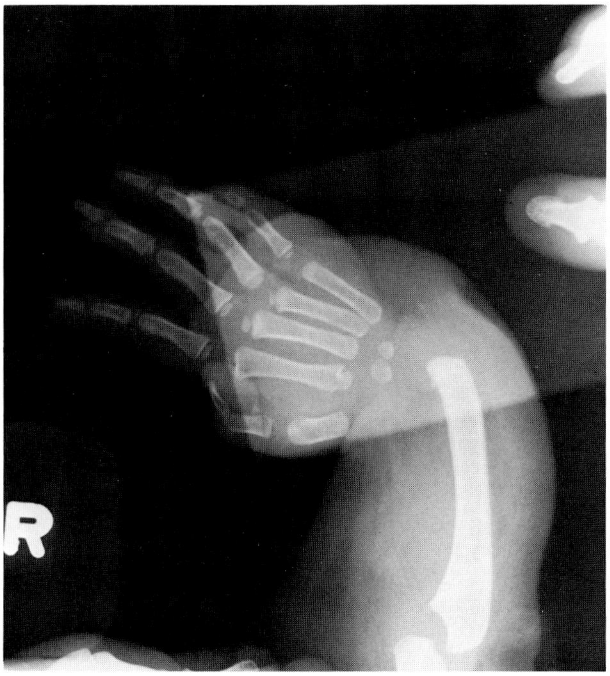

A

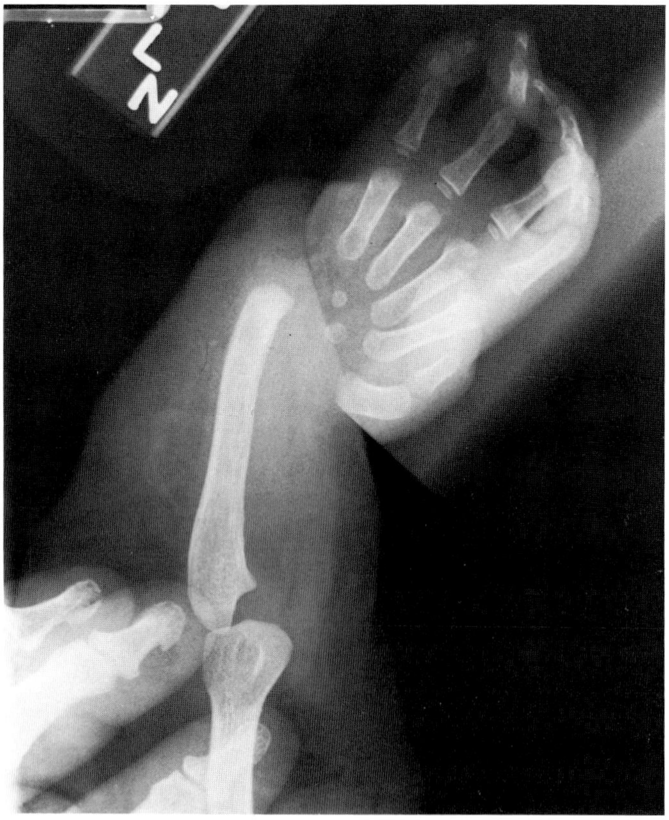

B

Thrombocytopenia with Absent Radii (TAR)

Clinical Information

This 2-year-old female with congenital anomalies of the upper extremities had experienced episodes of melena and nosebleeds in the past. There had been no bleeding episodes for several months. She had been treated since birth for very low platelet counts. Her platelet counts had slowly increased but were not yet normal. She was admitted for medical evaluation. No information is available regarding the presence of a similar condition in relatives.

Roentgen Findings

Anteroposterior films of both forearms and hands (A, B) show bilateral absence of the radii. The thumbs are present. Both hands are clubbed.

Comments

Thrombocytopenia with absent radii (TAR), or congenital hypomegakaryocytic thrombocytopenia, is a rare condition that is evident at birth. The radiologic appearance is unmistakable (2, 3). Patients with TAR are the only individuals who display absent radii in the presence of thumbs. There are many conditions in which absence of the thumbs is associated with absent radii, usually also with absence of the carpal scaphoid bones. It is the presence of the thumbs that distinguishes this condition. These patients invariably have clubbed hands but learn to use them remarkably well. TAR is an autosomal recessive trait. Thrombocytopenia has been associated with trisomy 18, but patients with TAR have a normal chromosomal pattern (4).

TAR is characterized by a decreased number or total absence of megakaryocytes in the bone marrow. Platelet counts range from 15,000 to 30,000 during infancy. No other blood coagulation defects have been noted. More than 90% of these patients have symptoms related to the thrombocytopenia ranging from purpura and petechiae to major bleeding. Bleeding episodes can be precipitated by infection, surgery, or other stresses. Steroids and splenectomy are not helpful. TAR was fatal in about 40% of patients before platelet transfusions were used in the treatment of this condition. Death usually results from bleeding. If a patient survives the first year of life there often is a spontaneous increase in the platelet count and a consequent decrease in bleeding tendencies.

The bony abnormalities are bilateral. There may be many additional congenital anomalies, although none of them are consistently present. One-third of these individuals have a cardiac anomaly, which most frequently is tetralogy of Fallot or an atrial septal defect. No significant differential diagnostic possibilities exist. Fanconi's anemia is usually cited as a differential diagnostic consideration, although the hematologic disorder in this condition is a pancytopenia due to bone marrow failure from a stem cell defect. The bony abnormalities are usually not bilaterally symmetrical and symptoms do not appear until 5–10 years of age. Males are affected more commonly than females. Fanconi's anemia is usually fatal within 3 years. The Holt-Oram syndrome is an autosomal dominant trait with thumb anomalies that are very different from those seen with TAR. TAR can be diagnosed before birth by use of ultrasound and fetoscopy. Intrapartum platelet counts can be obtained by fetal scalp blood sampling. Fetal platelet counts below 50,000 per cubic millimeter carry a serious risk of bleeding during vaginal delivery. Cesarean section must be considered in such patients (1).

Source Materials

1. Ayromlooi J. A new approach to the management of immunologic thrombocytopenic purpura in pregnancy. Am J Obstet Gynecol 130:235, 1978.
2. Fayen WT, Harris JW. Case Report. Thrombocytopenia with absent radii (the TAR syndrome). Am J Med Sci 280:95, 1980.
3. Gellis SS, Feingold M, Chudley AE. Thrombocytopenia and absent radii syndrome. Am J Dis Child 133:747, 1979.
4. Rabinowitz JG, Moseley JE, Mitty HA, Hirschhorn K. Trisomy 18, esophageal atresia, anomalies of the radius, and congenital hypoplastic thrombocytopenia. Radiology 89:488, 1967.

Case 94

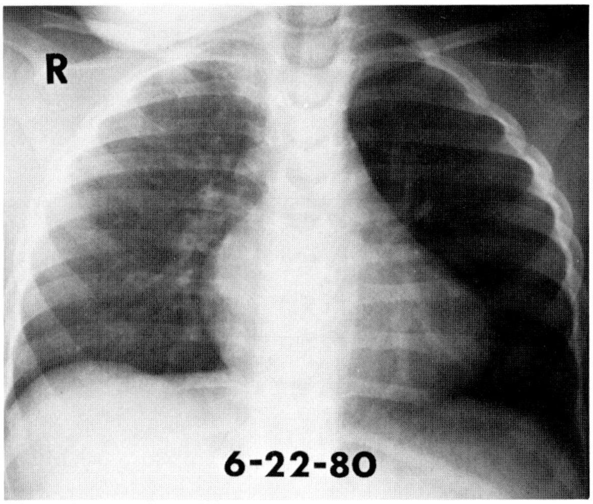

A

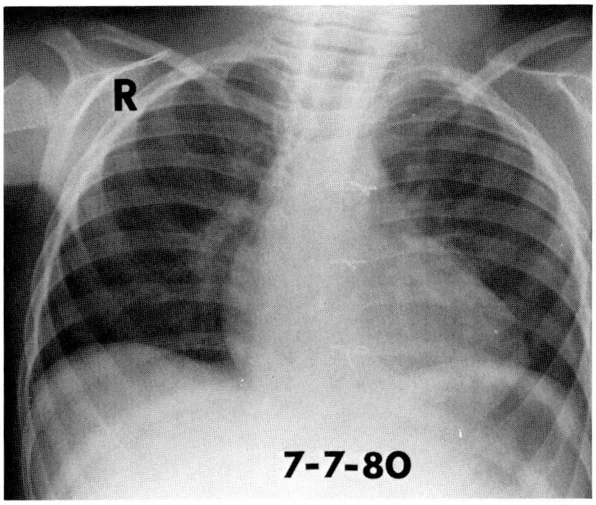

B

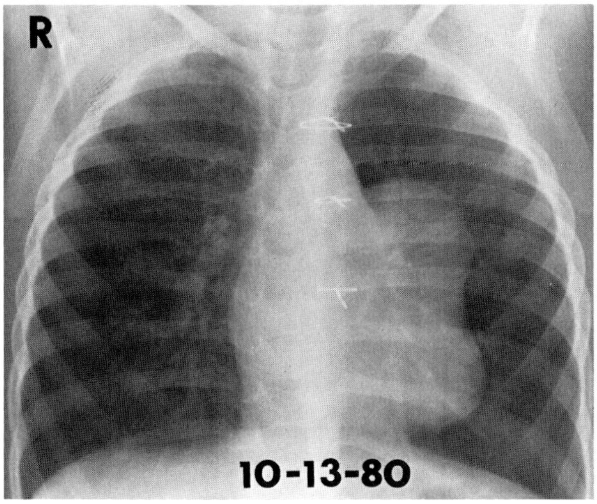

C

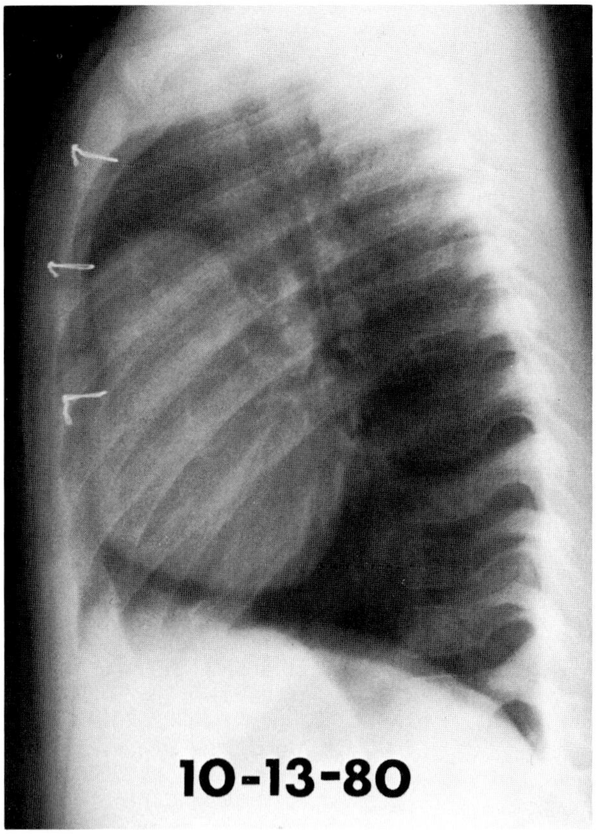

D

Ventricular Patch Aneurysm

Clinical Information

This black male was born 8-19-78. Tetralogy of Fallot was diagnosed at cardiac catheterization and angiocardiography on 6-30-80. He developed hypercyanotic spells which increased in severity. Total correction of his anomaly with insertion of a pericardial patch was performed in July of that year. Radiographic studies in October 1980 led to a diagnosis of aneurysmal dilatation of the pericardial patch, which was proved at subsequent surgery.

Roentgen Findings

A posteroanterior chest film (A) reveals a cocked-up apex, indicative of right ventricular hypertrophy. Film B, taken soon after the patient's repair, shows wire sutures in the sternum. The pulmonary blood flow may be a bit more prominent. Chest films dated 10-13-80 (C, D) show a large, smooth aneurysmal dilatation in the region of the main pulmonary artery. This abnormality is located anteriorly, immediately behind the sternum.

Comments

Total repair of tetralogy of Fallot requires surgical relief of the pulmonic stenosis and closure of the ventricular septal defect. An infundibulectomy is often needed to obtain a satisfactory right ventricular outflow tract. Total relief of the obstruction may be impossible without insertion of a patch. These patches have been made of synthetic plastic materials such as Ivalon, Dacron, and Teflon, but pericardium is now in common use. Total repair of tetralogy of Fallot is usually successful, but an aneurysm of the patch occasionally develops. This aneurysm can result from loosening of the sutures at one edge of the patch with creation of a false aneurysm. Such is more likely to occur with a plastic patch than with pericardium. Disruption of the suture line occurred in about 25% of the early operations of this type when Ivalon was used. Some improvement was experienced when Teflon was introduced. At the present time Dacron or pericardium is utilized.

An aneurysm may also develop when pericardium is used because the patch stretches and dilates. Less commonly, an aneurysm forms due to dilatation of myocardium that has been markedly thinned when an infundibulectomy is performed and no patch inserted. Several factors increase the likelihood of aneurysm formation. These include improper surgical technique, an inadequate blood supply to the involved area of the right ventricle, and infection. An elevated intraventricular pressure and forceful myocardial contractions tend to stretch the pericardial graft and abet the development of an aneurysm.

These aneurysms are usually asymptomatic. They most often are discovered on routine chest films obtained days, months, or years after the surgery. The course of most of these aneurysms is benign. Reoperation is usually not required unless there is evidence of congestive failure, systemic embolization, or impending rupture. A rapid increase in the size of an aneurysm over a short period of time is ominous and suggests the need for immediate surgery. The diagnosis is made from chest films, which show a large, obviously abnormal, additional convexity along the left heart border just below the normal location of the pulmonary artery. A lateral chest film reveals the aneurysm to be situated in an anterior position and to encroach upon the retrosternal space. Paradoxical movements of this area or absence of pulsations are seen at fluoroscopy. The wall of the aneurysm occasionally contains calcification. Angiocardiography shows the density to fill with the opaque medium.

Source Materials

1. Hipona FH, Bloom DL. Postoperative aneurysm of the right ventricle. AJR 95:642, 1965.
2. Littler WA, Meade JB, Hamilton DI. Ventricular aneurysms after cardiac surgery. Br Heart J 33:962, 1971.
3. Payne WS, Kirklin JW. Late complications after plastic reconstruction of outflow tract in tetralogy of Fallot. Ann Surg 154:53, 1961.

Case 95

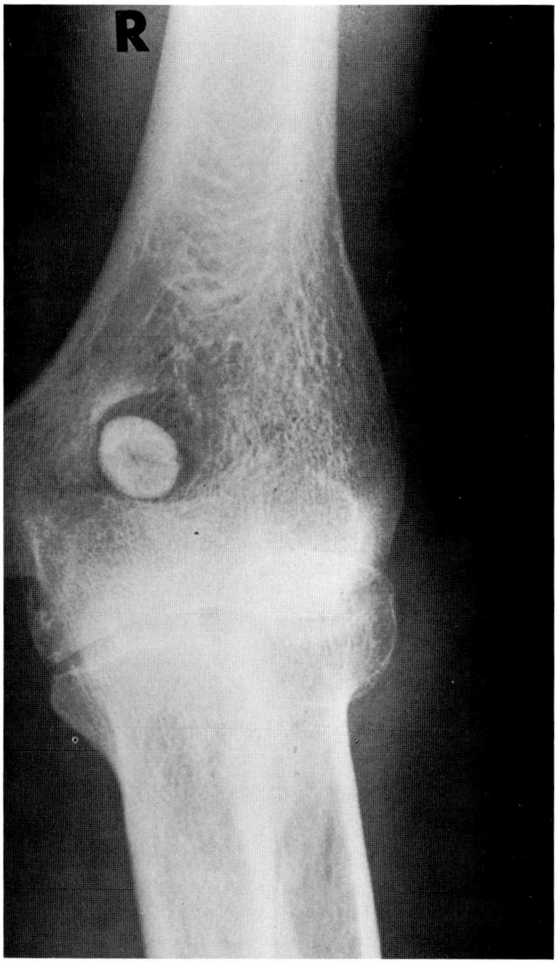

A

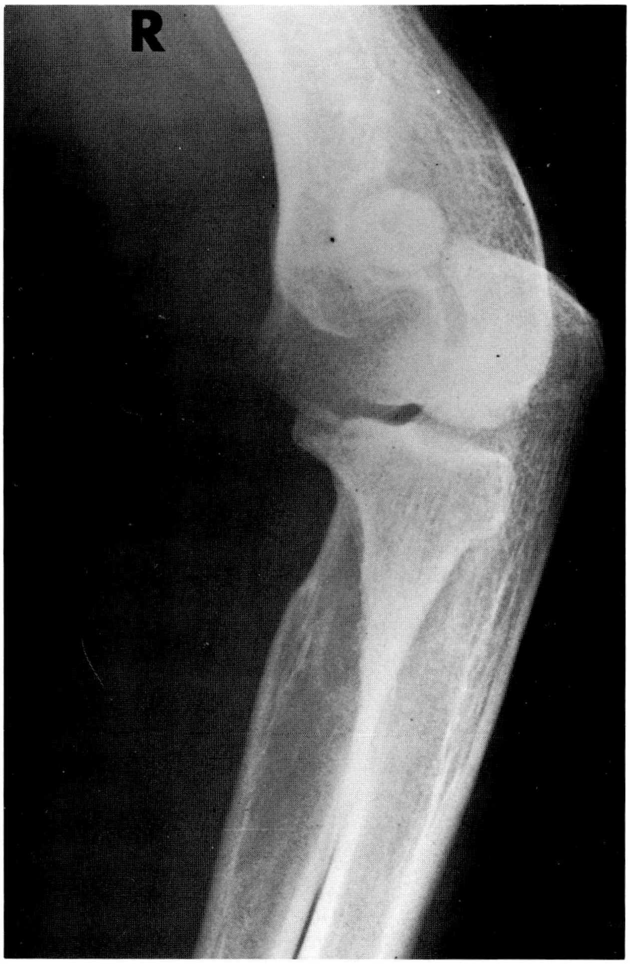

B

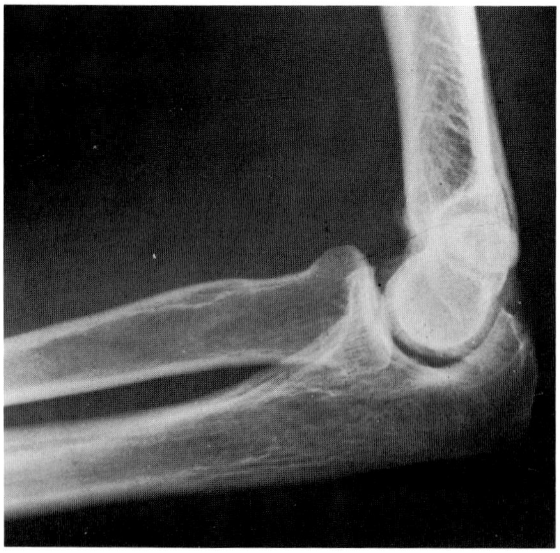

C

Supratrochlear Foraminal Bone

Clinical Information

Films of the right elbow of this adult male were obtained following injury. His symptoms of tenderness cleared with symptomatic therapy. There was no history of remote trauma.

Roentgen Findings

Anteroposterior (A), oblique (B), and lateral (C) views of the right elbow show no evidence of fracture. There is a rounded area of bony density, 1.2 cm in diameter, lying within the supratrochlear fossa of the distal humerus. This rounded separate bony ossicle is smoothly marginated and much denser than the surrounding bone. It is well corticated. This x-ray appearance is a characteristic of a supratrochlear foraminal bone (2).

Comments

This radiologic finding has been thought to be of varying significance. It has been described as an insignificant normal variant (2). Some of these ossicles that have been removed have been said to reveal a histologic pattern similar to that seen with osteochondritis dissecans elsewhere in the body (3). It is conceivable that a supratrochlear foramen is the end result of an inadequate vascular supply. Proponents of osteochondritis dissecans as the etiology of a supratrochlear foraminal bone believe it results from a local disturbance in the bone's blood supply. Others feel a supratrochlear foraminal bone results from remote trauma (1, 4). Some of the reported cases that are held to incriminate trauma have shown an additional loose body elsewhere within the elbow joint. This led to the conclusion that the large bony fragment within the supratrochlear fossa had migrated to this location after having been avulsed from intra-articular bone elsewhere within the joint (1, 3). Another explanation is that trauma leads to secondary chondrometaplasia, said to be evident pathologically, that accounts for the symptoms (4).

Many individuals with a supratrochlear foraminal bone, such as this patient, have no symptoms. It seems reasonable that an asymptomatic supratrochlear foraminal bone is a normal variant. Significant complaints may only develop in individuals who suffer a complication such as osteochondritis dissecans or other changes that may be the result of trauma. Symptoms can appear after relatively trivial injury. Individuals with a symptomatic supratrochlear bone have limitation of elbow joint extension. It is possible for these symptoms to result from a slight shift in the position of this ossicle. If symptoms persist, or if the ossicle becomes extruded from the supratrochlear fossa, the only reasonable treatment is surgical removal. Bone removed from symptomatic individuals often shows abnormal histologic changes.

The location and x-ray appearance of this ossicle are characteristic. The case shown is typical of those reported in the literature. The unusual bony structure lies within the fossa, which accommodates the coronoid process of the ulna anteriorly and the olecranon process posteriorly. The fossa is normally divided by a layer of almost transparent bone, which sometimes is perforated or indeed may be completely absent. The absence of this bony membrane in the supratrochlear fossa leads to formation of a supratrochlear foramen, which apparently is never present before 7 years of age. A supratrochlear foramen is only seen in mammals. It is common in gorillas and chimpanzees. A supratrochlear foraminal bone is less common in more privileged societies and, for some unknown reason, displays a left-sided predominance.

Source Materials

1. Bassett LW, Mirra JM, Forrester DM, et al. Post-traumatic osteochondral "loose body" of the olecranon fossa. An entity which can be mistaken for a normal anatomical variant or osteoid osteoma. Radiology 141:635, 1981.
2. Keats TE. An Atlas of Normal Roentgen Variants That May Simulate Disease, 2nd Ed. Year Book, Chicago, 1979, p. 142.
3. Martell W, Abell MR. Case report 46. Skeletal Radiol 2:173, 1978.
4. Obermann WR, Loose HWC. The os supratrochleare dorsale: A normal variant that may cause symptoms. AJR 141:123, 1983.

Case 96

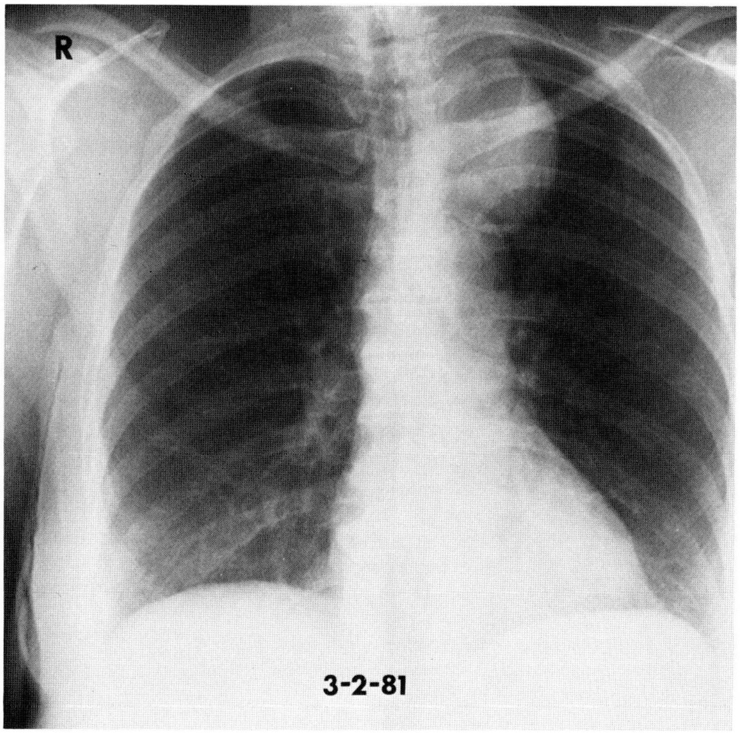

A

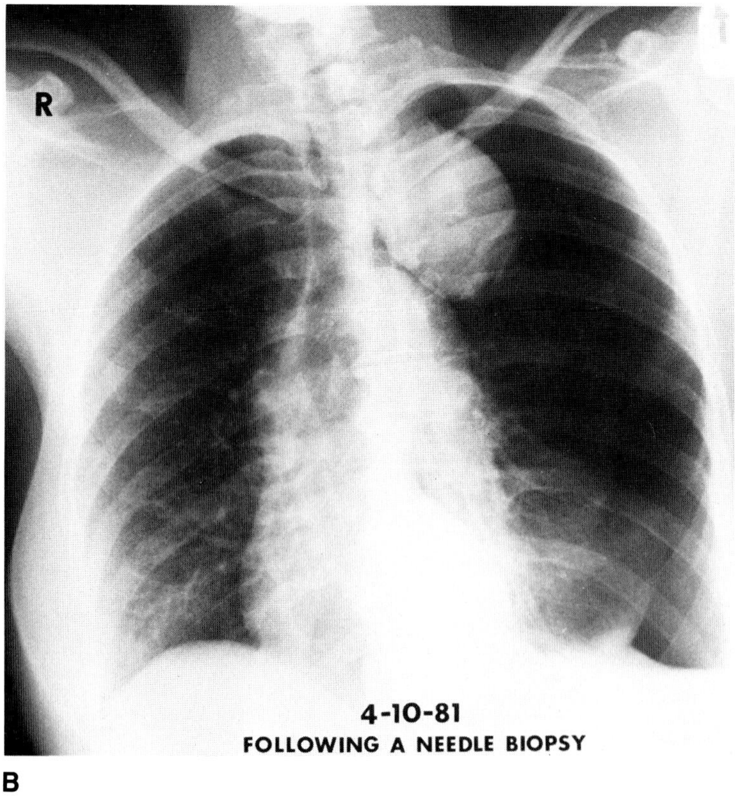

B

Bronchogenic Cyst of the Mediastinum

Clinical Information

This 59-year-old black female complained of a chronic nonproductive cough. A needle biopsy led to the diagnosis of a bronchogenic cyst.

Roentgen Findings

A posteroanterior chest film (A) shows a smoothly outlined soft tissue density along the left side of the mediastinum just above the aortic knob, which is not obscured by this lesion. A lateral film obtained at the same time revealed the lesion to be in the middle to posterior portions of the superior mediastinum. Film B immediately followed a needle biopsy of the lesion. There is a sizable pneumothorax on the left, and a fluid level is present in the left pleural space. The fluid is probably blood. The mediastinal origin of the mass density is clearly demonstrated.

Comments

Bronchogenic cysts are uncommon congenital anomalies that result from abnormal budding or branching of the tracheobronchial tree. The lesion supposedly commences during the first 2 months of intrauterine life. Bronchogenic cysts, like neurenteric cysts and duplication cysts of the gastrointestinal tract, develop from the primitive foregut (1). They are located in either the lungs or the mediastinum, in roughly equal frequency (4). These cysts are nearly always solitary, thin-walled, and unilocular. They are lined with ciliated columnar (respiratory) epithelial cells and contain dirty, milky, or brownish mucoid material. Although many are attached by a stalk to a major airway, open communication with the tracheobronchial tree is rare in the absence of infection. There is no sex predilection. The cysts are relatively prevalent in Yemenite Jews. They may be associated with certain other congenital anomalies such as absence of the left side of the pericardium.

Pulmonary bronchogenic cysts are more common in the lower lobes. Mediastinal cysts are most often found in the middle or superior mediastinum adjacent to a major airway. Another frequent location is subcarinally with the cyst projecting inferiorly and often toward the right or posteriorly. Bronchogenic cysts are usually asymptomatic unless they become infected, which occurs occasionally. A cyst in a subcarinal location can compress the major airways, especially in an infant, and become life-threatening (2).

Bronchogenic cysts are seen radiographically as a solitary, round or oval, water density mass with sharp borders (4). Lobularity is rare. Calcification is uncommon except in the rare presence of a "milk of calcium" cyst. The cysts can vary in size but rarely extend over more than two posterior ribs. They occasionally disappear spontaneously due to rupture into an airway. Air-fluid levels within the cyst imply previous infection which had led to a communication with an airway. These cysts are rarely located in the anterior mediastinum (3). Those in the superior mediastinum can be distinguished from goiters and cystic hygromas because the latter two entities are much more likely to displace the trachea. Aneurysms tend to pulsate. In contrast to neurenteric cysts, posterior mediastinal bronchogenic cysts do not have associated vertebral abnormalities. The presence of calcification in a posterior mediastinal mass points toward a neural tumor rather than a bronchogenic cyst. Lymphomas, which are common in the middle mediastinum, are much more likely to be lobulated than are bronchogenic cysts. Bronchogenic cysts at fluoroscopy change in size and shape with respiration and variations in posture. Fluoroscopy fails to reveal intrinsic pulsations.

Source Materials

1. Bronchogenic cyst: Case #5. AJR 140:1014, 1983.
2. Kagan AR, Steckel RJ. Diagnostic oncology case study. Symptomatic subcarinal mass in a child. AJR 135:633, 1980.
3. Mediastinal cyst. Case of the day. AJR 138:1202, 1982.
4. Rogers LF, Osmer JC. Bronchogenic cyst: A review of 45 cases. AJR 91:273, 1964.

Case 97

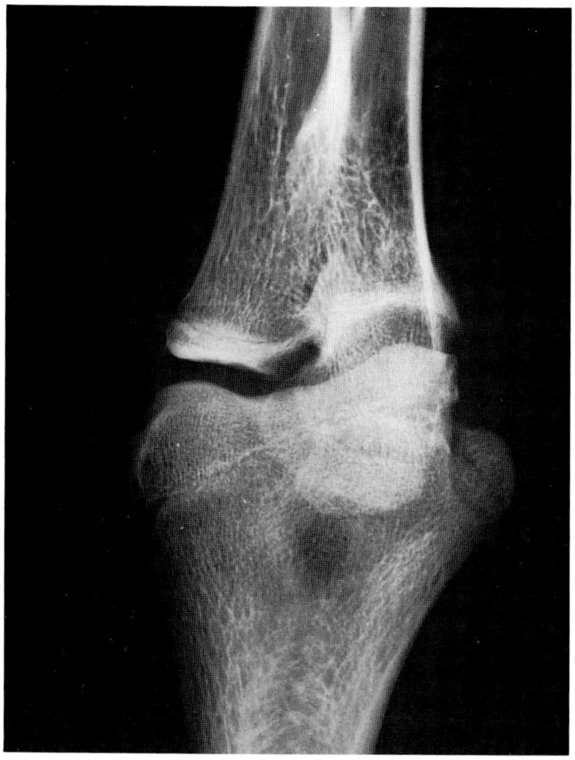

A

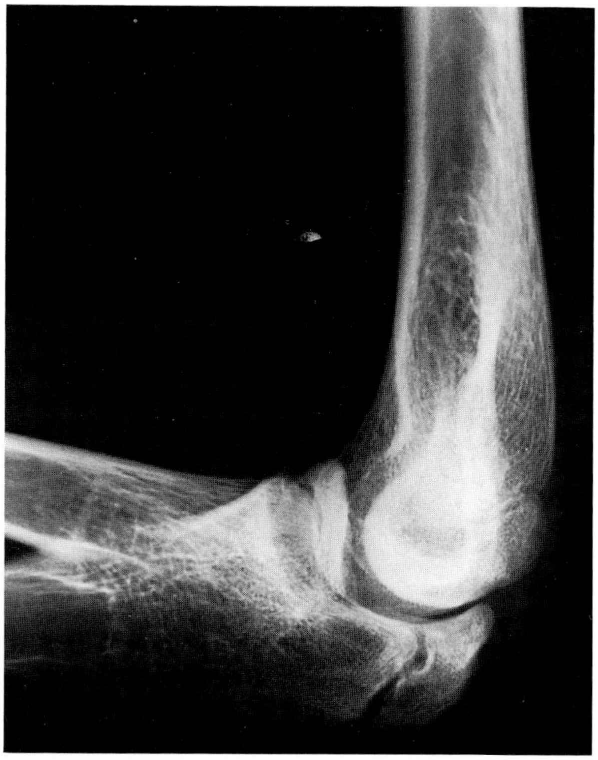

B

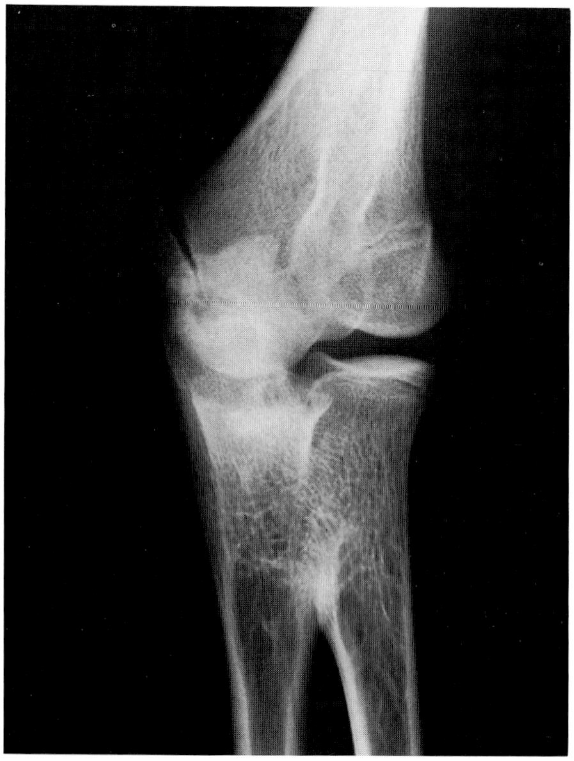

C

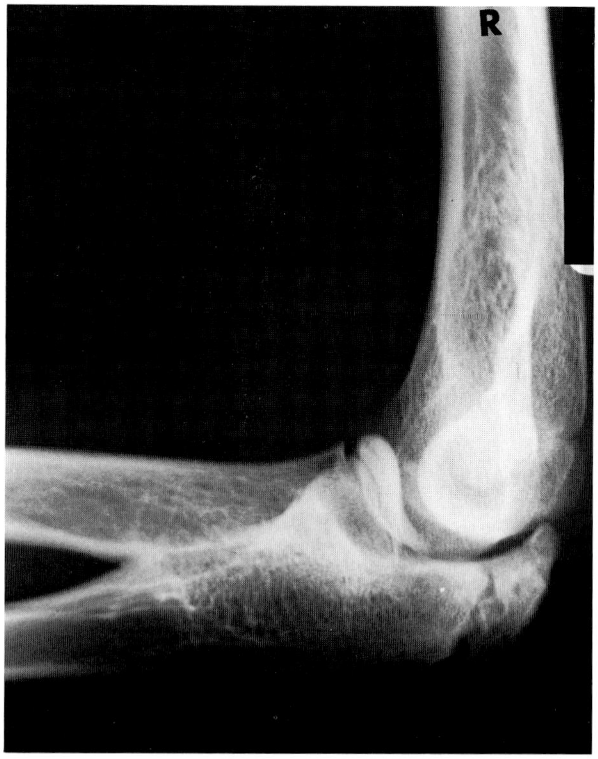

D

Congenital Radioulnar Synostosis

Clinical Information

This 16-year-old black male injured his right elbow in a fall. No fracture was evident, and all of the soft tissue swelling and tenderness caused by the injury disappeared with symptomatic therapy. He had always experienced difficulty in pronating and supinating his hands, especially supination. His hands were relatively fixed in a moderate amount of pronation.

Roentgen Findings

The radiologic appearance of each forearm is virtually identical (A–D). Osseous fusion is evident at the proximal end of the radius and ulna bilaterally. This synostosis extends from the elbow joint distally to the radial tuberosity. Neither of the radial heads is dislocated, and the olecranon processes have not fused with the ulnar shafts.

Comments

Congenital synostosis of the radius and ulna almost always occurs at their proximal ends. These two bones are formed from the same precartilaginous plate. Their perichondrium is continuous at their proximal ends during early development. Failure of separation, which normally occurs during the seventh intrauterine week, accounts for synostosis of these two bones. The normal embryonic attitude of the forearm prior to dissolution of the interzonal mesenchyme is in a variable amount of pronation. Therefore, congenital synostosis of these two bones leaves them fixed in pronation. Synostosis of the radius and ulna is the commonest developmental failure of segmentation that involves the long tubular bones. There are two types of congenital fusion of the radius and ulna. The fusion in type I, as in this case, extends from the proximal ends of the two bones for a distance of from 2 to 6 cm. In type II cases the fusion is localized to a smaller area just distal to the proximal radial epiphysis. Type II is more frequently associated with congenital anomalies of the hand. Disproportionate growth of the radial head and proximal ulna in individuals with localized synostosis can lead to dislocation of the radial head, which can become enlarged and may interfere with elbow extension (3).

Congenital radioulnar synostosis can be associated with many other skeletal anomalies (1). Some of these patients may have chromosomal aberrations. Congenital radioulnar synostosis is bilateral in about two-thirds of the patients. This type of fusion can vary from side to side. There is an equal male and female distribution. In some cases there is a familial predisposition. The condition appears to be transmitted primarily through the paternal side. Although there is more likely to be interference with elbow extension in type II fusion, these patients have somewhat more mobility of the forearm than do patients with type I fusion. All of these individuals have great difficulty in supinating the hands. This can be a significant handicap. Some patients with radioulnar synostosis have been treated with a rotational osteotomy (2). This leaves the hand in supination, which is a more functional attitude.

There is no significant differential diagnostic possibility. Fusion of the radius and ulna can occasionally follow trauma (4). Such patients may present a very similar radiologic appearance, although this is unusual.

Source Materials

1. Berant M, Berant N. Radioulnar synostosis and craniosynostosis in one family. J Pediatr 83:88, 1973.
2. Green WT, Mital MA. Congenital radio-ulnar synostosis: Surgical treatment. J Bone Joint Surg 61A:738, 1979.
3. Mital MA. Congenital radioulnar synostosis and congenital dislocation of the radial head. Orthop Clin North Am 7:375, 1976.
4. Watson FM, Eaton RG. Post-traumatic radio-ulnar synostosis. J Trauma 18:467, 1978.

Case 98

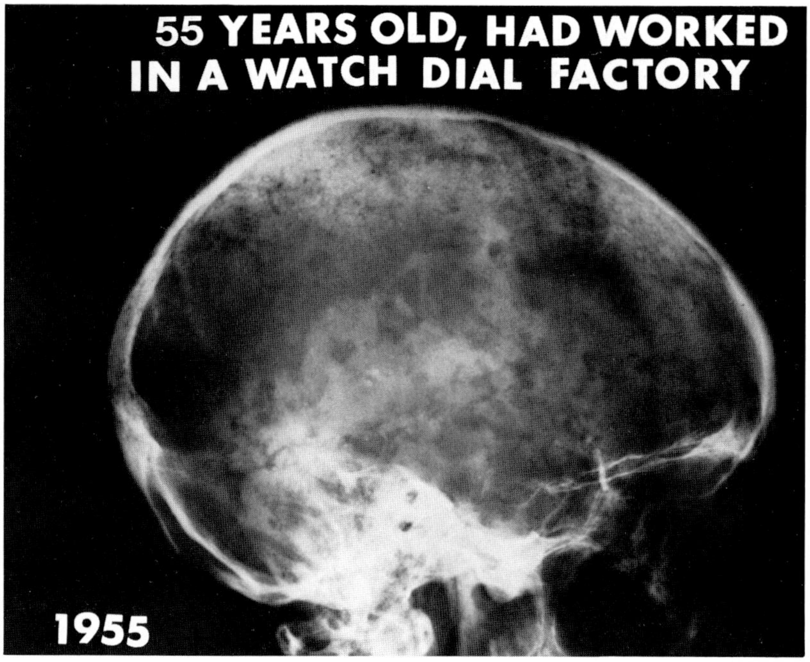

A

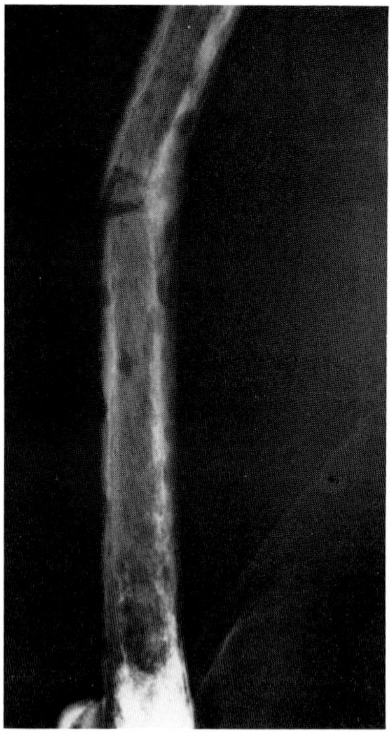

B

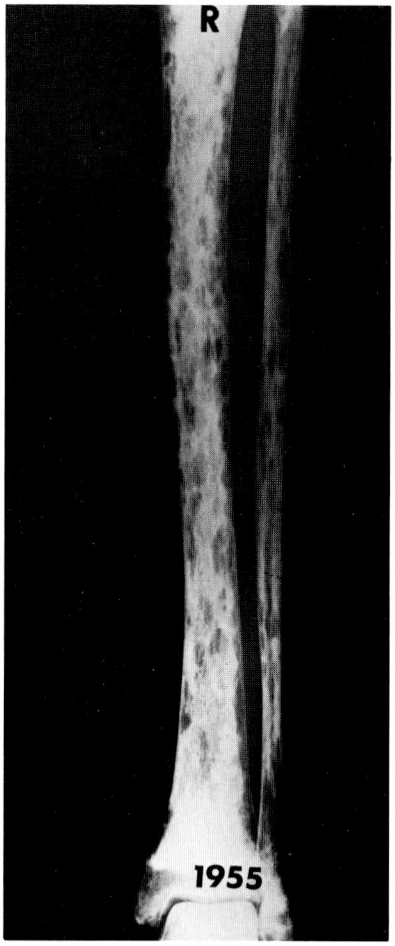

C

Radium Poisoning

Clinical Information

This 55-year-old white female had worked in a watch dial factory as a young girl. She painted the numerals with a radium-containing compound. Through the years she had experienced numerous problems, including pathologic fractures, from abnormalities caused by her excessive body burden of radium.

Roentgen Findings

A lateral film of the skull (A) shows rather extensive areas of bony destruction scattered throughout the cranium, but most marked in the posterior portions of the parietal bones. Zones of bony sclerosis are interspersed between the lytic areas. A lateral film of the left femur (B) shows many scattered moth-eaten areas of radiolucency and a transverse fracture with anterior angulation in its midshaft. No callus is evident. The right tibia and fibula (C) show similar moth-eaten lesions. An area of increased density in the distal end of the right tibia is consistent with avascular necrosis.

Comments

Radium poisoning is due to the ingestion, injection, or inhalation of radium or similar radioactive compounds. Such poisoning has come about from industrial exposure or from compounds that were administered for medical purposes. Radium compounds were prescribed by physicians for various abnormalities until about 1932, when their harmful effects became generally recognized. Most of the industrial exposures came from painting watch dials with radium compounds to make them luminous. The radium was ingested when the workers pointed their brushes with their lips and tongues. Hundreds of workers were involved. There still are many people alive who had exposure to toxic quantities of radium.

Radium behaves metabolically in the same manner as does calcium. Ingested radium is usually deposited with rather generalized distribution in the outer bony cortex. The deposited radium emits alpha particles, which bombard nearby cells. This can result in their death, cellular injury with recovery, arrested cellular division, or abnormal repair with neoplasm. The effects of alpha particles can lead to premature epiphyseal closure or to other growth disturbances. Bone resorption is extremely common. Longtime exposure frequently causes large resorption cavities that contain gelatinous osteoid tissue (2). The number and severity of the bony lesions generally parallel the body burden of radium (1, 3). These patients also may exhibit hematologic abnormalities, particularly anemia. Malignant tumors often develop 20–30 years after exposure. These most frequently are osteosarcomas and fibrosarcomas, which can be multicentric. Tumors of the paranasal sinuses and mastoids are quite frequent (4).

The radiologic manifestations of radium poisoning include a coarsened trabecular pattern and numerous sharply defined lytic lesions in the skull and long bones. These represent areas of bony resorption secondary to alpha particle bombardment. There also may be patches of sclerosis secondary to ischemia, particularly in the metaphyses. Zones of necrosis are especially common in weight-bearing areas. Pathologic fractures, bone infarcts, and malignant tumors are frequently encountered. Differential diagnostic considerations include multiple myeloma and aseptic necrosis. It usually is possible to identify radium poisoning, which leads to radiologic evidence suggestive of both aseptic necrosis and multiple myeloma—an unlikely event with other diseases.

Source Materials

1. Evans RD. The effect of skeletally deposited alpha-ray emitters in man. Br J Radiol 39:881, 1966.
2. Glenn JA Jr, Galindo J, Lawrence CE. Chronic radium poisoning in a dial painter. AJR 83:465, 1960.
3. Hasterlik RJ, Miller CE, Finkel AJ. Radiographic development of skeletal lesions in man many years after acquisition of radium burden. Radiology 93:599, 1969.
4. Littman MS, Kirsh IE, Keane AT. Radium-induced malignant tumors of the mastoid and paranasal sinuses. AJR 131:773, 1978.

Case 99

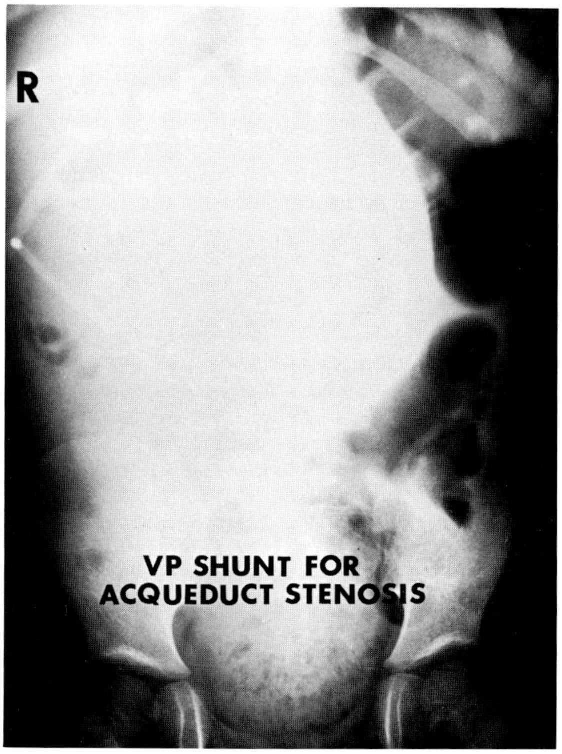

A

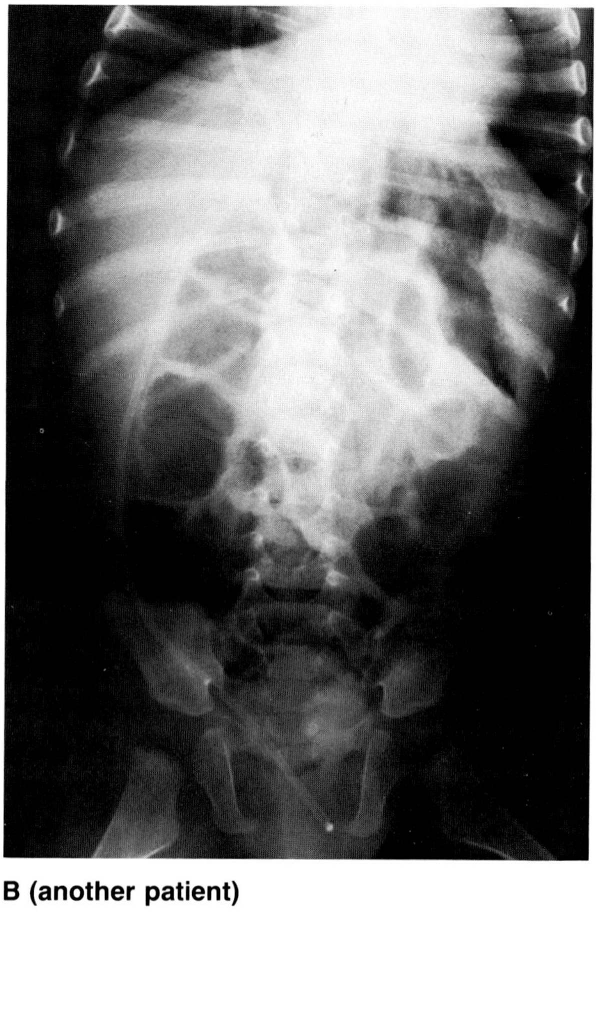

B (another patient)

Ventriculoperitoneal Shunt Complication: Peritoneal Cyst

Clinical Information

This 4-year-old girl had a ventriculoperitoneal shunt (VPS) inserted to relieve increased intracranial pressure and hydrocephalus from aqueductal stenosis. She subsequently developed a large right-sided abdominal mass that extended across the midline. This proved to be a peritoneal cyst filled with cerebrospinal fluid. The cyst was drained and a ventriculoatrial shunt was substituted for the VPS.

Roentgen Findings

An abdominal film (A) shows VPS tubing with its tip near a large homogeneous right upper quadrant soft tissue density, which displaces the intestines to the left and downward.

Comments

Various shunting procedures have been used in the treatment of hydrocephalus. Early VPS procedures, when the tubing was made of polyethylene, experienced a high revision rate because the peritoneal end often became occluded. Considerable success was achieved with ventriculoatrial shunts using Silastic tubing, although complications such as endocarditis, septicemia, and pulmonary hypertension were fairly frequent. The use of Silastic and a low-pressure slit valve at the peritoneal end overcame the distal obstruction problem with VPS procedures.

VPS malfunction can occasion increasing intracranial pressure with symptoms that include decreased levels of consciousness and vomiting. Abdominal complications may lead to distention and an abdominal mass with some associated pain. The tubing can kink or break. Its distal end often retracts as the patient grows. At least 15% of these patients develop inguinal hernias and hydroceles (4). The hernias are usually bilateral. It is felt that excessive peritoneal fluid while the processus vaginalis is still open creates the hernias. Shunt catheters may extend into the hernial sac (see B, from another patient) (2). Intestinal obstruction can occur. Only rarely does the VPS tubing perforate the bowel, although there have been reports of the tube passing out the rectum. Infection is seen in 10% of these patients. Some of the Silastic tubes incite a degree of inflammation. This may obstruct the end of the tubing. On rare occasions a sterile generalized peritonitis occurs, which can interfere with fluid absorption and lead to massive ascites. Regional inflammation near the tip of the catheter can cause peritoneal adhesions and produce regional cystic encapsulations as seen in this case. The cysts may contain over 1000 ml of fluid. Proper treatment is surgical drainage. Repositioning the catheter tip within the peritoneal cavity is fruitless, since recurrence is the rule.

An increased quantity of free peritoneal fluid is a normal concomitant of a satisfactorily functioning VPS, although absence of demonstrable fluid does not necessarily indicate shunt malfunction. X-ray examinations in the presence of fluid encapsulation show evidence of an abdominal mass with bowel displacement. There is always a close association between the mass and the tip of the VPS catheter. An injection of contrast agent through the VPS catheter will usually outline the pseudocyst. Similar information is obtained from the CT scanning (1). A satisfactory diagnosis can be made with ultrasound (3).

Source Materials

1. Chuang VP, Fried AM, Oliff M, et al. Abdominal CSF pseudocyst secondary to ventriculoperitoneal shunt: Diagnosis by computed tomography in two cases. J Comput Assist Tomogr 2:88, 1978.
2. Crofford MJ, Balsam D. Scrotal migration of ventriculoperitoneal shunts. AJR 141:369, 1983.
3. Fried AM, Adams WE Jr, Ellis GT, et al. Ventriculoperitoneal shunt function: Evaluation by sonography. AJR 134:967, 1980.
4. Kaufman HH, Carmel PW. Hydrocele after ventriculoperitoneal shunting. Am J Dis Child 135:359, 1981.

Case 100

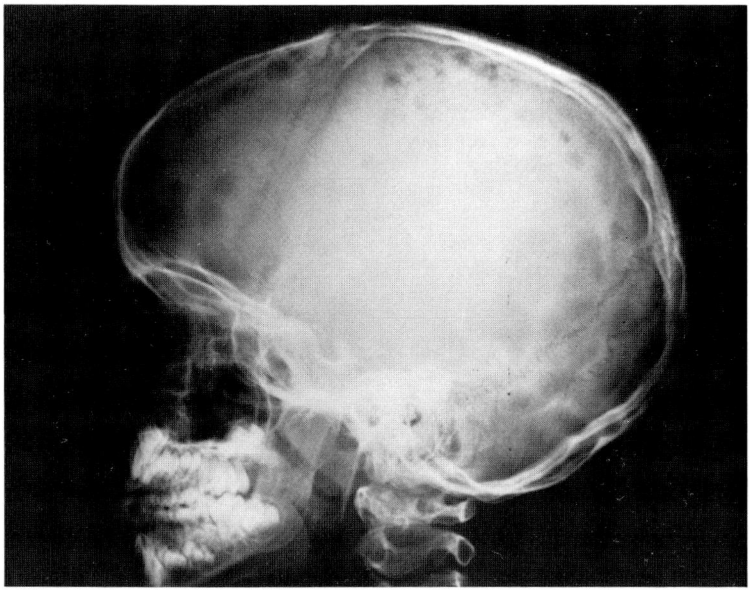

A

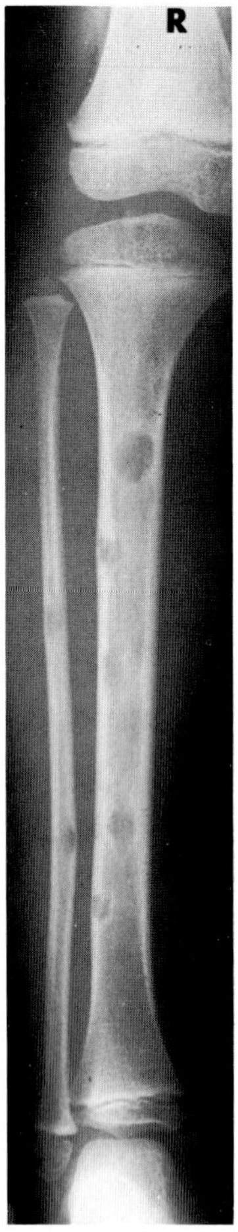

B

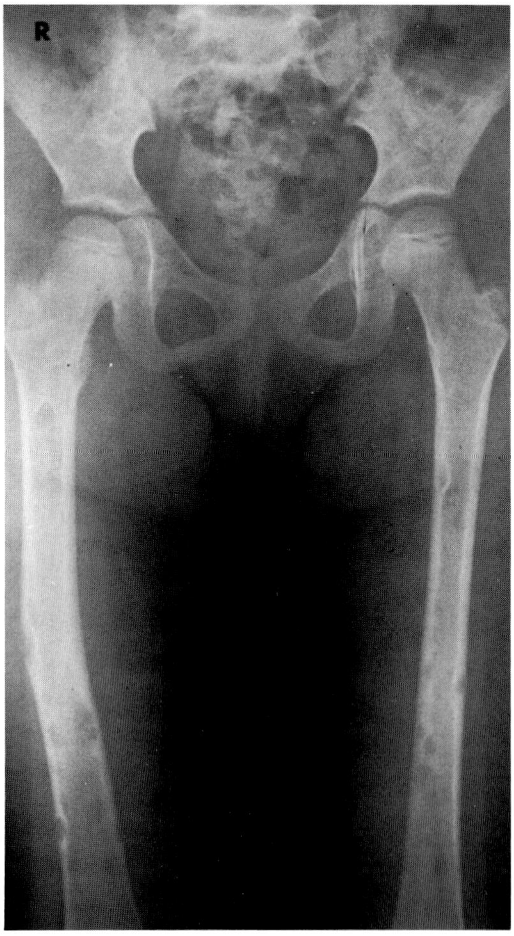

C

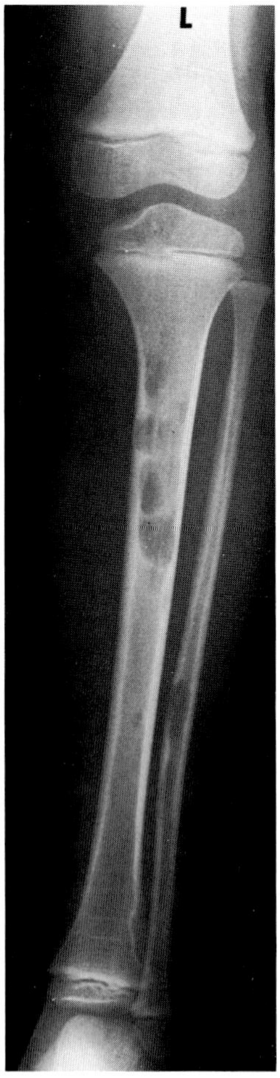

D

Cystic Angiomatosis of Bone

Clinical Information

Radiographs of the right leg of this asymptomatic white female were obtained following trauma. Cystic lesions were discovered, which led to a subsequent radiologic survey of her bones. No skin lesions were evident. An excision biopsy of an involved rib was diagnosed as cystic angiomatosis of bone.

Roentgen Findings

A lateral film of the skull (A) and anteroposterior films of the pelvis and both lower extremities (B–D) show many smoothly outlined, rounded lytic areas with thin sclerotic borders in all of the visualized bones. The lesions are particularly abundant in the right femur, both tibiae, and the skull. A few similar lesions were seen in the ribs and the upper extremities. The tubular bones of the hands and feet were spared. The cortices are not expanded. No periosteal reaction is seen. One area along the lateral aspect of the middle of the right femur shows slight lateral bowing. This may be the site of an old fracture.

Comments

Cystic angiomatosis of bone is a rare disease. Although various etiologies have been suggested, it probably is a hamartomatous condition that is not evident in the neonatal period (2). One patient is known to have had normal bones at birth (4). The condition does not appear to be a neoplasm nor related to an inborn error of tissue development. The lesions usually first become manifested about the 10th year of life. Cystic angiomatosis of bone is not familial, nor does it exhibit any sex predilection. Although almost any bone can be involved, the femur is most frequently affected. Progression of the condition is very slow. The condition has a good prognosis if only the bones are affected, although long-term follow-ups have not been reported. The only symptom if the lesions are limited to the bones is pain from pathologic fractures. This disease is very serious if there is visceral involvement. In fact, it is always eventually fatal when internal organs are affected. The most commonly involved viscera are the spleen, pleurae, and skin, although the liver, thymus, and many other internal organs have been affected.

A specific microscopic diagnosis of this condition is difficult from small biopsies. A confident identification is made more easily from an excision biopsy of a rib. Microscopic studies show cavities that are empty or filled with fluid and cellular material. The findings suggest either lymph vessels or blood vessels. Both types of vessels were present in one patient who had visceral involvement. Laboratory studies are negative.

Radiographs usually show the lesions to be located in the medullary portion of the bones. Cortical involvement is neither common nor extensive. The cortex remains intact and periosteal reaction is uncommon unless there has been a pathologic fracture. The lesions are characteristically lytic rounded areas with thin sclerotic margins. The long bones of the hands and feet are usually spared. Lesions vary in size from very tiny to several centimeters in diameter. Lymphangiograms show the injected opaque material within the lesions in cystic lymphangiomatosis (4). Several conditions can simulate cystic skeletal angiomatosis. Perhaps the most difficult to exclude is histiocytosis X, which unlike cystic angiomatosis of bone very infrequently affects the bones below the knees and the elbows. Other diseases, such as hyperparathyroidism, fibrous dysplasia, or congenital fibromatosis, that may lead to a similar x-ray appearance have distinctive clinical features or symptoms of systemic involvement.

Source Materials

1. Brower AC, Culver JE, Keats TE. Diffuse cystic angiomatosis of bone. Report of two cases. AJR 118:456, 1973.
2. Case records of the Massachusetts General Hospital. Case 30-1980. N Engl J Med 303:270, 1980.
3. Graham DY, Gonzales J, Kothati SM. Diffuse skeletal angiomatosis. Skeletal Radiol 2:131, 1978.
4. Nixon GW. Lymphangiomatosis of bone demonstrated by lymphangiography. AJR 110:582, 1970.

Alphabetical List of Cases